Anesthesiology - New Insights

Edited by Mark Ulrich Gerbershagen

Published in London, United Kingdom

Anesthesiology - New Insights
http://dx.doi.org/10.5772/intechopen.1003444
Edited by Mark Ulrich Gerbershagen

Contributors
Albert Tsai, Alexandra Roi, Amit Ahluwalia, Carlo Alessandro Locatelli, Ciprian Ioan Roi, Fabrizio G. Bonanno, Jatinder Bali, Kim K. Kutun, Larissa Kiwakyou, Lukas Hartmann, Mark Ulrich Gerbershagen, Merve Elgörmüş, Milo Vason, Mircea Riviş, Mohammed Khamis, Natalie Bodmer, Ojasvini Bali, Pallavi Ahluwalia, Perin Kothari, Robert Owen, Roberto Zoppellari, Tolga Koyuncu, Torsten Richter

First published in London, United Kingdom, 2025 by IntechOpen
IntechOpen is the global imprint of INTECHOPEN LIMITED, registered in England and Wales, registration number: 11086078, 167-169 Great Portland Street, London, W1W 5PF, United Kingdom

For EU product safety concerns: IN TECH d.o.o., Prolaz Marije Krucifikse Kozulić 3, 51000 Rijeka, Croatia, info@intechopen.com or visit our website at intechopen.com.

British Library Cataloguing-in-Publication Data
A catalogue record for this book is available from the British Library

Anesthesiology - New Insights
Edited by Mark Ulrich Gerbershagen
p. cm.
Print ISBN 978-1-83634-077-5
Online ISBN 978-1-83634-076-8
eBook (PDF) ISBN 978-1-83634-078-2

Meet the editor

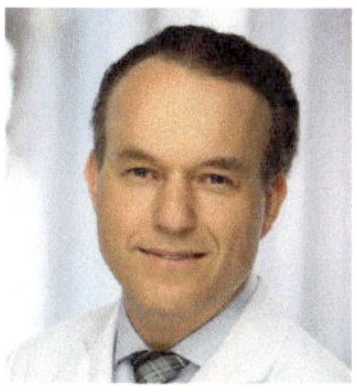

Prof. Dr. Mark U. Gerbershagen studied human medicine at the Christian Albrechts University in Kiel, Germany, from 1993 to 1999 and completed his residency at the University Medical Center Hamburg-Eppendorf. As he has always been interested in procedural and management issues, he completed a Master of Business Administration at the European Business School, Eltville, Germany. He habilitated on the subject of "Malignant hyperthermia" and has been an adjunct professor at the University of Witten Herdecke in Germany since 2013. Furthermore, he is a member of the Faculty Council of the Department of Health at Witten Herdecke University. Prof. Dr. Mark U. Gerbershagen has been head of the Department of Anesthesiology and Interdisciplinary Care Medicine at Cologne Holweide Hospital, Hospital Cologne, Germany, since 2016.

Contents

Preface

This book provides a thorough, comprehensive overview of contemporary developments in the field of anesthesiology. It encompasses a broad range of subjects, including the organization of anesthesiology services, individual surgical specialties, and medical education. Additionally, it places particular emphasis on the patient's perspective on our perioperative activities.

Each of these chapters is worth reading.

A critical issue for our young anaesthetists is, of course, continuing education and training. The question is how to make the profession of anaesthesia attractive in the future in terms of work-life balance and career opportunities. These topics are dealt with in the chapter "Current Perspectives in Anesthesiology Graduate Medical Education".

"Anesthesia for Robotic Surgeries in Children" confronts relatively new challenges in paediatric anaesthesia. Robotic laparoscopic surgery is becoming increasingly prevalent in the treatment of children, including neonates and infants. It provides the surgeon with a superior three-dimensional view and facilitates the procedure. It is imperative that anaesthetists are cognisant of the anaesthetic-related challenges that a child undergoing robotic surgery may encounter. These challenges encompass patient positioning, restricted airway and intravenous access, pressure damage to nerves and tissues, and the potential for hypothermia. Additionally, it is imperative to comprehend the physiological changes induced by pneumoperitoneum and their impact on the various organ systems. Ventilation strategies are required to maintain oxygenation and prevent hypercarbidemia and atelectasis.

The number of children undergoing surgery is increasing due to technological developments. The chapter "The Effect of Parental Anxiety on Postoperative Paediatric Cognitive Dysfunction" addresses potential adverse effects on the mental health of children undergoing surgery. These adverse effects may be exacerbated when families suffer from high levels of stress and anxiety. Unfortunately, parental stress and anxiety also alter the child's emotional state and have a negative impact on the child's recovery process during postoperative care. This situation can negatively impact the child's short- and long-term psychological and physiological outcomes. While the above negative effects in children may improve in the short term, unfortunately, they can also have lasting effects for up to a year. This article looks at the impact of parental anxiety on cognitive difficulties in children.

"Interdisciplinary Emergencies in the Delivery Room" require close collaboration between anesthetists and obstetricians to ensure the safety of both mother and baby.

Proper training and adherence to established protocols are essential for managing critical situations such as postpartum hemorrhage, preeclampsia, and emergency cesarean sections. Hypertensive pregnancy disorders, including eclampsia and HELLP syndrome, pose significant risks and require early diagnosis and intervention. Postpartum hemorrhage remains one of the leading causes of maternal mortality and requires prompt treatment with uterotonics, blood transfusions, or surgical interventions. Amniotic fluid embolism is a rare but severe complication that can lead to cardiovascular collapse and requires immediate resuscitation. Shoulder dystocia, a fetal emergency, can often be managed with the McRoberts maneuver but may require advanced obstetric and anesthetic interventions. Effective communication, structured emergency plans, and continuous training help improve outcomes and reduce maternal and neonatal mortality.

"Solutions for Insufficient Epidural Analgesia for Planned Vaginal Birth" introduces us to the problems and possible solutions for optimal pain therapy during labour. Epidural analgesia (EDA) is a common method for pain relief during childbirth, but it can sometimes fail or be contraindicated, requiring alternative options. Spinal analgesia provides quick pain relief but has a limited duration, while combined spinal-epidural analgesia (CSE) offers both immediate and prolonged effects. Intravenous opioids like remifentanil, pethidine, and fentanyl can be used, though they carry risks such as respiratory depression in both mother and baby. Pethidine is no longer preferred due to its severe side effects, while remifentanil is effective but requires continuous monitoring. Nitrous oxide offers moderate pain relief and is self-administered, making it a less invasive alternative, though it is less effective than EDA and has environmental concerns. Despite its lower analgesic effect, many women prefer nitrous oxide because it provides a sense of control during labor.

"Considerations and New Perspectives of Locoregional Anesthesia in Dentistry" points out that locoregional anaesthesia has been a fundamental component of dental pain management for over a century and has evolved with advances in clinical anatomy, anaesthetic techniques and patient-specific considerations. This chapter examines various methods of anaesthesia, including plexus and troncular techniques, highlighting their indications, benefits and challenges, particularly in patients with medical conditions that may complicate anaesthesia administration. Complications such as allergic reactions, nerve injury and anaesthetic failure, and emerging technologies such as computer-assisted anaesthesia and light-guided anaesthesia are discussed. The future of loco-regional anaesthesia in dentistry is focused on improving efficacy, reducing side effects, and enhancing patient comfort through innovative delivery systems and reversal agents.

Another very specialized and forward-looking topic is discussed in the chapter "Anesthetic Management of Bronchoscopic Lung Volume Reduction". Bronchoscopic lung volume reduction is a recently developed procedure with considerable potential for treating severe chronic obstructive pulmonary disease with hyperinflation. In comparison with open lung volume reduction, this procedure is associated with a significantly reduced risk of morbidity and mortality. However, there are still considerable risks associated with the procedure, particularly the risk of pneumothorax. A comprehensive understanding of the patient's pathophysiology and procedural steps is paramount to ensure a successful procedure and a safe outcome. Implementing a Bronchoscopic Lung Volume Reduction program requires a multidisciplinary team to prepare patients for the procedure and follow them safely until they are discharged from the hospital.

This book also addresses the topic of "Essentials of Ocular Anesthesia: Techniques, Indications, and Complications". This chapter discusses various types of anesthesia techniques, including topical, regional, and general anesthesia, highlighting their indications, techniques, and potential complications in ocular surgery.

"Fascial Plane Blocks" are regional anaesthetic techniques that relieve pain by injecting local anaesthetic into specific interfacial planes, indirectly targeting nerves rather than directly. These blocks, including transversus abdominis plane blocks, quadratus lumborum blocks, erector spinae blocks and pectoral nerve blocks, are commonly used for surgery of the abdominal wall, thorax and lower limbs. They offer an effective alternative to traditional regional anaesthetic techniques, such as epidural and paravertebral blocks, with advantages such as reduced complications and ease of use under ultrasound guidance. However, their efficacy and safety depend on precise anatomical knowledge, correct technique and an understanding of the spread of local anaesthetics within fascial compartments.

"General Anaesthesia in the Context of Haemorrhagic Shock and Trauma" underlines the negative effect of general anaesthesia on the already pathologically altered homeostasis of the trauma patient. Haemorrhagic shock is defined as a scenario of disturbed cardiovascular and cellular respiratory physiology manifested by hypotension and hypoperfusion. As studies evaluating the effects of standard general anaesthesia in haemorrhagic shock or trauma are not available, it is recommended that in any haemorrhagic shock situation with or without trauma, general anaesthesia tailored to the actual physiology of the patient, in particular titrated-to-response anaesthesia, should be performed.

The number of tracheostomized patients being treated outside of intensive care units in rehabilitation clinics and respiratory facilities is continuously increasing. As a result, we are also increasingly confronted with tracheostomy patients in the context of anesthesia services. The special features of these patients are described in the chapter "The Tracheotomized Patient for Anesthesia".

"Anesthesiologic Management of Patients with Opioids or Psychoactive Substance Use" focuses on patients who present unique challenges to the anaesthetist due to altered physiology and pharmacological interactions with anaesthetics that may increase perioperative risks. These substances can significantly affect anaesthetic requirements and responses. Preoperative assessment is critical and should include a thorough history, physical examination and toxicology screen to identify substance use, and careful scheduling of surgery to reduce the risk of withdrawal or intoxication. Intraoperative management must be tailored to the patient's substance use; regional anaesthesia is often preferred for opiate-tolerant patients to reduce additional opioid requirements, whereas general anaesthesia with close cardiovascular monitoring is recommended for stimulant patients, along with avoidance of contraindicated agents such as succinylcholine in those at risk of hyperkalemia from amphetamine-induced rhabdomyolysis.

I hope you enjoy reading this book and gain new insights.

Mark Ulrich Gerbershagen
Hospital Cologne,
University Witten Herdecke,
Cologne, Germany

Section 1

Medical Education in Anesthesiology

Chapter 1

Current Perspectives in Anesthesiology Graduate Medical Education

Natalie Bodmer, Perin Kothari, Albert Tsai and Larissa Kiwakyou

Abstract

This chapter explores the current state of anesthesiology graduate medical education (GME), highlighting recent program changes and innovations in education. We address the ongoing efforts to mitigate trainee burnout, promote diversity, equity and inclusion within anesthesiology training programs, and adapt to the changing educational landscape in the wake of the COVID-19 pandemic. The virtual and hybrid education strategies adopted during the pandemic continue to provide flexible education opportunities for graduate medical learners, while emerging immersive technologies hold promise as ways to increase access to simulation training in critical procedural and communication skills. By examining these trends, this chapter aims to inform and support anesthesiologists and GME program leaders as they navigate evolving educational paradigms and work to improve trainee experiences and outcomes.

Keywords: anesthesiology, graduate medical education, burnout, wellness, diversity equity and inclusion, simulation, augmented reality, virtual reality, artificial intelligence, COVID-19

1. Introduction

The anesthesiology training landscape is undergoing a transformation that began quietly before the COVID-19 pandemic and is now amplified by the clinical and social repercussions of the past several years. From increased recognition of the risks of trainee burnout and lack of diversity within graduate medical education (GME) programs to the tectonic changes brought by facing a global healthcare crisis, the current training environment is very different from the one experienced by anesthesiology learners even a decade ago. Disruption of the traditional progression through residency and fellowship, loss of clinical opportunities, and social distancing requirements accelerated the adoption of virtual education technologies while highlighting the critical importance of trainee well-being and support systems.

2. Updates in wellness for anesthesiology trainees

Physician burnout was recognized as a crisis at both personal and public health levels even before the COVID-19 pandemic highlighted the mental health risks of practicing in high-stakes, high-stress healthcare environments [1]. Burnout, a concept initially introduced in the 1970s and extensively studied by Maslach, is defined as a triad of emotional exhaustion, cynicism, and professional inefficacy in which depletion of emotional and physical resources leads to maladaptive detachment, depersonalization, and loss of fulfillment [2, 3].

Only in the last two decades has burnout been broadly accepted as an occupational hazard for resident physicians. In 2004, a Journal of the American Medical Association (JAMA) literature review on resident burnout reported a paucity of studies on the topic as well as ongoing debate over its importance [3]. A survey of U.S. anesthesiology residents by de Oliveira et al. in 2013 identified 41% of respondents as being at high risk for burnout; risk factors for burnout included working >70 hours per week, consuming >5 alcoholic drinks per week, and female gender [4]. In addition to the personal impact of burnout, residents at high risk of burnout and depression reported significantly higher rates of medication errors in the prior year (33% of high-risk respondents compared to 0.7% of lower-risk respondents) [4].

A growing understanding of the scope and impact of trainee burnout has led to changes to address treatable sources of workplace stress and to provide support in managing unavoidable stressors. Recently, burnout was officially added to the 11th revision of the International Classification of Diseases (ICD-11) as an occupational phenomenon. It has been described by the World Health Organization as "chronic workplace stress that has not been successfully managed" [5], highlighting that both addressing the root causes of stress and providing mechanisms for coping are essential. The Accreditation Council for Graduate Medical Education (ACGME) revised its common program requirements in 2017 with an expanded section on resident well-being that addresses the need for active involvement by programs and institutions. The group states that "[s]elf care is an important component of professionalism…[and] a skill that must be learned and nurtured in the context of other aspects of residency training," and that training places "have the same responsibility to address well-being as they do to evaluate other aspects of resident competence" [6].

2.1 Expansion of wellness programs and interventions

In response to these statistics and the ACGME mandate, anesthesiology programs have begun implementing wellness interventions ranging from mobile applications to longitudinal curricula spanning the duration of residency [7–10]. The earliest published study on a wellness program for anesthesiology residents, performed during 2006–2008, examined the impact of 16 weekly sessions teaching an evidence-based wellness intervention. Residents randomized to participate in the program showed an improvement in coping and their degree of social support at work, as well as a reduction in anxiety. Results further suggested a trend towards reduced avoidance coping (a coping mechanism involving avoiding or denying stressors) and alcohol consumption [11].

In 2014, after a survey of Canadian anesthesiology program directors found that most programs did not have a formal wellness curriculum, the University of Saskatchewan developed and implemented a curriculum that was well-received by their residents [12]. Although the program took time to implement and required establishing Department and Resident Wellness Committees, it was ultimately able to create a successful culture of peer support and self-care [12].

2.1.1 Equipping family and friends for support

Marriage and domestic partnerships have been identified as protective factors against burnout [13]. Since a lack of familiarity with the training experience may make it challenging for family and friends to effectively support trainees, some programs have begun holding educational anesthesia family days to help loved ones better understand the rigors of residency. The University of North Carolina instituted an annual Family Anesthesia Experience in 2017, where residents in their first year of anesthesiology training could participate together with their support persons in high-fidelity anesthesia simulations and didactic sessions on wellness, burnout, and substance use disorder. The experience continues to be held yearly, with a temporary move to a virtual format during the pandemic. Participating family and friends reported that the experience helped them better understand the residents' roles and stressors, and they felt that it would improve their communication and support at home [14].

2.1.2 Utilizing mobile applications

As technology becomes increasingly integrated into medical training and practice, smartphone applications present a promising modality for providing resources and support at the individual level. The University of Pittsburgh Medical Center studied whether providing free access to a meditation application could improve anesthesia resident well-being; participating residents were surveyed after 1 and 4 months of app use to assess wellness metrics including depression, stress, sleep quality, and burnout. Use of the meditation application was associated with reduced depression scores and an increased sense of personal achievement, but not with changes in the remaining two dimensions of burnout (depersonalization and emotional exhaustion) [7]. Although this study suggests positive trends with the use of a smartphone application as a wellness intervention, further investigation is needed to define the role of technology in addressing resident burnout and to optimize its implementation.

2.1.3 Reducing barriers to accessing mental health care

While the medical community has begun to normalize healthcare providers accessing mental health care, both physical and psychological barriers continue to persist. A recent review of studies assessing barriers to accessing mental health care found that residents most commonly cited lack of time as a factor, with other significant barriers including concerns about documentation, cost, and stigma associated with seeking care [15]. Many programs are working to dismantle structural barriers by offering mental health services staffed by providers who work primarily with residents, providing free care, and maintaining medical records that are separate from hospital electronic medical record systems [15]. Using an opt-out system, in which residents are provided with an appointment unless they actively elect not to participate, has been shown to increase utilization of mental health services among trainees. In a recent study examining an opt-out appointment system for residents across a variety of specialties, 59% of residents attended the appointments, with approximately one-third of these participating in additional sessions. The majority of residents in the study reported that opt-out appointments increased their willingness to engage with mental health services and were highly satisfied with the appointments; they also felt this approach demonstrated that their training programs cared about their well-being [16].

2.1.4 Work hour restrictions

A survey of U.S. anesthesiology trainees performed in 2021 as a 10-year follow up to the initial survey by de Oliveira et al. showed comparatively lower rates of burnout and depression. Despite being performed during the pandemic, the number of trainees identified as high risk for burnout had decreased from 41–24%, with 15% screening positive for depression compared to 22% in the original study [13]. These results suggest positive changes, potentially due to increased emphasis on addressing factors related to burnout and implementation of new programs. However, working >70 hours per week remained a significant risk factor for burnout, while >7 overnight calls per month was identified as a new risk factor [13].

Given concern over long work hours and sleep deprivation adversely impacting resident quality of life and patient safety, work hour restrictions have been implemented by many countries in the last two decades [17]. In 2003, the ACGME implemented duty hour restrictions for U.S. resident physicians, limiting work hours to no more than 80 hours of work per week, averaged over 4 weeks. A year later, the European Union limited resident physicians to 48 hours of work per week as part of the European Work Time Directive (EWTD) [17, 18].

An international comparison analysis published in 2023 examining resident working hours in 14 countries reported multiple strategies to reduce working hours, including limited day and/or night shift length, mandatory rest breaks, reduced night shift frequency, and weekly work hour limits. Of these, restriction of weekly work hours was the most common approach used to limit overall work hours, with maximum weekly working hours ranging from 40 to 48 hours/week in many European countries to 71.5 hours/week in Israel and 60–80 hours/week in North America. However, the study also found that residents often work more than the weekly maximum in many countries, and the authors recommend establishing mechanisms for monitoring and enforcing compliance with regulations [17].

A survey of internal medicine residents at the University of Colorado Health Science Center comparing burnout levels in 2003 (prior to ACGME duty hour restrictions) to levels in 2004 showed a reduction in emotional exhaustion and trends towards fewer residents with high depersonalization and positive depression screens, but no change in personal accomplishment or self-reported quality of care [19]. Additionally, residents reported attending fewer educational conferences after implementation of duty hour restrictions [19]. Subsequent studies continue to report mixed results: in a systematic review examining literature published in the U.S. during 2010–2013, nearly half of the studies reported that duty hour restrictions had no impact on resident wellness, with over half reporting negative impacts on resident education [20]. At best, studies have found modest improvements in U.S. resident well-being; at worst, some have found reduced quality of patient care which may be due to increased number of patient care handoffs and residents attempting to perform the same amount of work in less time [17].

Even after duty hour restrictions, the number of weekly hours worked by residents in U.S. training programs may still be twice those worked in some European programs. While studies on rates of resident burnout after implementation of the EWTD to work hours are lacking, a pilot study from the U.K. on patient safety found improved quality of care and patient safety after limiting work hours to 48 hours/week [21]. Further studies on the impact of work hour restrictions on resident well-being are needed, as is consideration of how to improve working conditions while preserving resident education and patient safety.

2.2 Impact of the COVID-19 pandemic on trainee wellness

During the pandemic, residents and fellows worldwide were redeployed to COVID-19 units, experienced disrupted training and examination schedules, and endured a period of intense personal and professional uncertainty. An early-pandemic survey of anesthesiology training programs across six continents described reduced exposure to key clinical training experiences such as airway management; junior trainees were disproportionately impacted as programs tried to protect them from aerosolizing procedures and minimize exposure to all providers involved. Survey respondents also described interruptions in the normal progression of training as elective case volume plummeted, certifying examinations were canceled, and educational activities were modified or suspended. During this time, programs worked to establish a variety of mental health resources ranging from stress recognition training to counseling sessions with trained faculty [22].

While the positive trends towards reduction in burnout noted in the 2021 follow-up survey of U.S. anesthesiology trainees are encouraging [13], rates of burnout and depression remain concerningly high. As we enter the post pandemic era, studies have yet to fully examine the impact of the last few years on anesthesiology trainees. A survey of U.S. attending anesthesiologists performed by the American Society of Anesthesiologists (ASA) in late 2022 reported that nearly 19% of respondents were experiencing burnout, with an additional 67% determined to be at high risk for burnout [23]. These numbers were higher than an initial survey conducted by the ASA in 2020, suggesting an increase in burnout among attending anesthesiologists during the 2 years of the pandemic. Major contributing factors included inadequate workplace support and staffing shortages [23]. While the stressors experienced by attending physicians may differ from those experienced by trainees, it is likely that increased burnout in the wake of the pandemic is not an isolated phenomenon. Furthermore, when the educators and role models for our next generation of physicians are suffering from burnout, it directly impacts the growth and development of their trainees. Ongoing attention should be given to the mental health of our healthcare providers at all levels of practice.

3. Diversity, equity and inclusion in anesthesiology training

Anesthesiologists care for patients of all backgrounds during their most vulnerable moments and serve as their advocates throughout the perioperative journey. From pre-operative optimization and intraoperative management to critical care and pain management, their actions have a broad impact across the healthcare system. Effectively caring for diverse patient populations requires understanding how diversity impacts healthcare as well as improving diversity within anesthesiology training programs.

3.1 Teaching diversity, equity, and inclusion

Research has consistently shown that gender and racial diversity significantly impact patient outcomes and contribute to healthcare disparities [24]. Despite overall national improvements in health outcomes, certain patient populations continue to receive lower quality health care [24]. Achieving health equity is a national priority, and incorporating diversity, equity, and inclusion (DEI) curricula into medical education is a key component of this goal. The ACGME has introduced requirements for training programs to address healthcare disparities, although it allows flexibility for programs to tailor the education based on each institution's patient population. These additional milestones emphasize the importance of evaluating trainees on their ability to provide patient-centered, culturally competent care [25]. Specialty accreditation bodies, such as the American Board of Anesthesiology (ABA), now also include DEI content in their competency examinations [26].

DEI education is a critical step towards achieving equity in healthcare, as trainees must be equipped with the tools and support needed to serve an increasingly diverse patient population. Such training also encourages the expansion of research to include more diverse groups and in areas which disproportionately affect certain populations, which is crucial for eliminating healthcare disparities [27]. The body of literature on DEI in medical education is sparse, but the awareness of its importance continues to expand. In response to the updated ACGME Common Program Requirements, residency and fellowship programs have begun incorporating these topics into their formal curricula; it is likely that additional educational interventions are occurring which have yet to be widely published.

Highlighting DEI education ensures intentionality in what is covered and taught to trainees. This approach helps address and alter the hidden curriculum, which is defined as the values and beliefs unintentionally taught during training. The hidden curriculum has been linked to worse care for all patients across medical specialties, contributing to persistent disparities in morbidity, mortality and access to healthcare among people of color [28]. By encouraging purposeful approaches for all patients, DEI training helps raise awareness of implicit biases and prompts learners to confront assumptions that might otherwise go unquestioned.

Programs have used various methods to incorporate DEI education into their curricula. Based on a review of current literature, the most common methods for teaching DEI are facilitated small group discussions and formal lectures [29]. Some programs have taken creative and learner-centric approaches to DEI education, including simulation cases, journal clubs, field trips, and self-reflective writing workshops [29]. Although most interventions are currently held as single sessions, some programs have adopted multi-year longitudinal curricula [29]. It is crucial to acknowledge that DEI topics are inherently nuanced and complex, therefore the effectiveness of delivering this content depends on each individual learner's unique background and life experiences. Overall, interactive educational methods are generally more effective than traditional lectures for complex topics, such as these related to DEI [30].

GME has a clear mandate to produce a generation of physicians who are firmly grounded in culturally competent care and committed to reducing healthcare disparities. While lectures, workshops, and simulations are valuable tools for integrating these topics in the resident education, it is crucial to avoid treating diversity and bias training as mere formalities. Effective DEI education should be implemented with the goal of reducing implicit biases [31]. Programs must ensure the delivery of meaningful DEI curricula that address cultural competency and health care disparities and assess residents' ability to provide culturally competent care.

Recent research suggests that the environment physicians train in can impact their care of patients. A retrospective review revealed that female patients treated by female physicians had over twice the survival rate after an acute myocardial infarction compared to those treated by male physicians [32]. Interestingly, upon further analysis, the data also suggested that female patients treated by male physicians who had greater exposure to female patients and colleagues had improved outcomes [32]. This suggests that a physician's exposure to a diverse environment can positively influence their care and treatment of diverse patient populations, highlighting the importance of cultivating diversity within GME training programs in addition to teaching about it.

Much remains to be studied about how to best integrate DEI education, and it is essential to determine whether increasing trainees' knowledge about healthcare disparities translates into more equitable care. There is still little published research examining how DEI-focused curricula impact patient care outcomes [33], and while further study is needed on methodology, the importance of addressing health disparities as part of GME is undeniable. By equipping physicians to deliver more culturally responsive care, the hope is that that it will ultimately translate into expanded access to high-quality healthcare for underserved populations.

3.2 Practicing diversity, equity and inclusion

While DEI education is an essential component of training, it is also critical to actively cultivate diversity within GME programs. In its Common Program Requirements for Residency, the ACGME mandates that programs practice "systematic recruitment and retention of a diverse and inclusive workforce of residents, fellows (if present), faculty members, senior administrative GME staff members, and other relevant members of its academic community" [25].

Despite advances over the years, women and minorities remain underrepresented in the field of anesthesiology. While women became the majority of U.S. medical school graduates as of 2020–2021 and made up nearly 52% of U.S. medical school graduates in 2022–2023, they comprised only 36% of anesthesiology residents that same year [34]. The Association of American Medical Collages (AAMC) reported that in 2022–2023, among anesthesiology residents, 0.8% were American Indian or Alaska Native, 7.7% were Black or African American, 7.6% were Hispanic, Latino or of Spanish origin, and 0.4% were Native Hawaiian or other Pacific Islander [35].

In 2021, a survey of residents across the U.S. found that 42% of respondents felt that having female/diverse faculty was somewhat to very important in their decision to pursue anesthesiology, with 67.2% reporting that role models and mentors were somewhat to very important in their decision [36]. In this same study, over one-third of the female respondents reported having experienced discrimination due to gender or gender identity, compared to less than 7% of male respondents. Approximately 19% of trainees also reported discrimination during the residency application process because of their race/ethnicity [36]. The results of this survey suggest that diversity among faculty is important in recruiting and preparing the next generation of anesthesiologists while also showing that much remains to be done in creating inclusive resident recruitment processes.

As systematically combating biases in recruitment and selection of residents represents an ongoing opportunity for improvement, it is important that programs are supported in this mission. Recently, a group at the Indiana University School of Medicine developed a DEI Toolkit for program directors, which was implemented during the 2021–2022 recruitment season at their institution. The toolkit contained a compilation of resources and guidelines, training on unconscious bias and allyship, as well as resources for reporting mistreatment. Approximately 63% of program directors in the study accessed the toolkit, and 31% made changes to their recruitment process by requiring unconscious bias training for faculty and residents involved in residency interviews and the rank process or created a standardized scoring rubric for interviews [37].

3.2.1 Improving access through virtual interviews

During the pandemic, GME programs shifted to virtual interviews to comply with social distancing requirements and reduce the risk of virus spread. Even though the height of the pandemic has passed, the AAMC continues to recommend that programs use virtual interviews to improve accessibility to programs and equalize the application process [38]. Traditional in-person interviews can impose a financial burden of hundreds to thousands of dollars from costs associated with travel, restricting access to those able to afford it or who are willing to take out additional loans. This financial barrier is reduced or eliminated when interviews are hosted virtually. By expanding access to all eligible applicants regardless of their financial situation, virtual interviews increase the equity and inclusivity of the selection process and have to potential to improve diversity within programs. For programs choosing to return to in-person interviews, the AAMC recommends offering financial support for travel to applicants who may need it [38].

3.2.2 Update on race-conscious admissions

In the U.S., the legal landscape surrounding race-conscious admission programs in higher education changed abruptly in June 2023, when the U.S. Supreme Court issued a ruling reversing decades of affirmative action policy. Prior policy had supported the consideration of race during admissions with the goal of recruiting a diverse student body, but colleges and universities are now barred from using race as a factor in the admission process. While this ruling was directed towards undergraduate admissions, it also carried repercussions for graduate medical admissions. The ACGME released a statement on July 12, 2023, reaffirming its commitment to promoting diversity and inclusion within all levels of GME while clarifying that this goal can be achieved through strategies other than race-based affirmative action [39].

While much remains to be accomplished, an important first step towards improving diversity within GME is increasing awareness. Providing training to reduce implicit bias during recruitment and evaluation, supporting trainees in cultivating relationships with role models, offering pathway programs, and creating equitable education systems are all strategies to promote diversity and prepare physicians to address inequalities in our healthcare systems [39]. Through such steps, programs can create more equitable and inclusive environments for both anesthesiology trainees and the patients they care for.

4. Education strategies in the post pandemic era

The COVID-19 pandemic drastically changed the landscape of medical education, impacting all levels of learners. While many educational activities were suspended worldwide as anesthesiology departments focused on keeping their physicians safe and adequately staffing COVID-19 units, education pioneers across the globe innovated methods to minimize exposure for learners while still preparing the next generation of physicians to care for patients [40].

In the years leading up to the pandemic, there were gradual shifts towards the use of technology and self-directed learning to decrease traditional didactic-based learning [41]. This was accelerated by the pandemic, with some changes requiring implementation before formal study could ensure their validity. In the years since, these techniques have been increasingly studied. While educators are researching and pushing the boundaries of education in all fields, this section focuses on concepts most relevant to anesthesiology training and education. Across all learner levels, learning management systems have become crucial for housing and organizing educational materials, and there is a renewed emphasis on the social functions of these tools [42].

As graduate medical learners are influenced by their exposure to clinical anesthesia during their undergraduate medical school training, the impact of COVID-19 on undergraduate medical education will also be addressed here.

4.1 Undergraduate medical education

Anesthesiology clerkships for medical students were significantly disrupted by the pandemic, both due to the cancelation of surgeries and the high-risk nature of aerosolizing procedures integral to the practice of anesthesia. In March 2020, the AAMC suggested pausing clinical rotations [41], and while some anesthesiology clerkships were transitioned to virtual formats, others were canceled altogether. With a lack of adequate personal protective equipment and reduced surgical volumes, medical students had few opportunities for exposure to clinical anesthesiology prior to starting residency.

In response to these challenges, some departments created virtual clerkship experiences. The University of Minnesota Medical School created a two-week virtual anesthesiology clerkship that used a variety of educational tools to create an experiential learning environment. Core anesthesia topics, such as the preoperative evaluation and airway management, were covered with prerecorded PowerPoint lectures and supplemental reading assignments. The operating room experience, which was most impacted by the pandemic, was replicated with sessions filmed in a high-fidelity simulated operating room with live monitors and a mannequin patient. Faculty-led case-based learning discussions (CBLDs) then expanded on the recorded curriculum in small-group virtual sessions. Medical students who participated in the virtual clerkship reported that the experience exceeded their expectations; the majority found the CBLDs to be informative, and all participants agreed that the virtual assignments facilitated their learning [43]. Other departments also used case-based learning and virtual sessions to educate their learners as clinical exposure decreased.

4.2 Graduate medical education

The greatest efforts to ensure adequate education during the COVID-19 pandemic were directed towards anesthesiology residents and fellows. As they would be called upon to practice as fully trained physicians on graduation, it was essential to create tools to supplement their clinical exposure and allow for the safe practice of anesthesiology. In particular, opportunities for airway management were drastically diminished as emphasis was placed on using the most experienced operator during procedures such as intubation. Many institutions shifted towards exclusive use of video laryngoscopy, rapid-sequence intubations without mask ventilation, and endotracheal intubation instead of supraglottic airways to minimize aerosolization and virus spread [44]. One single-center study from the United Kingdom noted a nearly 23% decrease in the number of intubations performed by trainees, with the number of supraglottic airways reduced by 44% [45]. In response to reduced hands-on experience in the clinical setting, techniques such as simulation, airway training courses, and mannequin-based practice emerged as supplemental educational tools [46].

Traditional didactics were also disrupted, and many programs developed online educational supplemental teaching and courses to allow continuation of didactic teaching as in-person sessions were canceled due to social distancing requirements. The flipped classroom model (FCM), which is based on providing learners with some foundational knowledge prior to class and then applying it to more advanced problem-solving scenarios in the classroom, has been utilized for decades and has become increasingly indispensable across all levels of learners [47–50].

A wave of research on the FCM indicates its efficacy for learners at the GME level, with one study noting that participants of the FCM had increased knowledge retention compared to traditional lectures [51]. The FCM, which allows for active and autonomous learning with individualized resources tailored to various learning styles [52], has been shown to be preferred by residents as well [49]. A European study of the FCM directly correlated increased retention of knowledge with the hours of pre-classroom worked assigned to the residents [47], while another study noted that faculty found increased student interaction and learning in FCM sessions [53].

4.3 A shift towards competency-based assessment

In 2020, the ACGME introduced major changes in milestone targets to emphasize competency-based training and objective performance measures, replacing long-standing time- and volume-based assessments of clinical mastery [54]. This shift in milestone criteria coincided with the onset of the pandemic, disrupting established medical training paradigms as institutions grappled with new assessment metrics in the midst of social distancing restrictions. In response, the Clinical Learning Environment Review (CLER) program was mobilized by the ACGME in 2022 to examine the impact of the pandemic on GME. The subsequent CLER report identified rapid adoption of virtual and hybrid education modalities by training institutions, a trend which appears to have permanently reshaped the landscape of medical education [55, 56].

5. Immersive simulation technologies: Augmented and virtual reality

Simulation-based medical education (SBME) in anesthesiology training has been shown to improve technical, communication, and leadership skills and has the potential to fulfill requirements for competency-based training assessments [57–59]. However, exposure to SBME in anesthesiology training remains limited. A survey of 45 anesthesiology residency programs in 2022 revealed that most programs (64%) had infrequent exposure to SBME due to social distancing (76%), scheduling (58%), and administrative barriers [60]. Additional barriers included costs associated with equipment and facility use, space constraints, and travel challenges. The authors concluded that although SBME was widely adopted by anesthesiology training programs, the frequency of exposure to simulation was limited by pandemic restrictions, scheduling constraints, and a lack of simulation staff. Although COVID-19-related challenges have subsided since the reported study, resident scheduling and costs associated with SBME programs are likely to persist as barriers to readily accessible simulation education in anesthesiology.

5.1 High fidelity simulation through mixed-reality technology

Immersive simulation technologies such as augmented reality (AR) and virtual reality (VR) have benefited from immense commercial interest over the past decade, with the likes of Apple, Google, and Meta all investing heavily in hardware and software development. The rise of these technologies, along with pandemic-driven innovations in healthcare education, have accelerated the adoption of mixed-reality technology in SBME [56].

AR and VR have the ability to digitally reconstruct aspects of the clinical environment and have been shown to improve clinical learning in anesthesiology [58]. They are also portable, customizable, and cost-effective, potentially lessening the financial and logistical barriers that have limited expanded exposure to SBME in anesthesiology. AR and VR headsets can be readily deployed in a wide range of physical settings, allowing learners to participate in interactive, high-fidelity simulations from the hospital, medical school, and home as well as in global-health applications [61].

Software customizations provide operational flexibility to learners utilizing AR and VR for SBME, as simulation scenarios can be created with vast permutations of variables to reflect the reality of clinical practice. Importantly, these technologies offer operational simplicity and cost-efficiency compared with traditional in-person, center-based simulations, which are generally labor-intensive and expensive to operate. With continued maturation of the immersive technology market, AR and VR are expected to become even more affordable and user-friendly.

Although AR and VR have already been adopted for procedural training in clinical practice, non-technical and communication skills are still largely taught by traditional in-situ simulations [62–64]. Recent investigations on the use of AR in non-technical skills assessment have yielded positive participant perception of the technology and may be further developed to expand the scope of training goals [65]. Many AR and VR headsets incorporate eye-tracking technology, which may be leveraged to provide gaze pattern analysis, reaction time, and other objective performance data [66–68]. Immersive technology presents an exciting opportunity for medical education and research, as its potential applications are broad and only beginning to be explored.

6. The rise of artificial intelligence

The rapid rise of artificial intelligence (AI) in healthcare represents the newest frontier for GME. Even as the era of COVID-19 subsides and social distancing comes to an end, AI has emerged as another global change, the implications which are yet to be understood. A 2021 cross-sectional survey of U.S. physician anesthesiologists found that 48% of respondents had a positive attitude towards using AI in clinical practice, believing that it could lead to more efficient, timely, and effective health care. Concerns about the implementation of AI in anesthesiology include the current lack of transparent algorithms, unclear malpractice implications, and the risk of medical errors. Respondents also expressed unease about potential decrease in demand for anesthesiologists and reduction in earnings. Although the survey had only a 4% response rate, it provides early insight into perceived benefits and barriers to implementing of AI in anesthesiology [69].

Areas that will need to be addressed by GME in the near future include policies on the use of generative AI (such as ChatGPT) in academic work, as well as guidance on how to evaluate and safely use emerging AI technologies. Current software programs and human reviewers alike are unable to consistently identify AI-generated content, and some publishers are beginning to issue guidelines on the use of generative AI in manuscript development [70]. AI now has the ability to create responses to clinical questions, generate treatment plans, and provide patient education [70]. A recent review identified applications involving AI and machine learning specific to anesthesiology, including depth of anesthesia monitoring, image-guided techniques, prediction of events such as hypotension, and control of drug administration [71]. The emergence of AI raises important questions about its use in both scholarly and clinical work, and today's trainees must learn to ethically and safely navigate this nascent but powerful technology.

7. Conclusion

From personal well-being and methods of learning to the ways in which trainees interact with their environment and individual patients, we can celebrate the progress made in anesthesiology GME while acknowledging that much remains to be done. The revised program requirements from the ACGME, along with statistics on the high rates of burnout among anesthesiology residents, have inspired multiple strategies for improving trainee wellness ranging from full curricula to family education days and mindfulness training. In contrast to the early 2000s, when the validity of trainee burnout was still being questioned, it is now expected that all programs address trainees' psychological, emotional and physical well-being as part of their development as physicians [6].

With recent surveys showing that women and minorities are still underrepresented in the field of anesthesiology [34, 35], GME programs must continue to work towards equitable recruiting processes for residents and fellows. The ACGME has outlined the need to create a diverse and inclusive workforce in all areas of GME, from trainees to faculty to staff, and to ensure residents practice cultural humility and respect for diversity when interacting with their patient populations [25]. While programs have begun incorporating DEI training into their education programs and examining the recruiting processes for residents and fellows, this remains an essential area for ongoing research and innovation.

Even as pandemic restrictions are lifted and clinical environments return to normal, the medical education landscape remains altered in ways that are likely to be permanent. From flipped classrooms to virtual education, educational tools continue to evolve and will require ongoing study to confirm their efficacy compared to traditional learning methods. The rapid development and adoption of novel teaching tools for anesthesiology training has also enabled educators to explore nontraditional methods in technical, communication, and knowledge-based instruction. Mixed-reality technologies such as AR and VR hold immense potential as valuable adjuncts to traditional in-situ simulation and possess operational advantages that may facilitate expanded access to SBME, while AI applications stand to further revolutionize training in the coming years.

The anesthesiology training landscape continues to transform. Like its physicians, who must constantly adjust to rapidly changing clinical situations, anesthesiology GME continues to adapt to evolving educational environments. Amid advances in technology and shifts in attitude and resources, the field of anesthesiology remains well-positioned to adapt to the educational needs of its current and future learners.

Conflict of interest

The authors declare no conflict of interest.

Author details

Natalie Bodmer†, Perin Kothari†, Albert Tsai† and Larissa Kiwakyou*
Division of Cardiothoracic Anesthesiology, Department of Anesthesiology Perioperative and Pain Medicine, Stanford University, Palo Alto, California, USA

*Address all correspondence to: lmiyachi@stanford.edu

†These authors share equal contributions to this work.

References

[1] Office of the Surgeon General. Addressing Health Worker Burnout: The U.S. Surgeon General's Advisory on Building a Thriving Health Workforce. Washington (DC): US Department of Health and Human Services; 2022 [Accessed: August 11, 2024]

[2] Maslach C, Leiter M. ch. 43. In: Behavior GF, editor. Burnout, in Stress: Concepts, Cognition, Emotion. Cambridge: Academic Press; 2016. pp. 351-357

[3] Thomas NK. Resident burnout, (in eng). JAMA. 2004;**292**(23):2880-2889. DOI: 10.1001/jama.292.23.2880

[4] de Oliveira GS et al. The prevalence of burnout and depression and their association with adherence to safety and practice standards: A survey of United States anesthesiology trainees, (in eng). Anesthesia and Analgesia. 2013;**117**(1):182-193. DOI: 10.1213/ANE.0b013e3182917da9

[5] World Health Organization. Burn-out an Occupational Phenomenon: International Classification of Diseases. Geneva: World Health Organization; 2019. Available from: https://www.who.int/news/item/28-05-2019-burn-out-an-occupationalphenomenon-international-classification-of-diseases [Accessed: August 9, 2024]

[6] Accreditation Council for Graduate Medical Education. Common Program Requirements Section VI with Background and Intent. Chicago: Accreditation Council for Graduate Medical Education; 2017. Available from: https://www.acgme.org/globalassets/PFAssets/ProgramRequirements/CPRs_Section-VI_with-Background-and-Intent_2017-01.pdf [Accessed: August 9, 2024]

[7] Carullo PC, Ungerman EA, Metro DG, Adams PS. The impact of a smartphone meditation application on anesthesia trainee well-being, (in eng). Journal of Clinical Anesthesia. 2021;**75**:110525. DOI: 10.1016/j.jclinane.2021.110525

[8] Repine KM, Bawmann O, Mendlen M, Lowenstein SR. Investigating wellness and burnout initiatives for anesthesiology resident physicians: Time for evidence-based investigation and implementation, (in eng). Anesthesiology Clinics. 2022;**40**(2):275-285. DOI: 10.1016/j.anclin.2022.01.004

[9] Brainard AJ, Ziniel SI, Zuk J, Dingmann C, Janosy NR. Evaluation of a formal wellness curriculum to reduce burnout in anesthesia residents: A pilot study, (in eng). The Journal of Education in Perioperative Medicine. 2019;**21**(1):E631

[10] Thornton KC, Sinskey JL, Boscardin CK, Sullivan KR. Design and implementation of an innovative, longitudinal wellness curriculum in an anesthesiology residency program, (in eng). A & A Practice. 2021;**15**(2):e01387. DOI: 10.1213/XAA.0000000000001387

[11] Saadat H, Snow DL, Ottenheimer S, Dai F, Kain ZN. Wellness program for anesthesiology residents: A randomized, controlled trial, (in eng). Acta Anaesthesiologica Scandinavica. 2012;**56**(9):1130-1138. DOI: 10.1111/j.1399-6576.2012.02705.x

[12] Chakravarti A, Raazi M, O'Brien J, Balaton B. Anesthesiology resident wellness program at the University of Saskatchewan: Concept and

development, (in eng). Canadian Journal of Anaesthesia. 2017;**64**(2):185-198. DOI: 10.1007/s12630-016-0772-1

[13] Bui D, Winegarner A, Kendall MC, Almeida M, Apruzzese P, De Oliveira G. Burnout and depression among anesthesiology trainees in the United States: An updated National Survey, (in eng). Journal of Clinical Anesthesia. 2023;**84**:110990. DOI: 10.1016/j.jclinane.2022.110990

[14] Martinelli SM, Tran TN, Chidgey BA, Isaak RS, Teeter EG, Chen F. Family anesthesia experience: Improving social support of residents through education of their family and friends, (in eng). MedEdPORTAL. 2023;**19**:11370. DOI: 10.15766/mep_2374-8265.11370

[15] Slavin S, Cheong J, Bienstock J, Bernstein C. Overcoming barriers to mental health care for residents, (in eng). Journal of Graduate Medical Education. 2024;**16**(3):374-378. DOI: 10.4300/JGME-D-24-00409.1

[16] Kevern T, Davies DR, Stiel K, Raaum S. Impact of opt-out therapy appointments on resident physicians' mental health, well-being, stigma, and willingness to engage, (in eng). Journal of Graduate Medical Education. 2023;**15**(6):734-737. DOI: 10.4300/JGME-D-22-00898.1

[17] Maoz Breuer R et al. Work like a doc: A comparison of regulations on residents' working hours in 14 high-income countries, (in eng). Health Policy. 2023;**130**:104753. DOI: 10.1016/j.healthpol.2023.104753

[18] Temple J. Resident duty hours around the globe: Where are we now? (in eng). BMC Medical Education. 2014;**14** (Suppl. 1):S8. DOI: 10.1186/1472-6920-14-S1-S8

[19] Gopal R, Glasheen JJ, Miyoshi TJ, Prochazka AV. Burnout and internal medicine resident work-hour restrictions, (in eng). Archives of Internal Medicine. 2005;**165**(22):2595-2600. DOI: 10.1001/archinte.165.22.2595

[20] Bolster L, Rourke L. The effect of restricting residents' duty hours on patient safety, resident well-being, and resident education: An updated systematic review, (in eng). Journal of Graduate Medical Education. 2015;7(3):349-363. DOI: 10.4300/JGME-D-14-00612.1

[21] Cappuccio FP et al. Implementing a 48 h EWTD-compliant Rota for junior doctors in the UK does not compromise patients' safety: Assessor-blind pilot comparison, (in eng). QJM. 2009;**102**(4):271-282. DOI: 10.1093/qjmed/hcp004

[22] Sneyd JR et al. Impact of the COVID-19 pandemic on anaesthesia trainees and their training, (in eng). British Journal of Anaesthesia. 2020;**125**(4):450-455. DOI: 10.1016/j.bja.2020.07.011

[23] Afonso AM, Cadwell JB, Staffa SJ, Sinskey JL, Vinson AE, U.S. Attending anesthesiologist burnout in the postpandemic era, (in eng). Anesthesiology. 2024;**140**(1):38-51. DOI: 10.1097/ALN.0000000000004784

[24] Institute of Medicine, Board on Health Sciences Policy, Committee on Understanding and Eliminating Racial and Ethnic Disparities in Health Care. Unequal Treatment: Confronting Racial and Ethnic Disparities in Health Care. Washington (DC): National Academies Press; 2003

[25] Accreditation Council for Graduate Medical Education. Common Program

Requirements (Residency). Available from: www.acgme.org/globalassets/pfassets/programrequirements/cprresidency_2023.pdf [Accessed: August 19, 2024]

[26] American Board of Anesthesiology. Board Statement on DEI Work, Mission and Milestones. Available from: https://www.theaba.org/2021/06/board-statement-on-growing-dei-work-mission-and-milestones-2/ [Accessed: August 1, 2024]

[27] Ellinas H, Trimm F, Kountz D, Bienstock J. Implementing systematic culture change to improve diversity in graduate medical education, (in eng). Journal of Graduate Medical Education. 2022;**14**(2):235-236. DOI: 10.4300/JGME-D-22-00086.1

[28] Hall WJ et al. Implicit racial/ethnic bias among health care professionals and its influence on health care outcomes: A systematic review, (in eng). American Journal of Public Health. 2015;**105**(12):e60-e76. DOI: 10.2105/AJPH.2015.302903

[29] Chung AS et al. Educational outcomes of diversity curricula in graduate medical education, (in eng). Journal of Graduate Medical Education. 2023;**15**(2):152-170. DOI: 10.4300/JGME-D-22-00497.1

[30] Pluta WJ, Richards BF, Mutnick A. PBL and beyond: Trends in collaborative learning, (in eng). Teaching and Learning in Medicine. 2013;**25**(Suppl 1):S9-S16. DOI: 10.1080/10401334.2013.842917

[31] Sukhera J, Watling C. A framework for integrating implicit bias recognition into health professions education, (in eng). Academic Medicine. 2018;**93**(1):35-40. DOI: 10.1097/ACM.0000000000001819

[32] Greenwood BN, Carnahan S, Huang L. Patient-physician gender concordance and increased mortality among female heart attack patients, (in eng). Proceedings of the National Academy of Sciences of the United States of America. 2018;**115**(34):8569-8574. DOI: 10.1073/pnas.1800097115

[33] Borum ML, Onumah C. To the editor: Assessing outcomes of diversity curricula in graduate medical education is necessary to decrease health care disparities, (in eng). Journal of Graduate Medical Education. 2023;**15**(5):610-611. DOI: 10.4300/JGME-D-23-00576.1

[34] Lautenberger D, Dandar V. The State of Women in Academic Medicine 2023-2024: Progressing Towards Equity. Washington DC: Association of American Medical Colleges; 2024

[35] Association of American Medical Colleges. Table B5. Number of Active MD Residents, by Race/Ethnicity (Alone or In Combination) and GME Specialty. Washington (DC): Association of American Medical Colleges; 2023. [Online]. Available from: www.aamc.org/data-reports/students-residents/data/report-residents/2023/table-b5-md-residents-race-ethnicity-and-specialty [Accessed: August 19, 2024]

[36] Patel S et al. Diversity, equity, and inclusion among anesthesiology trainees, (in eng). Womens Health Reports (New Rochelle). 2022;**3**(1):414-419. DOI: 10.1089/whr.2021.0123

[37] Nabhan ZM et al. Advancing equity in graduate medical education recruitment through a diversity equity and inclusion (DEI) toolkit for program directors, (in eng). Journal of Medical Education and Curricular Development. 2023;**10**:23821205231203136. DOI: 10.1177/23821205231203136

[38] Association of American Medical Colleges. Interviews in GME: Where Do We Go From Here? Available from: https://www.aamc.org/about-us/mission-areas/medical-education/interviews-gme-where-do-we-go-here [Accessed: September 6, 2024]

[39] Nasca T. Follow-up to Dr. Nasca's June 13 Letter to the Community after Supreme Court Decision Regarding College Admissions and Race. Chicago: Accreditation Council for Graduate Medical Education; 2023. Available from: https://www.acgme.org/newsroom/2023/7/letter-to-the-community-july-12/ [Accessed: August 27, 2024]

[40] Anwar A, Seger C, Tollefson A, Diachun CAB, Tanaka P, Umar S. Medical education in the COVID-19 era: Impact on anesthesiology trainees, (in eng). Journal of Clinical Anesthesia. 2020;**66**:109949. DOI: 10.1016/j.jclinane.2020.109949

[41] Rose S. Medical student education in the time of COVID-19, (in eng). JAMA. 2020;**323**(21):2131-2132. DOI: 10.1001/jama.2020.5227

[42] Martinelli SM, Chen F, Isaak RS, Huffmyer JL, Neves SE, Mitchell JD. Educating anesthesiologists during the coronavirus disease 2019 pandemic and beyond, (in eng). Anesthesia and Analgesia. 2021;**132**(3):585-593. DOI: 10.1213/ANE.0000000000005333

[43] Nguyen W, Fromer I, Remskar M, Zupfer E. Development and implementation of video-recorded simulation scenarios to facilitate case-based learning discussions for medical students' virtual anesthesiology clerkship, (in eng). MedEdPORTAL. 2023;**19**:11306. DOI: 10.15766/mep_2374-8265.11306

[44] Raithel S, Fields KG, Wu Y, Yao D. Adoption of airway management guidelines during COVID-19 pandemic improved endotracheal intubation success, (in eng). Journal of Clinical Anesthesia. 2022;**76**:110556. DOI: 10.1016/j.jclinane.2021.110556

[45] Hughes L, Murphy O, Lenihan M, Mhuircheartaigh RN, Wall TP. Impact of the COVID-19 pandemic on anaesthesia specialty training: A single-Centre quantitative analysis, (in eng). BJA Open. 2023;**5**:100117. DOI: 10.1016/j.bjao.2022.100117

[46] Pereda E, De Hert S, El Tahan M, Romero CS. Retailoring training programmes in anaesthesia and intensive care after the coronavirus disease 2019 outbreak, (in eng). Current Opinion in Anaesthesiology. 2023;**36**(3):369-375. DOI: 10.1097/ACO.0000000000001260

[47] Marchalot A et al. Effectiveness of a blended learning course and flipped classroom in first year anaesthesia training, (in eng). Anaesthesia Critical Care & Pain Medicine. 2018;**37**(5):411-415. DOI: 10.1016/j.accpm.2017.10.008

[48] Martinelli SM et al. Results of a flipped classroom teaching approach in anesthesiology residents, (in eng). Journal of Graduate Medical Education. 2017;**9**(4):485-490. DOI: 10.4300/JGME-D-17-00128.1

[49] Martinelli SM, Chen F, Mcevoy MD, Zvara DA, Schell RM. Utilization of the flipped classroom in anesthesiology graduate medical education: An initial survey of faculty beliefs and practices about active learning, (in eng). The Journal of Education in Perioperative Medicine. 2018;**20**(1):E617

[50] Zhang D, Xiang J, Wei Y. Effects of flipped classroom teaching in

anaesthesiology residents: A protocol for systematic review and meta-analysis, (in eng). BMJ Open. 2024;**14**(5):e084362. DOI: 10.1136/bmjopen-2024-084362

[51] Chen F, Lui AM, Martinelli SM. A systematic review of the effectiveness of flipped classrooms in medical education, (in eng). Medical Education. 2017;**51**(6):585-597. DOI: 10.1111/medu.13272

[52] Wang Y, Su WJ, Li JC, Yang MC. Flipped classroom model in the standardized training of anesthesiology residents, (in eng). Asian Journal of Surgery. 2023;**46**(11):4899-4900. DOI: 10.1016/j.asjsur.2023.05.177

[53] Kurup V, Sendlewski G. The feasibility of incorporating a flipped classroom model in an anesthesia residency curriculum-pilot study, (in eng). The Yale Journal of Biology and Medicine. 2020;**93**(3):411-417

[54] Ambardekar AP et al. The anesthesiology milestones 2.0: An improved competency-based assessment for residency training, (in eng). Anesthesia and Analgesia. 2021;**133**(2):353-361. DOI: 10.1213/ANE.0000000000005499

[55] Nasca TJ, Wagner R, Weiss KB. Introduction to the CLER national report of findings 2022: The COVID-19 pandemic and its impact on the clinical learning environment, (in eng). Journal of Graduate Medical Education. 2023;**15**(1):140-142. DOI: 10.4300/JGME-D-22-00938.1

[56] Remtulla R. The present and future applications of technology in adapting medical education amidst the COVID-19 pandemic, (in eng). JMIR Medical Education. 2020;**6**(2):e20190. DOI: 10.2196/20190

[57] Higham H, Baxendale B. To err is human: Use of simulation to enhance training and patient safety in anaesthesia, (in eng). British Journal of Anaesthesia. 2017;**119**(suppl_1):i106-i114. DOI: 10.1093/bja/aex302

[58] Samadbeik M, Yaaghobi D, Bastani P, Abhari S, Rezaee R, Garavand A. The applications of virtual reality technology in medical groups teaching, (in eng). Journal of Advances in Medical Education & Professionalism. 2018;**6**(3):123-129

[59] Lorello GR, Cook DA, Johnson RL, Brydges R. Simulation-based training in anaesthesiology: A systematic review and meta-analysis, (in eng). British Journal of Anaesthesia. 2014;**112**(2):231-245. DOI: 10.1093/bja/aet414

[60] Chen MJ et al. Defining and addressing anesthesiology needs in simulation-based medical education, (in eng). The Journal of Education in Perioperative Medicine. 2022;**24**(2):1-15. DOI: 10.46374/volxxiv_issue2_mitchell

[61] Hess O et al. Communication skills training using remote augmented reality medical simulation: A feasibility and acceptability qualitative study, (in eng). Medical Science Educator. 2022;**32**(5):1005-1014. DOI: 10.1007/s40670-022-01598-7

[62] Casso G, Schoettker P, Savoldelli GL, Azzola A, Cassina T. Development and initial evaluation of a novel, ultraportable, virtual reality bronchoscopy simulator: The computer airway simulation system, (in eng). Anesthesia and Analgesia. 2019;**129**(5):1258-1264. DOI: 10.1213/ANE.0000000000003316

[63] Moo-Young J, Weber TM, Kapralos B, Quevedo A, Alam F. Development of

unity simulator for epidural insertion training for replacing current lumbar puncture simulators, (in eng). Cureus. 2021;**13**(2):e13409. DOI: 10.7759/cureus.13409

[64] Huang VW, Jones CB, Gomez ED. State of the art of virtual reality simulation in anesthesia, (in eng). International Anesthesiology Clinics. 2020;**58**(4):31-35. DOI: 10.1097/AIA.0000000000000298

[65] Tsai A et al. Participant perceptions of augmented reality simulation for cardiac anesthesiology training: A prospective, mixed-methods study, (in eng). The Journal of Education in Perioperative Medicine. 2023;**25**(3):E712. DOI: 10.46374/volxxv_issue3_Tsai

[66] Caruso TJ et al. Integrated eye tracking on magic leap one during augmented reality medical simulation: A technical report, (in eng). BMJ Simulation & Technology Enhanced Learning. 2021;**7**(5):431-434. DOI: 10.1136/bmjstel-2020-000782

[67] Chen HE et al. Can eye tracking be used to predict performance improvements in simulated medical training? A case study in central venous catheterization, (in eng). Proceedings of the International Symposium on Human Factors and Ergonomics in Health Care. 2019;**8**(1):110-114. DOI: 10.1177/2327857919081025

[68] Ashraf H, Sodergren MH, Merali N, Mylonas G, Singh H, Darzi A. Eye-tracking technology in medical education: A systematic review, (in eng). Medical Teacher. 2018;**40**(1):62-69. DOI: 10.1080/0142159X.2017.1391373

[69] Estrada Alamo CE, Diatta F, Monsell SE, Lane-Fall MB. Artificial intelligence in anesthetic care: A survey of physician anesthesiologists, (in eng). Anesthesia and Analgesia. 2024;**138**(5):938-950. DOI: 10.1213/ANE.0000000000006752

[70] Patel SJ et al. The year in graduate medical education: Selected highlights from 2022, (in eng). Journal of Cardiothoracic and Vascular Anesthesia. 2023;**37**(9):1568-1578. DOI: 10.1053/j.jvca.2023.04.040

[71] Lopes S, Rocha G, Guimarães-Pereira L. Artificial intelligence and its clinical application in anesthesiology: A systematic review, (in eng). Journal of Clinical Monitoring and Computing. 2024;**38**(2):247-259. DOI: 10.1007/s10877-023-01088-0

Section 2

Pediatric Anesthesiology

Chapter 2

Anesthesia for Robotic Surgeries in Children

Pallavi Ahluwalia and Amit Ahluwalia

Abstract

Robot-assisted laparoscopic surgery is increasingly popular in children, including newborns and infants, because it provides a better three-dimensional (3D) view for the surgeon, making the procedure easier. Anesthetists should be aware of the anesthesia-related challenges that a child undergoing robotic surgery may face. Some of these challenges are related to patient positioning, restricted airway and intravenous access, pressure damage to nerves and tissues, and the potential for hypothermia In addition, it is important to understand the physiological changes caused by pneumoperitoneum (PNP) and what effects they have on the different organ systems. Lung ventilatory strategies are needed to maintain oxygenation and prevent hypercarbia and atelectasis, such as limiting peak airway pressure to 25 cm H_2O, applying positive end-expiratory pressure (PEEP) of 5 mm Hg, and delivering a tidal volume of 6–7 ml/kg.

Keywords: anesthesia management, laparoscopic surgery, minimally invasive surgery, pediatric anesthesia, robot-assisted surgery, postoperative pain, complications

1. Introduction

Robot-assisted surgery has experienced significant growth in the recent decades. The use of minimally invasive surgical techniques in pediatric surgery has increased dramatically in the last 10 to 15 years, primarily due to the numerous benefits they offer (**Box 1**). Robotic surgery provides improved precision, eliminates operative tremors, offers better ergonomics, ensures improved accuracy of movements, seven degrees of freedom, and three-dimensional views, and reduces surgeon fatigue.

1. Smaller scars, better healing
2. Reduced surgical stress and fluid shifts
3. Reduced blood loss
4. Less need for postoperative analgesia
5. Lesser postoperative respiratory and wound complications
6. Earlier ambulation
7. Decreased length of stay in hospital

Box 1.
Adv antages of robotic-assisted and laparoscopic surgery over open surgery.

Although robotic surgery is more costly, takes longer, and has a steeper learning curve, it is essentially an extension of laparoscopic surgery. Its primary purpose is to improve accessibility and surgical quality for complex treatments that would otherwise require open surgery. Consequently, robotics has been incorporated into every medical specialty, including pediatric surgery.

The use of robotic surgery in pediatric cases has become more common, with procedures ranging from urological surgeries such as pyeloplasty, nephrectomy, and ureteric transplantation to gastrointestinal surgeries such as cholecystectomy and colonoscopy [1]. Some surgeons have also performed choledochal cyst excision, Kasai's portoenterostomy, repair of tracheoesophageal fistula, and congenital diaphragmatic hernia using robotic techniques. However, performing robotic surgery on newborns and neonates is challenging due to limited space for maneuvering robotic tools. Therefore, specific guidelines for pediatric robotic surgery are needed. In response to this, the Italian Society of Pediatric and Neonatal Anesthesia and Intensive Care (SARNePI) and the Italian Society of Pediatric Surgery (SICP) have issued a joint consensus statement to guide the management of children undergoing robot-assisted surgery [2]. Pediatric anesthesiologists must understand the robotic system and its impact on anesthetic management, considering the increased use of robotic surgery in young patients. Some challenges include positioning difficulties, limited airway and IV access, longer surgery durations, potential hypothermia, and physiological changes resulting from pneumoperitoneum (PNP) to ensure a safe perioperative outcome for children undergoing robot-assisted surgery. Additionally, prolonged steep inclination during surgery may lead to airway and brain edema [3].

1.1 What is an robotic system?

The robotic system uses three-dimensional (3D) imaging devices to improve vision in the operating field and instrument action by providing seven degrees of freedom of motion that replicate the movement of the wrist, leading to improved control of delicate motions and avoiding handshakes by using a computerized scaling system. Several robotic systems are currently available for commercial use; however, one of the first and most extensively used robotic systems globally is the Da Vinci system from Intuitive Surgical (Sunnyvale, CA, USA) [4].

There are four primary parts of the Da Vinci system: (1) optical vision cart (**Figure 1**); (2) surgeon console (**Figure 2**); (3) Endo Wrist instruments; and (4) patient cart that may be moved to surround the patient during surgery. It moves and has four robotic arms for endoscopic instruments (**Figure 3**). During the process, this is docked over the patient (**Figure 4**). The patient cart is positioned against the side of the table, allowing unrestricted access to the patient's head and feet. When the four arms are finally docked, the anesthetist has to confirm again where the cart is about the airway and the I.V. infusion lines. In pediatric patients, this might be a major problem that needs to be actively discussed with the surgeon. The surgeon's console is located in the same room as the operation table, but it is separated from it. The surgeon should be able to see the console directly. It should be appropriately placed so that he is always able to see the patient. The console is used to move the surgical tools docked inside the patient and provides 3D inside picture of the operating field. Most robotic systems have a twin console, the second console utilized for help and education. The video tower that holds the insufflator and display is called the vision cart. It also has energy sources and a central computer. The anesthetist and surgical assistant utilize the vision cart to view the process and coordinate with the surgeon.

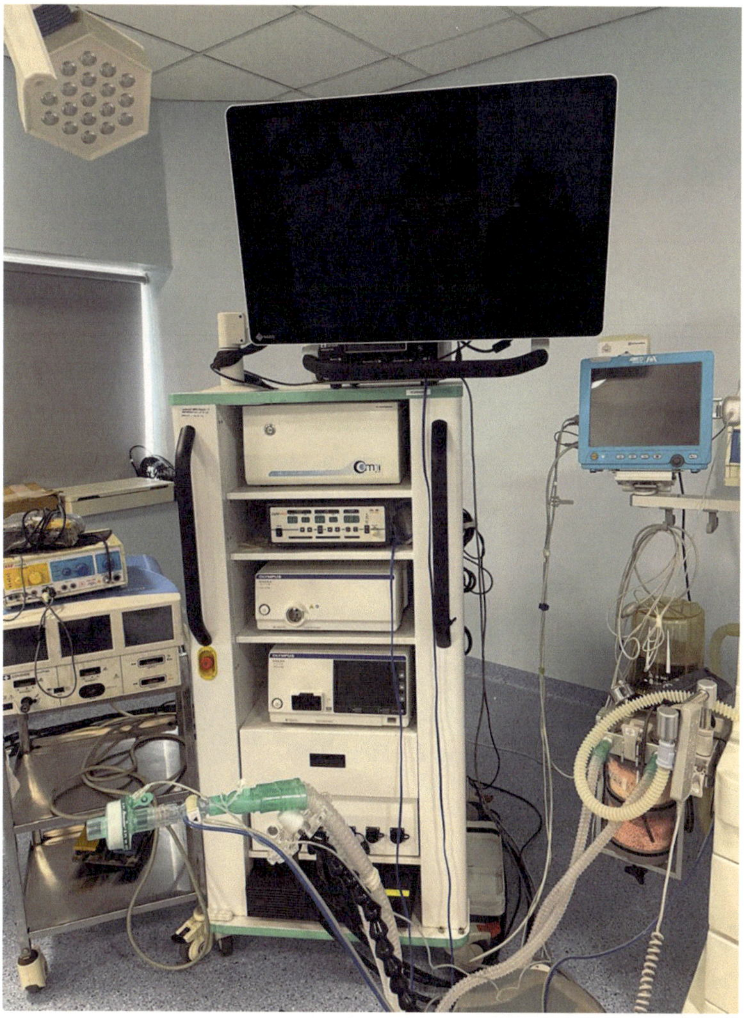

Figure 1.
Vision cart.

1.1.1 Anesthesia considerations in robotic surgery

- Because the patient is surrounded by so much hardware during robotic surgery, safety is of paramount importance. In addition to robotic arms, there are also concerns about access to the airway, IV lines, and extreme positions.

- During minimally invasive surgery, the patient is first placed in a supine position and later, the surgical area is aligned in the Trendelenburg position. For the upper abdominal surgeries (spleen, liver, and stomach), the patient is positioned head-up. Conversely, during pelvic procedures, the head is positioned low. The main part of the robotic system is docked to rest on the side of the operation table, and the pillar housing of the robot can be rotated to match the operative site. The robotic arms can impede airway access. The anesthetist has to actively watch, while the surgeon is docking the robot and check for access to the patient from various sides during arm adjustment.

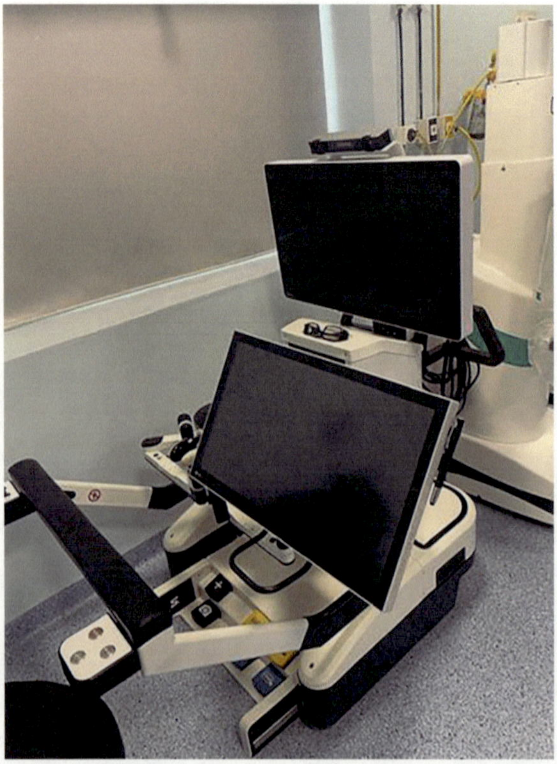

Figure 2.
Surgeon console.

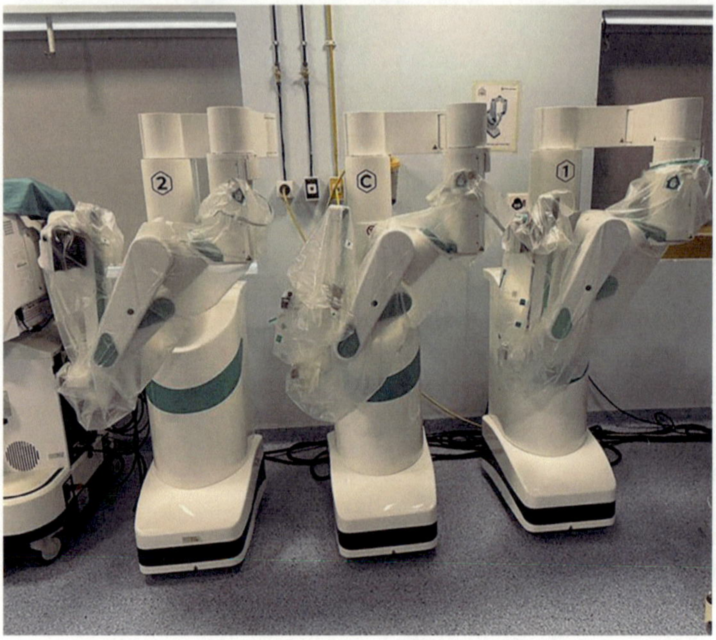

Figure 3.
Patient cart and robotic arms.

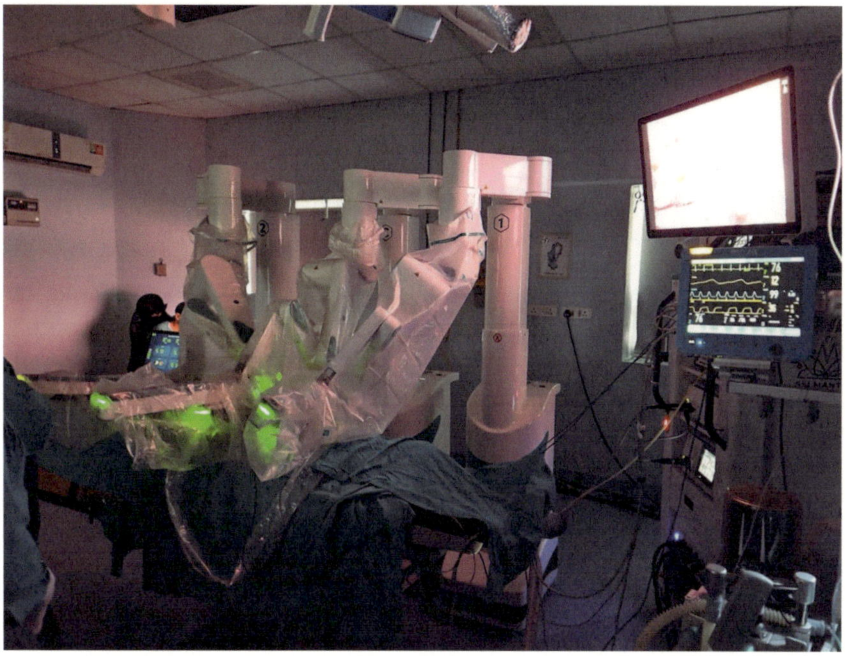

Figure 4.
Robotic surgery ongoing.

- After docking, the robot arms move and bend over the patient's body. There is a risk that one of the arms can press against the patient's face, chest, or other body regions. The surgical assistant should actively control the patient's pressure points and protect them with soft padding. If there is any excessive movement of the robotic arms that could strike the patient's body parts, the assistant needs to notify the console surgeon.

- Due to bleeding or significant vascular damage, an immediate change to an open surgical technique may be necessary. Hepatobiliary system procedures are highly susceptible to emergency conversions. Immediately, the lead surgeon must get ready to open the patient and the assistant surgeon on the patient's side and the scrub nurse can quickly undock the robot. To preserve hemodynamic stability in such situations, the anesthetist needs to be prepared with a massive transfusion protocol utilizing fluids and vasopressors.

2. Laparoscopic surgery

Carbon dioxide gas is insufflated into the abdomen during laparoscopic surgery to increase the field of vision and facilitate the surgeon's ability to work through tiny incisions. The most widely utilized gas is carbon dioxide for PNP because it almost perfectly satisfies all the requirements for the perfect gas for insufflation (**Box 2**). One disadvantage of carbon dioxide is that it passes through the peritoneum and is absorbed intravascularly. Various advantages and disadvantages of other gases are listed in **Table 1**. Additionally, laparoscopic surgery raises the frequency of nausea and vomiting following surgery (PONV).

- Not inflammable, inexplosive
- It should have limited systemic absorption
- If absorbed, it should have limited systemic effects, non-toxic
- It should be easily removed by the body
- It should have limited physiological effects if intravascular embolism occurs
- It should be highly soluble in blood
- Increase working and viewing space

Box 2.
Characteristics of an ideal gas for pneumoperitoneum [5] properties.

Gas	Advantages	Disadvantages
Air, oxygen	• Inexpensive • Easily available • Limited physiological effects	Support combustion
Nitrogen	• Poorly absorbed avoids hypercapnia • Does not support combustion	• Low blood gas solubility • Risk of gas embolism
Helium	• Poorly absorbed avoids hypercapnia • Does not support combustion	• Low blood gas solubility • Risk of gas embolism • Expensive
Argon	• Poorly absorbed avoids hypercapnia • Does not support combustion	• Low blood gas solubility • Risk of gas embolism • Decreases hepatic blood flow • Not cost-effective
Nitrous oxide	• Cheap	• Supports combustion • Dilates bowel • Risk of embolism

Table 1.
Advantages and disadvantages of various gases.

2.1 Effects of pneumoperitoneum on various systems

PNP causes pathophysiological alterations in several organ systems through the absorption of carbon dioxide (CO_2) into the body and physical pressure. The duration of the pressure application and the pressure exerted determine the absolute pressure.

2.1.1 Effects due to intra-abdominal pressure (IAP)

2.1.1.1 Central nervous system

Head down position, hypercarbia, increased SVR, and elevated IAP can increase intracranial pressure and decrease cerebral perfusion pressure. The creation of PNP causes an increase in the middle cerebral artery blood flow velocity even if CO_2 reactivity is normal in younger children. Preterm infants may be at risk for intraventricular hemorrhage in these situations [6].

2.1.1.2 Cardiovascular system

When the IAP rises above 15 mm Hg, the inferior vena cava and its surrounding collateral arteries are compressed, which lead to a decrease in preload and an increase in afterload. In healthy patients with normal cardiovascular function, this reduces venous return and cardiac output (CO), causes hypotension, and leads to an increase in systemic vascular resistance (SVR) and blood pressure. These hemodynamic alterations can cause the re-opening of prenatal shunts (either temporarily or permanently) in children. Laparoscopic surgery may be difficult in newborns and infants with congenital abnormalities [7]. There is a "squeezing" out of blood from the splanchnic venous bed even at IAP levels <15 mm Hg, which raises the venous return and CO. The CO may also increase because of sympathetically mediated peripheral vasoconstriction.

2.1.1.2.1 Considerations in children

Due to their immature cardiac fibers, newborns and infants under 3 months of age have a relatively constant cardiac output and are unable to increase contractility. The only way they can raise the CO is by raising the heart rate. These changes also depend upon the patient's position and IAP. Head-down positions, as used for pelvic procedures, can increase venous return and preload with an increase in central venous pressure (CVP), pulmonary capillary wedge pressure (PCWP), and mean arterial pressure. In contrast, head-up positions during laparoscopy, as for a cholecystectomy, can increase venous pooling, thereby reducing venous return and CO followed by hypotension in a hypovolemic child. A rapid PNP or insertion of trocars causes stimulation of the peritoneum, which can provoke bradycardia or asystole in children because of higher-resting vagal tone [8]. An increase in CBF and ICP while the reduction in renal and splanchnic blood flow can occur due to an increase in IAP and intrathoracic pressure.

2.1.1.3 Pulmonary system

In laparoscopic surgeries, PNP is created, which raises IAP. Elevated IAP causes reduced diaphragmatic excursion, a cephalic shift of the diaphragm causing atelectasis, and reduced lung compliance and functional residual capacity (FRC) [9]. Additionally, it raises airway pressure and lowers thoracic compliance. Ventilation-perfusion (V/Q) mismatch can cause preferential ventilation of non-dependent areas. Intermittent positive pressure ventilation (IPPV) can increase the risk of barotrauma, hypoxia, hypercarbia, and variations in ventilatory pressure [10]. Trendelenburg's position further worsens these effects. Hyperventilation is limited in robotic surgery due to higher ventilator-inspired pressure. Transpulmonary pressure (Ptp) is the difference between intrapleural and alveolar pressure. As the Ptp rises, it causes lung parenchymal injury and raises the risk of acute lung injury and respiratory distress syndrome. PNP increases the external and intrapleural pressures, but decreases the Ptp value, so that the ventilation pressure can be safely increased in proportion to the applied pressure.

2.1.1.3.1 Considerations in children

Infants are more susceptible to hypoxia because they require more oxygen (6–8 ml/kg/min) than adults (2–3 ml/kg/min). Children with respiratory diseases may not be able to tolerate hypoxia and hypercarbia, but the impact of these respiratory changes is minimal in otherwise healthy children and can be countered by adjusting the ventilatory parameters [11]. Children with respiratory diseases are at high risk of atelectasis due to low FRC, which makes them more susceptible to hypercarbia. In rare cases, CO_2 emboli can enter the arterial circulation *via* the patent foramen ovale and lead to hemodynamic collapse.

2.1.1.4 Renal system

By compressing the renal parenchyma and arteries, the PNP raises renovascular resistance and reduces flow in the renal vein. Moreover, it results in elevated antidiuretic hormone secretion, an increase in plasma concentration of catecholamines, and activation of the renin-angiotensin system [12]. During the laparoscopic procedure, patients may experience oliguria, which may last for several hours after the procedure.

2.1.1.5 Gastrointestinal system

Splanchnic circulation receives 30% of cardiac output and has a regional storage function. It is known that the first signs of increased intraabdominal pressure arise with the impairment of splanchnic perfusion. Intestinal ischemia, decreased gastric perfusion, and decreased portal circulation have been reported due to increased IAP [13]. Hypercapnia can also cause dilation of the splanchnic vessels, so the net effect on blood flow in the splanchnic circulation is insignificant [14].

2.1.1.6 Ophthalmic system

The intraocular pressure (IOP) can rise with PNP and Trendelenburg position, and in adults, this effect may remain for 45–60 minutes following surgery [15]. A steep Trendelenburg posture in an adult might cause an uncommon but severe side effect such as blindness, particularly if the procedure takes a long time. However, there is little literature indicating possible blindness in children. In contrast, children with glaucoma are at risk of having their vision loss worsened by an increase in intraocular pressure.

2.1.1.7 Other effects

Particularly during extended procedures, a rise in IAP can raise static venous blood flow and raise the risk of deep vein thrombosis. Research has demonstrated that a laparoscopy results in a decreased release of acute stress mediators. In comparison with laparotomy, there is a reduced surge in the plasma concentrations of catecholamine, cortisol, epinephrine, insulin, prolactin, and growth hormones as well as in glucose, leucocyte, and CRP and interleukins.

2.1.1.8 Carbon dioxide absorption

The amount of CO_2 that diffuses determines how the body reacts to systemic CO_2 uptake. According to Fick's law [Vgas α A/t.D (Pl-P2)] [16], the amount of CO_2 that diffuses through the peritoneum and into the bloodstream is determined. This equation states that the area of the membrane in contact with the gas (A), the difference in the partial pressure of the gas across the membrane (P1-P2), and a diffusion constant (D) all relate to the diffusion of gas across a membrane. As a result, the diffusion is inversely proportional to the square root of the molecular weight and the membrane thickness and directly relates to the solubility of the gas.

A longer surgical operation (>1 hour) causes hypercarbia due to higher absorption of CO_2. This hypercarbia increases systemic blood pressure and pulse rate by activating the sympathetic nervous system, leading to hypertension, and myocardium's sensitivity to catecholamines' arrhythmogenic effects when utilizing volatile anesthetics.

To restore end-tidal carbon dioxide ($ETCO_2$) levels to baseline, a higher-minute ventilation volume is required. Following abdominal deflation, CO_2 falls for roughly 10 minutes, resulting in a discrepancy between the arterial and end-tidal CO_2 (0.33–8.8 mm Hg). In children, hypercarbia is greater due a reduced distance between arteries and the serous surface, an increased ratio of peritoneal surface area to mass, and less peritoneal thickness. Even an IAP of <10 mm hg causes CO_2 absorption [17].

3. Selection criteria for robotic surgery

There are no set criteria for selecting children for robot-assisted surgery. The consensus from the Italian Societies of Pediatric and Neonatal Anesthesia and Intensive Care (SARNePI) and the Italian Society for Pediatric Surgery (SICP) was that robotic surgery is very expensive and ought to be reserved for complicated pediatric reconstructive operations such as choledochal cyst excision, fundoplication, and pyeloplasty [2]. The use of robotic surgery in patients under 1 year or under 10 kg is technically difficult. However, patients who are younger or lighter can undergo robotic surgery, depending on the surgeon's expertise. Robot-assisted surgery can perform all procedures that can also be performed using laparoscopic techniques. The patient's body measurements are crucial because the robotic system requires at least 8 to 10 cm of space between two nearby ports. Enhanced Recovery After Surgery (ERAS) guidelines should be adhered to in all robotic surgeries for economic benefits.

4. Preoperative assessment and investigations

A thorough preoperative assessment is done to stratify the risk and rule out any congenital anomalies involving CNS, respiratory system, and CVS. IAP and CO_2 absorption affect the cardiorespiratory system and may lead to pulmonary hypoperfusion and hypoxia. Thus, minimally invasive surgery is avoided in pediatric patients with congenital heart disease (CHD). Research concerning these problems in children with CHD [18] younger than 5 years of age has not demonstrated any negative effects when the IAP is maintained between 8 and 12 mm Hg. However, transesophageal echocardiography monitoring is crucial for children with serious heart disease. Thorough assessment and tailored perioperative care improve outcomes. Limitation of intercostal space, the smaller size of the thoracic cavity, lung isolation techniques, and physiological changes during one-lung ventilation are a few challenges in Robotically Assisted Thoracic Surgery (RATS) [19]. It is prudent to confirm the placement of the airway device bronchoscopically before draping and docking of robot. IOP stabilization is necessary for children with glaucoma before robotic surgery.

Laboratory tests are done based on the child's clinical condition. Typically, very little blood is lost during robotic laparoscopic surgeries. Blood should be easily available if blood loss is expected. Baseline investigations may include a preoperative hemoglobin value, liver function tests for liver dysfunction, renal function tests, and electrocardiography (ECG) and echocardiogram (ECHO) in children with heart disease.

4.1 Preoperative preparation

The child should follow the fasting 6-4-2/1 rule before surgery. ERAS protocol advocates that drinking clear fluids up to 1–2 hours before surgery improves perioperative outcomes [20].

Premedication is not necessary for neonates but is advisable for children older than 1 year to reduce anxiety. Midazolam is commonly used and can be given intravenously or orally based on the accessibility of vascular access. α-adrenergic antagonists such as dexmedetomidine and clonidine can also be used as premedication. Children with reactive airways should be nebulized with anticholinergic and bronchodilators. Aspiration prophylaxis with metoclopramide and H_2 antagonists might be necessary. An anticholinergic medication to reduce cholinergic-mediated airway responsiveness and avoid bradycardia may be required. Intravascular volume should be assessed in neonates undergoing surgery.

4.2 Monitoring

ETCO, temperature, urine output, heart rate, noninvasive blood pressure (NIBP), oxygen saturation (SpO_2) both pre- and post-ductal, particularly in newborns and children, and other vital signs are monitored. Oxygen, air, and anesthetic agent concentration during inspiration and expiration are also monitored. To find any ventilatory leaks before and after insufflation, measurements of the exhaled tidal volume and peak inspiratory pressure (PIP) should be made. It is recommended to employ entropy or the Bispectral Index (BIS) to facilitate the titration of anesthetic drugs for early recovery. Monitoring neuromuscular blockade helps avoid patient movement during surgery, preventing vascular or organ injury. Although not required, invasive blood pressure (IBP) measurement may be helpful. ABG can be done to measure arterial carbon dioxide partial pressure ($PaCO_2$), and difference between $ETCO_2$ and $PaCO_2$ can be recorded during PNP. ABG will also determine base deficit and electrolytes. The optional placement of a central venous catheter should also be considered. The indication should be strictly defined. Central venous access can be helpful in the administration of antibiotics, vasoactive drugs, and hyperosmolar fluids as well as the transfusion of blood products. It can be inserted *via* the internal jugular, subclavian, brachiocephalic, or axillary vein under ultrasound guidance, depending on the child's age and the anesthesiologist's experience. Children are more likely to experience hypothermia during anesthesia because they have a higher body surface area-to-mass ratio and less subcutaneous fat. This is exacerbated by the injection of cold, dehumidified CO_2 into the abdominal cavity, and a longer operating time. Hypothermia can be prevented by using warm infusion fluids, a warm air blanket, a heated humidifier, and a warming mattress. It is also recommended to use warm inflation gas at a flow of less than 2 l/min. It is therefore important to keep the child's core body temperature within the normal range.

4.2.1 Intraoperative concerns

Perioperatively, there is always a risk that an intravenous access will dislocate. Since it would be difficult to create another intravenous access in an emergency, it is recommended to insert two intravenous accesses with long extensions into the upper extremity before docking the surgical robot. To avoid a delayed onset of drug action, veins in the upper limbs should preferably be used, since venous return from the legs can be impaired by increased IAP. In the case of bleeding, one of these IV lines can also be utilized for checking intraoperative electrolytes or hematocrit. Infusion lines need to be exceptionally long and free from kinking or obstructions. IV lines' injection ports must be simple to reach. It is best to leave one arm free so the anesthetist can access it if necessary. To prevent injury to the vessel wall, care should be used when fixing the IV, arterial, and central venous access lines. Erosion, thrombosis, inflammation, blockage, dysfunction, and exit-site infections could potentially occur.

Decompressing the stomach is necessary to introduce the trocars without obstructing the surgeon's surgical view or causing gastric damage. This is done by placing a nasogastric tube. Also, it lessens the possibility of regurgitation, due to elevated IAP. Judicious fluid management is crucial to maintaining urine output. It is also advisable to empty the bladder using a bladder catheter to avoid injury during installation or when maneuvering the trocar.

Optimal patient positioning during robot-assisted surgery is a dynamic process and aims to optimize the view of the surgical field, allow the anesthesiologist access to the patient, and at the same time minimize the occurrence of compression injuries. It is important to ensure that straps do not compromise blood supply. Anesthesia becomes more challenging due to patient positioning in either Trendelenburg, reverse Trendelenburg, or in a lateral decubitus position for robotic surgery along with PNP.

The operating table is tilted sideways to facilitate surgical visualization. Patients have to be firmly fastened to the operation table, ideally with a foam ring and soft cushions to prevent slipping on the mattress. Padding should be done to shield the patient's pressure points and the head. It is important to ensure that the patient is not touched by robotic arms in motion. Eye protection, lubricating drops, and tools to avoid nerve damage should be used (e.g., Heel and elbow pads, cotton padding, and pillows).

4.3 Anesthetic management

Anesthesia management is not specific to robotic surgery. Depending on the accessibility of intravenous access, induction can take place *via* inhalation or intravenous route. Modified rapid sequence induction may be utilized in children undergoing emergency surgery. A cuffed endotracheal tube is recommended to minimize the risk of leakage and subsequent drop in tidal volume. The ETT needs to be positioned accurately and firmly. Arms should be positioned on the side of the body and fastened.

A balanced anesthetic technique with inhalational agents (isoflurane, desflurane, and sevoflurane), or TIVA (propofol and opioids (fentanyl and remifentanil), and non-depolarizing drugs (vecuronium or atracurium) with IPPV is preferred.

The Holliday-Segar formula should be followed in pediatric patients, while choosing IV fluids for surgical procedures. This formula uses patient's weight to calculate water and caloric loss. (4 ml/kg for 0–10 kg, 2 ml/kg for 11–20 kg, and 1 ml/kg for >20 kg) [21]. Balanced salt solutions are the recommended choice.

The administration of fluids should be directed to maintain euvolemia and prevent anuria and hypotension following PNP. During the first hour following surgery, the estimated fluid deficit is replaced followed by maintenance fluids. This fluid resuscitation reduces the incidence of hypotension and maintains urine output throughout the surgical procedure. About 10 ml/kg/hr. of buffered Isotonic solution with 1–2.5% glucose can be used as background infusion.

The infusion regimen can be titrated based on the duration of surgery, blood loss, acid-base balance, and glucose levels. After the surgical treatment, the peritoneum should be deflated. To reverse the neuromuscular blockade, combine neostigmine with atropine or glycopyrrolate. Postoperative nausea and vomiting prevention with dexamethasone (0.15–0.2 mg/kg) or ondansetron (0.2 mg/kg) are also advised.

4.4 Ventilation strategies during robotic surgery

Controlled ventilation reduces the FRC drop caused by increased IAP and patient position while facilitating CO_2 removal. Respiratory compliance is reduced. A 25–30% increase in minute ventilation and peak inspiratory pressure is necessary to avoid hypercarbia. PEEP, or positive end-expiratory pressure, mitigates the effects of elevated IAP in the lower lung zones and prevents the atelectasis development. An increase in Fi02 may be required to maintain the Oxygen saturation. For pediatric laparoscopies, a moderate-to-low IAP of 6-l0 mm Hg (compared to 12–15 mm Hg in adults) is advised as it has negligible impact on splanchnic perfusion and organ function.

In addition, due to the lower compliance of the abdominal wall in children, good operating conditions can be achieved at lower IAP values. Furthermore, insufflation pressures that exceed 10 mm Hg cannot enhance the workspace in infants; hence, the pressure created by the PNP should be maintained between 6 and 10 mm Hg in children under 2 years old and 10–12 mm Hg in 2–10 years old, and 12 mm Hg in those over 10 years old [2]. Carbon dioxide is insufflated into the peritoneal cavity at a rate of 4–6 liter/ min to a pressure of 10–20 mm Hg in adults, but flow rate is limited to <2 liter/ minute in children. The PNP is maintained by a constant gas flow of 200–400 ml/min.

Volume-controlled and volume-targeted pressure-controlled ventilation (PCV) can be used. Cuffed ETT prevents leaks and can be used to give high PEEP during PNP. PC-inverse ratio ventilation (IRV) can be used as an alternative with an inspiratory to expiratory ratio in the range of 2:1 to 4:1 [22]. The advantage of PC-IRV is that a lower TV is required to achieve normal PaO_2 and $PaCO_2$ values.

Kim et al. investigated that the mean airway pressure and dynamic compliance were substantially greater with PCV with 5 cm of water PEEP in comparison with volume-controlled ventilation (VCV) with 5 cm H_2O. The authors found no differences in other ventilatory parameters and oxygen saturation, so they recommended that VCV and PCV can be safely used in children undergoing laparoscopic procedures [23].

General anesthesia causes loss of FRC, resulting in pulmonary atelectasis. The effect of GA on FRC is exacerbated in children due to their compliant chest wall and quickly collapsible airways. PNP increases the shunt fraction and dead space. The lung-protective ventilation technique (LPVS) involves administering low TV, optimal PEEP, and a lower Fio_2 to prevent lung barotrauma induced by high IAP. However, this can lead to gradual fall in FRC and alveolar collapse. The incidence of atelectasis in infants has been reported to exceed 50% within the first minute of induction of GA, and the incidence increases further during laparoscopic surgeries [24]. Various studies have shown that applying a recruitment maneuver/sustained higher-positive pressure can help decrease atelectasis in the dependent portions of the lungs.

4.4.1 Extubation

The overall incidence of reintubation after robotic surgery is nearly 0.7% (including both adults and children) and delayed extubation is 3.5%. The incidence of airway edema is around 26% [25].

4.4.2 Complications

Complications are mainly related to positioning and include peripheral neuropathies, corneal abrasions, soft tissue injury, hypothermia, and perioperative visual loss. Vascular complications include compartment syndrome, rhabdomyolysis, and thromboembolic disease. There can be cerebral, ocular, and airway edema. Cardiovascular complications include hypotension, hypertension, and arrhythmias. Respiratory complications are hypoxia, hypercarbia, atelectasis, bronchospasm, subcutaneous emphysema, pneumothorax, and endobronchial intubation. Bolenz et al. [26] found a substantial difference in the proportion of nerve-sparing procedures across robotic (85%), laparoscopic (96%), and open (90%) approaches ($P < 0.001$). There were differences in lymphadenectomy rates (robotic 11%, laparoscopic 22%, open 100%; $P < 0.001$), blood transfusion rates (robotic 4.6%, laparoscopic 1.8%, open 21.0%; $P = 0.001$), median operating room time (robotic 235 minutes, laparoscopic 225 minutes, open 198 minutes; $P < 0.001$), and median length of hospital stay (robotic 1 day, laparoscopic 2 days, open 2 days; $P < 0.0001$). In the hands of laparoscopic surgeons, complication rates in pediatric robotic-assisted laparoscopic surgery are low even during the learning phase. Fabrizio et al. documented that there were no robotic technology-related complications [27].

4.5 Postoperative pain relief

Laparoscopic surgery typically has less postoperative pain than open surgery. The pain may be caused by a laparoscopic port incision or by the PNP. The cause of shoulder pain could be related to the diaphragm surface irritation and desiccation of the peritoneum with the inflated dry CO_2 gas. To alleviate the incisional pain, local anesthetic injection into the port site, caudal block, nonsteroidal anti-inflammatory medications (NSAIDS), such as Ketorolac, and mild doses of opioids can be used. Nerve block such as the transversus abdominis plane (TAP), paravertebral block, and erector spinae block can be performed using local anesthesia alone or with additives such as clonidine and dexmedetomidine [28].

4.5.1 Future applications of robotic surgery

Nonrigid, flexible "snake-like" articulating arms will likely replace present models and facilitate fewer and smaller incisions and less invasive surgeries. With artificial intelligence and better imaging modalities, we may have semi-automated robots guiding surgical instruments with computer algorithms. Neural integration is being developed to allow robots to derive information from their surgeon *via* EEGs, magnetic EEGs, and near-infrared spectroscopy (NIRS), allowing them to (i) use machine learning algorithms to help record the steps of an operation and (ii) potentially modify the surgical environment to improve surgical precision, accuracy, and safety.

5. Conclusion

The use of robots in pediatric surgery presents challenges for both surgeons and anesthesiologists. To ensure a successful surgery, the anesthesiologist must understand the configuration of the robot and its physiological effects. Anesthesia management requires focusing on the issues created by patient placement, limited airway, and IV access, hypothermia, PNP, and ventilation.

Author details

Pallavi Ahluwalia[1*] and Amit Ahluwalia[2]

1 Department of Anaesthesia, Teerthanker Mahaveer Medical College, Moradabad, India

2 Department of Orthopaedic Surgery, Shri Siddhi Vinayak Medical College and Hospital, Sambhal, Uttar Pradesh, India

*Address all correspondence to: drpallaviahluwalia@yahoo.com

References

[1] Ostlie DJ, Miller KA, Woods RK, Holcomb GW. Single cannula technique and robotic telescopic assistance in infants and children who require laparoscopic Nissen fundoplication. Journal of Pediatric Surgery. 2003;**38**(1):111-115

[2] Tesoro S, Gamba P, Bertozzi M, Borgogni R, Caramelli F, Cobellis G, et al. Pediatric robotic surgery: Issues in management-expert consensus from the Italian Society of Pediatric and Neonatal Anesthesia and Intensive Care (SARNePI) and the Italian Society of Pediatric Surgery (SICP). Surgical Endoscopy. 2022;**36**(11):7877-7897

[3] Kaye AD, Vadivelu N, Ahuja N, Mitra S, Silasi D, Urman RD. Anesthetic considerations in robotic-assisted gynecologic surgery. The Ochsner Journal. 2013;**13**(4):517-524

[4] Intutive surgical I.da Vinci Gynecology. 2018. Available from: http://davincisurgery.com/da-vinci-gynecology/

[5] Yang X, Cheng Y, Cheng N, Gong J, Bai L, Zhao L, Deng Y. Gases for establishing pneumoperitoneum during laparoscopic abdominal surgery. Cochrane Database of Systematic Reviews. 15 Mar 2022;**3**(3):CD009569

[6] Kamata M, Hakim M, Walia H, Tumin D, Tobias JD. Changes in cerebral and renal oxygenation during laparoscopic pyloromyotomy. Journal of Clinical Monitoring and Computing. 2020;**34**(4):699-703

[7] Kim J, Sun Z, Englum BR, Allori AC, Adibe OO, Rice HE, et al. Laparoscopy is safe in infants and neonates with congenital heart disease: A National Study of 3684 patients. Journal of Laparoendoscopic & Advanced Surgical Techniques. Part A. 2016;**26**(10):836-839

[8] De Waal EEC, Kalkman CJ. Haemodynamic changes during low-pressure carbon dioxide pneumoperitoneum in young children. Pediatric Anesthesia. 2003;**13**:18-25

[9] Davarcı I, Karcıoğlu M, Tuzcu K, İnanoğlu K, Yetim TD, Motor S, et al. Evidence for negative effects of elevated intra-abdominal pressure on pulmonary mechanics and oxidative stress. The Scientific World Journal. 2015;**2015**:612642

[10] Tobias JD. Anaesthesia for minimally invasive surgery in children. Best Practice & Research. Clinical Anaesthesiology. 2002;**16**(1):115-130

[11] Acosta CM, Sara T, Carpinella M, Volpicelli G, Ricci L, Poliotto S, et al. Lung recruitment prevents collapse during laparoscopy in children: A randomised controlled trial. European Journal of Anaesthesiology. 2018;**35**(8):573-580

[12] Dunn MD, McDougall EM. Renal physiology. Laparoscopic considerations. Urology Clinical North America. 2000;**27**(4):609-614

[13] Kominsky HD, Cadeddu JA, Moschovas MC, Leveillee RJ. Pneumoperitoneum physiology. In: Wiklund P, Mottrie A, Gundeti MS, Patel V, editors. Robotic Urologic Surgery. Cham: Springer; 2022. DOI: 10.1007/978-3-031-00363-9_16

[14] Meierhenrich RMD, Gauss AMD, Vandenesch PMD, Georgieff MMD, Poch BMD, Schütz WMD. The effects of intra abdominally insufflated carbon dioxide on hepatic blood flow during laparoscopic surgery assessed

by transesophageal echocardiography. Anesthesia & Analgesia. 2005;**100**(2):340-347

[15] Karabayirli S, Çimen NK, Muslu B, Tenlik A, Gözdemir M, Sert H, et al. Effect of positive end-expiratory pressure administration on intraocular pressure in laparoscopic cholecystectomy: Randomised controlled trial. European Journal of Anaesthesiology. 2016;**33**(9):696-699

[16] Lasersohn L. Anaesthetic considerations for paediatric laparoscopy. South African Journal of Surgery. 2011;**49**(1):22-26

[17] Pennant JH. Anesthesia for laparoscopy in the pediatric patient. Anesthesiology Clinics of North America. 2001;**19**(1):69-88. DOI: 10.1016/S0889-8537(05)70212-1

[18] Gillory LA, Megison ML, Harmon CM, Chen MK, Anderson SA, Chong AJ, et al. Laparoscopic surgery in children with congenital heart disease. Journal of Pediatric Surgery. 2012;**47**(6):1084-1088

[19] Mattioni G, Palleschi A, Mendogni P, et al. Approaches and outcomes of robotic-assisted thoracic surgery (RATS) for lung cancer: A narrative review. Journal of Robotic Surgery. 2022;**17**:797-809

[20] Shinnick JK, Short HL, Heiss KF, Santore MT, Blakely ML, Raval MV. Enhancing recovery in pediatric surgery: A review of the literature. The Journal of Surgical Research. 2016;**202**(1):165-176

[21] Mathew A, Rai E. Pediatric perioperative fluid management. Saudi Journal of Anaesthesia. 2021;**15**(4):435-440

[22] Schick V, Dusse F, Eckardt R, Kerkhoff S, Commotio S, Hinkelbein J, et al. Comparison of volume-guaranteed or -targeted, pressure-controlled ventilation with volume-controlled ventilation during elective surgery: A systematic review and meta-analysis. Journal of Clinical Medicine. 2021;**10**(6):1276

[23] Kim JY, Shin CS, Lee KC, Chang YJ, Kwak HJ. Effect of pressure- versus volume-controlled ventilation on the ventilatory and hemodynamic parameters during laparoscopic appendectomy in children: A prospective, randomized study. Journal of Laparoendoscopic & Advanced Surgical Techniques. Part A. 2011;**21**(7):655-658

[24] Acosta CM, Lopez Vargas MP, Oropel F, Valente L, Ricci L, Natal M, et al. Prevention of atelectasis by continuous positive airway pressure in anaesthetised children: A randomised controlled study. European Journal of Anaesthesiology. 2021;**38**(1):41-48

[25] Maerz DA, Beck LN, Sim AJ, Gainsburg DM. Complications of robotic-assisted laparoscopic surgery distant from the surgical site. British Journal of Anaesthesia. 2017;**118**:492-503

[26] Bolenz C, Gupta A, Hotze T, Ho R, Cadeddu JA, Roehrborn CG, et al. Cost comparison of robotic, laparoscopic, and open radical prostatectomy for prostate cancer. European Urology. 2010;**57**:453-458

[27] Di Fabrizio D, Alizai NK, Najmaldin AS. Early and long-term complications of robotic assisted laparoscopy in infants and children. Journal of Pediatric Surgery. 2023;**58**(9):1832-1837

[28] Tao B, Liu K, Wang D, Ding M, Yang N, Zhao P. Perioperative effects of caudal block on pediatric patients in laparoscopic upper urinary tract surgery: A randomized controlled trial. BMC Pediatrics. 2019;**19**(1):427

Chapter 3

The Effect of Parental Anxiety on Postoperative Paediatric Cognitive Dysfunction

Tolga Koyuncu and Merve Elgörmüş

Abstract

Thanks to today's developing technologies, the number of paediatric patients undergoing surgery is increasing. The possible negative effects on the psychological health of children undergoing surgery have been previously documented in the literature. These undesirable effects may be exacerbated, especially when families stress and anxiety levels are high. Unfortunately, parents stress, and anxiety also changes the child's emotional state and negatively affect the child's recovery process during postoperative follow-up. This situation may have a negative impact on the child's short- and long-term psychological and physiological outcomes. While the negative effects we have mentioned may improve in children in the short term, unfortunately, they may also have effects that can last up to 1 year. In this article, we aimed to talk about the effects of parental anxiety on paediatric cognitive disorders.

Keywords: cognitive dysfunction, parental anxiety, paediatric patients, general anaesthesia, paediatric surgery

1. Introduction

The question of what emotion is has been the subject of considerable philosophical debate for over a century. The James-Lange theory of emotion suggests that physical changes in the body take place prior to the experience of the relevant emotion. According to this theory, witnessing an external stimulus leads to a physiological response. Your emotional response depends on how you interpret these physical reactions [1]. As an example, imagine that the plane you are boarding suddenly enters a violent turbulence. You start to tremble and your heart starts beating fast. The James-Lange theory suggests that you will interpret your physical reactions and conclude that you are afraid ("I'm trembling. Therefore I'm afraid").

You might be mistaken to think that James-Lange theory is something that should only be studied because of its historical significance. Researchers continue to find evidence that supports at least some parts of James and Lange's original ideas [1]. Clearly, this theory had both supporters and critics. The Cannon-Bard theory of emotion, coined by Walter Cannon and Philip Bard in the 1920s, challenged James-Lange theory directly. Cannon and Bard's theory suggests instead that our physiological responses, such as crying and trembling, are due to our emotions [2, 3].

It is possible to observe divergent perspectives on the same theory. It can be observed that uncertainty (the unknown) is something that humans do not readily accept. As a result, there is a tendency to seek certainty in uncertainty. The concept of uncertainty is not a pleasant one for humans; however, they tend to feel comfortable when they are able to gain a sense of certainty or when they are engaged in the act of prediction. Occasionally, however, humans may fail to recognise a crucial detail. The world we live in is full of uncertainties. It is therefore wise to cultivate the ability to live with uncertainty rather than to try to provide certainty in the face of uncertainty. As Jeremy Bentham said, "The power of the lawyer lies in the uncertainty of the law".

Underlying almost every type of anxiety is the concept of uncertainty. We should not forget some important points here. First of all, it is useful to learn how to deal with and manage uncertainties in order to manage anxiety. Therefore, to manage anxiety, it should be remembered that it can contain uncertainties, it can be more difficult to manage when it comes to children, each child is special and different in itself. Therefore, the outward manifestation of anxiety can be different in each child. It is very important to observe the child and his family at this stage. Also anxiety like any other disease. Do not underestimate anxiety observe, identify and treat it. The slightest mistake in handling a child's anxiety can have a psychological impact that will affect the child's entire life.

As the developmental psychologist Jean Piaget put it: "Children are not miniature adults". In order to ascertain the most appropriate manner in which to interact with children, it is first necessary to gain an understanding of their nature. It is essential to comprehend the physical, neurological and psychological development stages of children, as well as to recognise their potential and limitations. So It is erroneous to consider children as miniature versions of adults. One of the most striking differences between children and adults is the disparity in cognitive development. The human brain continues to mature throughout childhood, and children may encounter difficulties with tasks that adults find relatively simple, such as planning, problem-solving, and regulating emotions.

2. Paediatric anxiety

According to American Psychological Association (APA) Anxiety is defined as feelings of tension, apprehension, nervousness, fear, discomfort, and high autonomic activity with varying degrees of intensity resulting from anticipation of danger or a threatening event or something [4, 5], and it is a subjective feeling of tension, nervousness, worry and loss of sleep associated with an increased autonomic nervous system activity [6]. Preoperative anxiety in children is a common condition associated with a number of negative behaviours related to the surgical experience (e.g. restlessness, crying, spontaneous urination and the need for physical restraint during anaesthetic induction). This can lead to increased blood pressure, high heart rate and increased sensitivity, which can result in a lowered pain threshold, clinically increased postoperative pain, increased analgesic requirements, and increased agitation and delirium during recovery, all of which can seriously affect the patient's surgical outcome and rehabilitation [7].

Anxiety is a series of emotional states that people experience when they are in real danger or when they feel at risk. Suspicion is often a mechanism that helps us survive and protects us from danger. However, when there is no danger, anxiety is more frequent and intense, which suggests that the function of anxiety is impaired. For example, when walking down the road, an individual may experience distress when encountering an aggressive dog running at a fast pace in their direction. This is a typical response. Nevertheless, in the absence of any tangible threat, it is not a typical reaction for an individual to exhibit signs of anxiety and restlessness, such as expressing concerns about the possibility of being bitten by the dog.

A considerable number of children undergo surgery each year, and it is estimated that up to 70% of these children experience significant fear and anxiety before the operation [8]. Previous experiences related to the hospital, the environment of the operating theatre, being away from the child's safe area, the absence of parents, the presence of strange faces around, surgical equipment, an antiseptic smell, exposure to the hospital environment, the patient visualising people in pain, including the fact that feel abandoned, have a significant impact on the child's mind. Any negative experience of this condition not only creates a fear of the hospital and everything associated with it, but also sometimes leads to serious psychological consequences, such as post-traumatic stress disorder. This is especially important for 2- to 7-year olds, who are generally more volatile, impulsive and unintentional. They are aware of their parents presence and are more likely to experience fear and separation anxiety [4]. Children may look scared and/or agitated, breathe deeply, tremble, stop talking or playing and/or start to cry. Other children may become nauseous, wet themselves, have increased motor tone and/or attempt to run away from the operating room staff [4].

For children, preoperative anxiety can be more harmful than in adults [9]. Children's physiological, anatomical and pharmacological characteristics are very different from adults, and because of their developmental status.

There are many anatomical differences that affect ventilation and intubation. The tongues are large, the nasal passages are narrow because of not yet developed, hard, V- or U-shaped epiglottis, neck and trachea are short, the narrowest part of the larynx is the cricoid cartilage, both bronchi are separated at equal angles to the midline, O_2 consumption is greater than in adults, dead space and closing volumes are high, so there is a high risk of atelectasis in infants. Paediatric patients have a very low tolerance for hypoxia. Cardiovascular problems occur if hypoxia is not eliminated early.

In cardiac terms, children have a higher basal heart rate than adults. Cardiac output is directly related to heart rate. Conditions such as anaesthetic overdose, excessive effects of opioids and hypoxia can cause severe bradycardia. This triggering situation is much more dangerous in child whose general condition is bad. In an adult patient, we can observe a pre-existing hypovolemia characterised by tachycardia and hypotension. However, this is not the case in paediatric cases. This is because the vascular structures cannot respond to hypovolemia with vasoconstriction. As a result, intravascular losses will manifest in the clinical picture with hypotension without tachycardia.

Renal blood flow and glomerular filtration rate are low in the first 2 years of life due to high renal vascular resistance, and they have a lower tubular concentrating capacity, resulting in higher mandatory fluid losses.

Liver function is initially immature with decreased function of liver enzymes. This may require dose adjustment of some medications. For example, barbiturates and opioids have a longer duration of action due to slower metabolism. They are sensitive to hypoglycaemia due to low glycogen stores.

Hypothermia is a risk to be considered as infants and babies because they have a large surface area to weight ratio with minimal subcutaneous fat. Heat loss is exaggerated in children due to their poorly developed mechanisms for shivering, sweating and vasoconstriction.

Because babies have less adipose tissue, the effect of drugs that are eliminated by redistribution to adipose tissue may be prolonged. Paediatric patients are a group of patients who require special doses of medicines and whose approach principles are specific. Therefore, it requires pharmacological preparation, which is characterised by greater dilution of drugs and appropriate adjustment to weight also, higher pH of gastric fluid, longer gastric emptying and complete lack of intestinal function may delay the absorption of oral medications.

Children's anxieties and reactions to surgery are different from adults' and vary with age. Babies <9 months old are less likely to experience separation anxiety—they may respond positively to soothing sounds, gentle rocking and being held on another person's lap. Children aged 1–3 years are susceptible to separation anxiety. Between 3 and 6 years of age, children may have concerns about physical injury. Children between 7 and 12 years of age need further explanation and may benefit from a face mask for anaesthesia or from being allowed to hold the mask during the induction procedure [4]. The physiological, anatomical and pharmacological characteristics of children are very different from adults, not only is the management of anaesthesia different, but the complications that can occur are more dangerous in children. Therefore, it is useful to eliminate all factors that can cause postoperative problems. This will reduce postoperative complications. Studies have shown that these negative behaviours can continue to be observed even a year after leaving hospital [8], such as nightmares, restlessness, separation anxiety, sleep disturbances, night crying, incontinence, anger attacks, eating disorders, and fear of medical personnel.

Over time, all these negative changes in the situation begin to damage the child's self-confidence and social relationships. Social relationships become weaker and weaker. The child may find it difficult to make friends, or their friends may drift away from them; they may not be able to defend themselves, they may avoid being in social environments, the child may not be able to communicate comfortably, may have difficulty initiating or maintaining communication, and so its ability to cope with problems becomes weaker and weaker. Unfortunately, this situation tends to become more severe over time and can have an impact on the child's entire life.

The induction of anaesthesia appears to represent the most stressful moment for the child during the perioperative period, based on an analysis of children's behavioural and physiological parameters [6]. It is to be expected that a child will be fearful of undergoing anaesthesia. The stress and anxiety experienced by children during the induction of anaesthesia are associated with a range of factors, including those related to the child and the environment. The child-related factors includethe child's response to medical procedures include the child's age, developmental stage, previous experience with medical procedures, the child's mood, and the parental anxiety. The environment-related risk factors are the sound of the devices, brightness, noise levels made by health personnel, and operating theatre instruments and sounds. When a child is attempting to cope with a multitude of stressful situations, the administration of intravenous medication may exacerbate the child's distress. It has been proved that intravenous induction is more stressful for children than inhalation induction [10, 11].

It has been demonstrated that elevated preoperative anxiety is associated with an increased risk of postoperative pain, a higher consumption of analgesics, general anxiety, and sleeping problems [12, 13]. Anxiety during the induction of anaesthesia is also associated with emergence distress and postoperative behavioural problems.

Children who are extremely anxious before the operation are at a 3.5-fold higher risk of exhibiting negative postoperative behavioural patterns in comparison with those who showed lower anxiety levels [13]. Also, children who have previously experienced negative outcomes associated with medical procedures and illness are at an elevated risk of developing high anxiety during the preoperative period and demonstrate suboptimal cooperation during the induction of anaesthesia [10, 14]. It can be demonstrated that repeated surgeries do not represent a risk factor in themselves [14]. A series of studies have demonstrated that children who are shy and inhibited by temperament experience greater levels of fear and anxiety on the day of surgery compared to their counterparts. Conversely, children who display a more socially adaptive temperament tend to exhibit lower levels of anxiety when undergoing surgical preparation [15].

The management of preoperative anxiety in children can be achieved through a combination of psychological and pharmacological approaches, or a combination of both. These include preoperative preparation programmes and the presence of parents during the induction of anaesthesia.

Nowadays, there is a lot of research on postoperative anxiety and its causes in children. Not all of this research, but most of it, has shown a correlation between postoperative distress and anxiety levels in children, with these levels being affected by the preoperative period and the induction of anaesthesia. Children with pre-operative anxiety are at risk in many ways in the postoperative period.

3. Parental anxiety

The term “parental anxiety” is defined as a state of worry, fear, and stress related to the role of a parent or carer. Such concerns may be related to a child’s learning development, health, or relationships with others. The avoidance of negative situations and thoughts, as well as the manifestation of physical symptoms of anxiety, can be attributed to parental anxiety. Recent studies have indicated that up to 75% of children [16, 17] and 74% of parents experience preoperative anxiety prior to a paediatric surgical procedure [18]. It has been established that parental anxiety represents a significant modifiable risk factor for children’s preoperative anxiety [14]. The majority of existing literature on the impact of perioperative anxiety in children on clinical and healthcare systems has focused on the child’s anxiety. However, parental anxiety is also a significant factor that should not be overlooked, as it can have adverse effects on the child’s emotional state. Parents frequently express anxiety about their child’s surgery. Some of these concerns include the possibility of their child’s death, the potential for pain during and after surgery, the occurrence of unexpected complications during the child’s surgery, or the development of an incurable defect following surgery. Such concerns can impair the ability of parents to function normally and surgical staff to resolve the child’s health problems. Alot of studies have demonstrated a correlation between parental anxiety and children’s preoperative anxiety [11, 19, 20]. The anxiety experienced by parents prior to their child’s surgery has been identified as a significant predictor of preoperative anxiety in children [21]. The extent to which each parent experiences anxiety related to their child’s anaesthesia and surgery is contingent upon a multitude of factors, both intrinsic to the parents and intrinsic to the child. Studies have shown that mothers, parents of smaller (<1 year of age) children, with male child, higher level of education, exhibited greater levels of anxiety than other parents [22].

When the anxiety of the parents reaches an excessive level, this situation impedes the healthy communication between the parents and the healthcare personnel, as well as the child's care. The child who is already anxious during the operation is negatively affected by this condition of the parents such as delay in returning to normal activity and damage to the developing nervous system [23]. It has been demonstrated that preoperative parental anxiety can influence postoperative pain scores in children. Children whose parents exhibited moderate or severe preoperative anxiety exhibited higher pain scores [24].

High levels of parentsanxiety affect the severity of child's postoperative pain by increasing the sensitivity to pain. The postoperative recovery period is more complex in children with higher preoperative levels of anxiety [8] such as higher postoperative pain, increased analgesic consumption and higher rates of emergence delirium [19], postoperative maladaptive behaviours such as sleeping and eating disturbances [25], physiologically, the levels of blood cortisol heighten as a result of stress response that is associated with surgical anxiety. This may consequently increase the risk of infection and delay the healing process postoperatively [26].

4. Cognitive functions of children

The term 'Cognitive Function'is used to describe the abilities that enable an individual to process and utilise information, including awareness, perception, logical thinking, language, memory and reasoning. The six major categories of cognitive processes are memory and learning, complex attention, language and language processing, executive functions, social cognition, and perceptual and motor functions. Cognitive functions are defined as the mental processes that enable individuals to engage in meaningful activities on a daily basis. It is important to note that not all daily actions are the result of conscious thought. In fact, many of our daily tasks are based on established habits, which ultimately become part of our routine. Cognitive functions are not only instrumental in facilitating the completion of routine tasks, but they also play a pivotal role in the execution of non-routine tasks. Routine tasks are those that are performed without conscious thought or attention. To illustrate this point, consider the example of an individual who has developed the habit of brushing their teeth every morning upon waking. In this case, the act of brushing teeth has become a routine, and the individual no longer engages in conscious thought regarding the necessity of doing so. In contrast, non-routine tasks necessitate the allocation of attention to maintain focus. The application of practical processes is required until such time as the non-routine processes in question become established.

A substantial body of research indicates that working memory represents the most crucial of the perceptual and cognitive functions. Our capacity to learn new abilities, whether it be driving, playing tennis, or mathematics and meditation, is contingent upon our ability to retain information and make effective use of our working memory. The ability to achieve goals, plan, make decisions, and withstand the demands of an effective and efficient working memory is also dependent upon our ability to learn new skills.

4.1 Working memory

Working memory is the limited capacity for information processing that enables the execution of cognitive tasks. It is distinct from long-term memory, which stores vast amounts of information accumulated throughout an individual's lifespan. Working memory is a temporary storage system and is vital for many day-to-day tasks including intelligence, information, processing, executive function, comprehension, problem-solving, and learning. Its development and function have been studied in humans from infancy to old age and in various animal species. Working memory enables the retention of multiple pieces of information for immediate use, which is crucial for a range of activities, including reading, conversation, learning new concepts and decision-making between different options.

The terms "working memory" and "short-term memory" are often used interchangeably. Short-term memory is defined as the capacity to retain information for a limited period of time, typically associated with verbal or visual tasks. These may include, for instance, recalling a phone number, blending sounds into words while reading, or remembering objects, colours, locations, and directions. The term "employee memory" encompasses the processing and conversion of verbal and visual information. This may include, for instance, the retention of instructions and their accompanying details, which are then executed, the recollection of the appropriate response when called upon, the maintenance of one's position on a page when reading, and the retention of sequences of objects or numbers in reverse order.

Working memory is a vital component in the integration of new information with existing long-term memory. In order to focus, organise and problem-solve new information, it is necessary for the working memory to maintain the information in an active state. Maintaining information in an accessible format ensures that skills and knowledge are automated, thereby reducing the necessity for active thought to be given to each step of a task. Working memory is of great consequence to academic performance, as it constitutes an essential component of executive functions (such as planning, initiation, task tracking and organisation). In an educational setting, the academic disciplines that are most significantly influenced by deficiencies in working memory are mathematics, reading comprehension, complex problem-solving, and examination performance. The greatest impact on academic performance is observed in mathematics and reading comprehension.

To illustrate, consider a hypothetical scenario wherein a bucket of working memory is coupled with a reservoir that can be filled. Each addition of water contributes to the filling of the reservoir. However, if no further water is introduced over an extended period, the memory is subject to evaporation due to the lack of repeated utilisation.

In children with poor working memory, the lack of knowledge accumulation is evident; despite the continued addition of water to the pool metaphor, the pool remains empty.

In the event that a child is experiencing difficulties with working memory, they may:

- Forget needed materials at home and at school
- Require prompts to complete homework
- They miss the details in the instructions
- Often forget what was going to say
- Showing low language skills

- Need to re-read text and difficulties with reading
- Poor academic performance
- Need for more time and repetition
- Have difficulty following multistep directions
- Make mistakes writing and counting in class
- Has difficulty solving mathematical calculations from the head
- Having poor organisational skills (e.g. losing items easily)
- It is easily distracted when it does not take a lot of interest in an activity done in class.
- Despite best efforts, progressing at a slower rate than its contemporaries.

4.1.1 Working memory and attention

There is a substantial body of evidence indicating that working memory and attention are closely interrelated [27, 28]. The act of paying attention enables the individual to receive and process information. Working memory facilitates the brain's ability to process and make sense of the information. Attention and working memory are essential for the successful navigation of everyday life and the acquisition of knowledge. Both are components of executive functions that facilitate the acquisition and interpretation of novel information. However, although they are closely associated, these functions are not identical.

The process of attention is defined as the manner in which information is received. Furthermore, it enables the selection of pertinent information. One might conceptualise this process as a funnel. It gathers the information required and transmits it to the brain.

There are four key elements to consider when discussing the concept of care. It is possible that children may experience difficulties with any or all of these components.

Alertness: The capacity to be aware of one's surroundings and to respond appropriately to external stimuli. It is essential that children are adequately prepared to engage in focused attention.

Sustaining: It is reasonable to expect that children will demonstrate an ability to remain careful over time. This may be in the form of either a three-minute presentation or a 40-minute lecture.

Selection: It is essential that children are able to discern which stimuli warrant their attention. For instance, they must be capable of focusing on the teacher's instructions rather than the external noise in the hallway.

Shifting: It is beneficial for children to be able to shift their attention briefly when new information of importance is introduced. For example, children should be capable of focusing their attention on a brief announcement made via the intercom. Subsequently, the pupils should be able to resume their attention on the teacher.

4.2 The relation between cognitive development and anxiety

Anxiety disorders are among the most prevalent psychological disorders, affecting nearly 6.5% of children and adolescents worldwide [29]. Anxiety is a future-oriented emotional state, the intensity and severity of which varies from person to person. Furthermore, the capacity to perceive threats is a fundamental aspect of anxiety, and a child must develop the capacity to perceive the threat in order to experience anxiety. In accordance with Beck's cognitive theory, anxiety encompasses a considerable future-oriented element, as it is predominantly perceived as encompassing the anticipation of prospective future threats [30]. In other words, anxiety is the result of an excessive processing of threatening stimuli that are encountered during the continuation of actions that require sustained attention. At this juncture, it is feasible to discuss the concept of an overdeveloped threat processing mechanism. The capacity for children to engage in future-oriented thought and prediction emerges during the period spanning approximately 3 years of age. In a study on this subject, was to assess the capacity of preschoolers to anticipate future states of the self. A comparison was made between children between the ages of 3, 4 and 5 and their future self-status. In this study, children were requested to envisage participating in a relatively novel variety of events (e.g. walking in a sunny desert, walking in a snowy forest) and then select one of three items they would be required to bring with them to the aforementioned event. To illustrate, when the children were invited to envisage walking in a sunny desert, they were provided with sunglasses, soap, and seashells. The wearing of sunglasses was perceived as a prudent choice that could be made in anticipation of a future situation, such as the sun coming into one's eyes. The results demonstrated that the three age groups in question selected the correct items 61, 75, and 92% of the time, respectively. When prompted to provide rationale for their selections, 3-, 4-, and 5-year olds offered future-oriented justifications (e.g. "The sun can damage my eyes") in 44, 40, and 59% of the trials, respectively [31]. Individuals with an anxious disposition tend to adopt a pessimistic outlook with regard to future events, anticipating potential threats in both the near and distant future. It can be reasonably deduced that children who demonstrate deficiencies in future thinking are less prone to experiencing anxiety.

The number of studies examining the relationship between cognitive development and anxiety is increasing on a daily basis. One of these studies has demonstrated that children with typical cognitive abilities report higher levels of anxiety than children with below-average intellectual abilities [32]. Furthermore, there was a positive correlation between cognitive development and the level of anxiety [32]. A growing body of evidence indicates that anxiety has a detrimental impact on both the working memory area and cognitive processes, with varying degrees of impairment and associated negative consequences and also ıt has been demonstrated with a high degree of certainty that individuals experiencing anxiety are more likely to perceive threats in their environment, which can result in the disruption of essential ongoing tasks [33]. This is also referenced in Beck's anxiety theory, which posits that individuals experiencing anxiety tend to overestimate the threat posed by various situations, leading them to perceive a greater number of potential threats [30]. This theory posits that the inclination to perceive circumstances as inherently counterproductive represents a core tenet of cognitive models of anxiety. An individual experiencing severe anxiety is also prone to difficulty disengaging from distressing images and language, which can impede their ability to resume the task at hand [34].

Working memory has a profound impact on cognitive functions. Anxiety negatively affects working memory. Working memory is a transient capacity that enables us to retain essential information for processing, such as dialling a new telephone number or recalling the location of a misplaced item. This type of memory is also of significance for everyday reasoning and decision-making processes. As is the case with numerous other aspects of cognitive function, our working memory develops and improves during our early years, attains its peak in our twenties, and then declines at a gradual rate. Factors such as stress and fatigue can impair moment efficiency. Furthermore, numerous diseases and pharmaceuticals have been demonstrated to exert a detrimental impact on working memory. Examples of daily working memory errors include forgetting the reason for entering a room or the intended content of a forthcoming utterance, or sending an email without the requisite attachment. The effective and efficient completion of working memory tasks, the blocking of distractions, the switching from one sub-task to another, the strategic online monitoring of performance, the instant detection and correction of errors, and so forth, require the utilisation of numerous complex cognitive processes, including the updating of ongoing information. The effective and efficient completion of working memory tasks, the blocking of distractions, the switching from one sub-task to another, the strategic online monitoring of performance, the instant detection and correction of errors, and so forth, require the utilisation of numerous complex cognitive processes, including the updating of ongoing information. Anxiety has been demonstrated to exert a deleterious impact on working memory, which encompasses the capacity to retain and manipulate information within one's conscious awareness. Anxiety has been demonstrated to diminish the resources required for optimal working memory performance, while simultaneously elevating the probability of negative information being integrated into working memor [34].

5. Effects of maternal anxiety on children

Children are inclined to emulate the conduct of their parents. To illustrate, if the mother responds to a given situation with elevated levels of vocalisation, the child will often mirror this behaviour when confronted with a similar scenario. The tenets of social learning theory posit that children's problematic behaviours are acquired through observation of their parents' behaviours [35]. It would be beneficial to ascertain whether this also applies to anxiety.

A review of the literature reveals that parental anxiety is one of the principal predictors of childhood anxiety. Two meta-analysis studies on this topic demonstrated that parents with anxiety disorders exhibited a markedly elevated risk of childhood anxiety among their offspring [36, 37]. Micco et al. [32] revealed that children of parents with anxiety disorders are at an elevated risk of developing non-psychiatric anxiety and depressive disorders compared to the general population. Conversely, children of parents with psychiatric disorders are at an increased risk of developing anxiety disorders compared to the general population. Lawrence et al. [33] found that the comprehensive findings indicated a heightened risk for anxiety disorders, particularly in children with generalised anxiety disorder, separation anxiety, and specific phobia. Another study that assessed the impact of parental anxiety on child psychological functioning also identified a correlation between parental anxiety and child anxiety symptoms [38]. In addition, studies have shown that maternal anxiety is significantly associated with the problematic behaviours of preschool children and also it has been established that the more children are exposed to maternal anxiety, the more externalisingly problematic their behaviours will be [39]. Furthermore, children of mothers with elevated anxiety symptoms have been found to exhibit a heightened risk of developing attention deficit hyperactivity disorder (ADHD) symptoms, with a threefold increased likelihood compared to children of mothers with normal anxiety levels [40, 41]. It has been demonstrated that children with anxiety disorders also exhibit deficiencies in memory, specifically in the domains of visual-spatial working memory and semantic memory. This has been linked to a reduction in performance in language-related areas, including oral and written communication [42].

Anxiety has also an adverse impact on children's academic performance. Elevated levels of study anxiety, along with perceived rejection and distancing in parent-child relationships, have been associated with diminished academic achievement among school-aged children [42]. It is also important to consider the role of gender in this context. The findings indicate that the correlation between maternal anxiety and the maladaptive behaviours exhibited by preschool-aged children is more pronounced girls than boys [39], also girls exhibited higher levels of both academic anxiety and academic achievement than boys. Additionally, boys reported experiencing greater parental rejection than girls. Additionally, the data indicate that a child's age is a significant variable. The observed mother-controller behaviour and negativity in the preschool years predict the presence of anxieties 1 year later. In contrast, no such prediction was observed during the early adolescent period. This indicates that parental responses may exert a more pronounced influence on anxiety during the early childhood period.

6. Parents with an anxious child

It can be challenging for parents to recognise that their child is experiencing anxiety. This is due to the fact that it can be difficult for parents to ascertain what constitutes the typical or "normal" level of anxiety in children and to discern when additional assistance is required. Also, anxiety can impact a child's thoughts and emotions to a greater extent than it affects their behaviour, and it can manifest in a multitude of ways. Furthermore, if the family is excessively controlling or anxious, and even if the child displays such behaviour, it may prove challenging to identify, given that the child's atypical conduct is perceived as the norm within the family unit. It is extremely important for the family to recognise that their child is behaving differently. If it is left untreated, anxiety disorders among young people tend to follow a chronic and unremitting course, continuing into adulthood. Furthermore, adolescents with anxiety disorders are at an increased risk of developing subsequent anxiety disorders, depression, substance abuse and poor educational attainment as young adults.

To illustrate this, consider an anxious child. The child's anxiety may cause him or her to be angry or shy at times. Such behaviour will not be welcomed by schoolmates. After a while, the anger of the child, who begins to feel lonely, will increase, from time to time the child will become uncontrollable and become an individual who is excluded by its friends, complaints will come from the school and will also receive the reaction of the family. Over time, the child's condition will worsen. When the child reaches adolescence, with the consequences of being excluded from society, the possibility of becoming an introverted, asocial individual with bad habits will increase. It is therefore incumbent upon parents to observe their children closely and to seek professional assistance when they believe that their offspring are exhibiting behaviours that are outside the normal range. A variety of treatment modalities are available, including psychotherapy, pharmacotherapy, and combined treatment approaches. Cognitive behavioural therapy (CBT) and selective serotonin reuptake inhibitors (SSRIs) are regarded by many as the preferred first-line treatments.

It is evident that further research is required on certain topics. Such as:

- Prioritising trials with larger sample sizes,
- Comparing the effects of specific parental anxiety disorders on child anxiety,
- Effects on the child in case of treatment of anxious parents,
- Role of cognitive function as a predictor of anxiety treatment outcome.

Nevertheless, it is possible to derive certain inferences from the available data. There is a positive correlation between parental anxiety and the likelihood of anxiety in children. Furthermore, maternal anxiety is a significant risk factor for the emergence of problematic behaviours in children. Irritability,hard to concentrate, increase heart rate, being clingy, especially in young children,long-term and persistent anxiety, anger, and overly critical problems such as obsessions or compulsions,are among the symptoms that can be observed in these children. In addition, tantrums, regression (e.g., bedwetting), extreme sadness, fear of anxiety, making mistakes, or shame before something happens may also exist. In addition, lack of self-esteem and low self-esteem may be observed.

Author details

Tolga Koyuncu* and Merve Elgörmüş
Medical Faculty, Department of Anesthesiology and Reanimation, Recep Tayyip Erdogan University, Rize, Turkey

*Address all correspondence to: tolga.koyuncu@erdogan.edu.tr

References

[1] Barrett LF. Emotions are real. Emotion. 2012;**12**(3):413-429. DOI: 10.1037/a0027555

[2] Dror OE. The Cannon–Bard thalamic theory of emotions: A brief genealogy and reappraisal. Emotion Review. 2014;**6**(1):13-20

[3] Vanden Bos GR. APA Dictionary of Psychology. American Psychological Association; 2007

[4] Drasković B, Simin JM, Kvrgić IM. Psychological aspects of pediatric anesthesia. Medicinski Pregled. 2015;**68**(1-2):29-34. DOI: 10.2298/mpns1502029d

[5] Britteon P, Cullum N, Sutton M. Association between psychological health and wound complications after surgery. The British Journal of Surgery. 2017;**104**:769-776

[6] Kain ZN, Mayes LC, Caldwell-Andrews AA, Karas DE, McClain BC. Preoperative anxiety, postoperative pain, and behavioral recovery in young children undergoing surgery. Pediatrics. 2006;**118**(2):651-658. DOI: 10.1542/peds.2005-2920

[7] Wright K, Stewart S, Finley A, Buffett-Jerrott S. Prevention and intervention strategies to alleviate preoperative anxiety in children. Behavior Modification. 2007;**31**(1):52-79

[8] Liang Y, Huang W, Hu X, Jiang M, Liu T, Yue H, et al. Preoperative anxiety in children aged 2-7 years old: A cross-sectional analysis of the associated risk factors. Translational Pediatrics, North America. 2021;**10**

[9] Kain ZN, Caldwell-Andrews AA, Mayes LC, Weinberg ME, Wang S-M, MacLaren JE, et al. Family-centered preparation for surgery improves perioperative outcomes in children. Anesthesiology. 2007;**106**:65-74

[10] Karling M. Child behaviour and pain after hospitalization, surgery and anaesthesia [dissertation]. Umeå: Umeå University; 2006

[11] Aguilera I, Patel D, Meakin G, Masterson J. Perioperative anxiety and postoperative behavioural disturbances in children undergoing intravenous or inhalation induction of anaesthesia. Paediatric Anaesthesia. 2003;**13**:501-507

[12] Dave NM. Premedication and induction of anaesthesia in paediatric patients. Indian Journal of Anaesthesia. 2019;**63**(9):713-720. DOI: 10.4103/ija.IJA_491_19

[13] Getahun AB, Endalew NS, Mersha AT, Admass BA. Magnitude and factors associated with preoperative anxiety among pediatric patients: Cross-sectional study. Pediatric Health, Medicine and Therapeutics. 2020;**11**:485-494. DOI: 10.2147/PHMT.S288077

[14] Ayenew NT, Endalew NS, Agegnehu AF, Bizuneh YB. Prevalence and factors associated with preoperative parental anxiety among parents of children undergoing anesthesia and surgery: A cross-sectional study. IJS Open;**24**:18-26. DOI: 10.1016/j.ijso.2020.03.004

[15] Chow CHT, Wan S, Pope E, Meng Z, Schmidt LA, Buckley N, et al. Audiovisual interventions for parental preoperative anxiety: A systematic review and meta-analysis. Health Psychology. 2018;**37**(8):746-758. DOI: 10.1037/hea0000627

[16] Fortier MA, Del Rosario AM, Martin SR, Kain ZN. Perioperative anxiety in children. Paediatric Anaesthesia. 2010;**20**:318-322. DOI: 10.1111/j.1460-9592.2010.03263.x

[17] Malik R, Yaddanpudi S, Panda NB, Kohli A, Mathew PJ. Predictors of Pre-operative Anxiety in Indian Children. Indian Journal of Pediatrics. 2018;**85**(7):504-509. DOI: 10.1007/s12098-018-2606-3 Epub 2018 Jan 25

[18] Fortier MA, Kain ZN. Treating perioperative anxiety and pain in children: A tailored and innovative approach. Paediatric Anaesthesia. 2015;**25**(1):27-35. DOI: 10.1111/pan.12546. Epub 2014 Sep 30

[19] Rabbitts JA, Palermo TM, Zhou C, Mangione-Smith R. Pain and health-related quality of life after pediatric inpatient surgery. The Journal of Pain. 2015;**16**(12):1334-1341. DOI: 10.1016/j.jpain.2015.09.005. Epub 2015 Sep 28

[20] Rosenberg RE, Clark RA, Chibbaro P, Hambrick HR, Bruzzese JM, Feudtner C, et al. Factors predicting parent anxiety around infant and toddler postoperative and pain. Hospital Pediatrics. 2017;**7**(6):313-319. DOI: 10.1542/hpeds.2016-0166. Epub 2017 May 16

[21] Fortier MA, Del Rosario AM, Rosenbaum A, Kain ZN. Beyond pain: Predictors of postoperative maladaptive behavior change in children. Paediatric Anaesthesia. 2010;**20**:445-453

[22] Draskovic B, Stanic D, Uram-Benka A, Fabri I. Stress indicators during general anesthesia with opioid analgesics in children. Turkish Journal of Medical Sciences. 2014;**44**:1095-1102

[23] Kiyonaga A, Egner T. Working memory as internal attention: Toward an integrative account of internal and external selection processes. Psychonomic Bulletin and Review. 2013;**20**(2):228-242. DOI: 10.3758/s13423-012-0359-y

[24] Kane MJ, Bleckley MK, Conway AR, Engle RW. A controlled-attention view of working-memory capacity. Journal of Experimental Psychology. General. 2001;**130**(2):169-183. DOI: 10.1037//0096-3445.130.2.169

[25] Polanczyk GV, Salum GA, Sugaya LS, Caye A, Rohde LA. Annual research review: A meta-analysis of the worldwide prevalence of mental disorders in children and adolescents. Journal of Child Psychology and Psychiatry. 2015;**56**(3):345-365. DOI: 10.1111/jcpp.12381. Epub 2015 Feb 3

[26] Beck AT, Emery G, Greenberg RL. Anxiety Disorders and Phobias: A Cognitive Perspective. New York, NY, US: PsycNET; 2005

[27] Atance CM, Meltzoff AN. My future self: Young children's ability to anticipate and explain future states. Cognitive Development. 2005;**20**:341-361. DOI: 10.1016/j.cogdev.2005.05.001

[28] Muris P, Merckelbach H, Luijten M. The connection between cognitive development and specific fears and worries in normal children and children with below-average intellectual abilities: A preliminary study. Behaviour Research and Therapy. 2002;**40**(1):37-56. DOI: 10.1016/s0005-7967(00)00115-7

[29] Bar-Haim Y, Lamy D, Pergamin L, Bakermans-Kranenburg MJ, van IJzendoorn MH. Threat-related attentional bias in anxious and nonanxious individuals: A meta-analytic study. Psychological Bulletin. 2007;**133**(1):1-24. DOI: 10.1037/0033-2909.133.1.1

[30] Grant D, White E. The Influence of Anxiety on Cognitive Control

Processes2016. DOI: 10.1093/acrefore/9780190236557.013.74

[31] Weldon S, Gilchrist E. Implicit theories in intimate partner violence offenders. Journal of Family Violence. 2012;**27**:761-772. DOI: 10.1007/s10896-012-9465-x

[32] Micco JA, Henin A, Mick E, Kim S, Hopkins CA, Biederman J, et al. Anxiety and depressive disorders in offspring at high risk for anxiety: A meta-analysis. Journal of Anxiety Disorders. 2009;**23**(8):1158-1164. DOI: 10.1016/j.janxdis.2009.07.021. Epub 2009 Aug 6

[33] Lawrence PJ, Murayama K, Creswell C. Systematic review and meta-analysis: Anxiety and depressive disorders in offspring of parents with anxiety disorders. Journal of the American Academy of Child and Adolescent Psychiatry. 2019;**58**(1):46-60. DOI: 10.1016/j.jaac.2018.07.898. Epub 2018 Nov 1

[34] Burstein M, Ginsburg GS, Tein JY. Parental anxiety and child symptomatology: An examination of additive and interactive effects of parent psychopathology. Journal of Abnormal Child Psychology. 2010;**38**(7):897-909. DOI: 10.1007/s10802-010-9415-0. Erratum in: J Abnorm Child Psychol. 2010 Oct;38(7):895

[35] Song Z, Huang J, Qiao T, Yan J, Zhang X, Lu D. Association between maternal anxiety and children's problem behaviors: A systematic review and meta-analysis. International Journal of Environmental Research and Public Health. 2022;**19**(17):11106. DOI: 10.3390/ijerph191711106

[36] Ayano G, Betts K, Tait R, Dachew BA, Alati R. Maternal depressive and anxiety symptoms and the risk of attention deficit hyperactivity disorder symptoms in offspring aged 17: Findings from the Raine study. Journal of Affective Disorders. 2021;**284**:149-156. DOI: 10.1016/j.jad.2021.02.024. Epub 2021 Feb 8

[37] Sbicigo JB, Toazza R, Becker N, Ecker K, Manfro GG, Salles JF. Memory and language impairments are associated with anxiety disorder severity in childhood. Trends in Psychiatry and Psychotherapy. 2020;**42**(2):161-170. DOI: 10.1590/2237-6089-2019-0051. Epub 2020 Jul 17

[38] Najmussaqib A, Ijaz T. Impact of Study Anxiety, Parent Child Relationship on Academic Achievement of School Children. 2021

[39] Edwards SL, Rapee RM, Kennedy S. Prediction of anxiety symptoms in preschool-aged children: Examination of maternal and paternal perspectives. Journal of Child Psychology and Psychiatry. 2010;**51**(3):313-321. DOI: 10.1111/j.1469-7610.2009.02160.x. Epub 2009 Sep 21

[40] Johnco CJ, Magson NR, Fardouly J, Oar EL, Forbes MK, Richardson C, et al. The role of parenting behaviors in the bidirectional and intergenerational transmission of depression and anxiety between parents and early adolescent youth. Depression and Anxiety. 2021;**38**(12):1256-1266

[41] Woodward LJ, Fergusson DM. Life course outcomes of young people with anxiety disorders in adolescence. Journal of the American Academy of Child and Adolescent Psychiatry. 2001;**40**(9):1086-1093. DOI: 10.1097/00004583-200109000-00018

[42] Manassis K, Russell K, Newton AS. The Cochrane library and the treatment of childhood and adolescent anxiety disorders: And overview of reviews. Evidence-Base Child Health: A Cochrane Review Journal. 2010;**5**:541-554. DOI: 10.1002/ebch.508

Section 3

Obstetric Anesthesiology

Chapter 4

Interdisciplinary Emergencies in the Delivery Room

Kim K. Kutun and Mark Ulrich Gerbershagen

Abstract

Obstetric risks and difficulties are part of an anaesthetist's everyday life and require close interdisciplinary collaboration with obstetricians. To manage these situations, routine and regular training is essential, as is knowledge of common algorithms. There is no time to lose when mother and baby are at risk and immediate action is necessary. In order to reduce obstetric injuries, every anaesthesiologist working in obstetric care should deal with the most common emergencies and have a good overview of concepts for these scenarios. Knowledge of absolute emergencies with high mortality such as postpartum haemorrhage, through to less drastic complications such as hypertensive diseases of pregnancy, is necessary to increase patient safety. An overview of the main interdisciplinary emergencies in the delivery room is provided in this chapter.

Keywords: anaesthesia, obstetrics, interdisciplinary emergencies, delivery room, peripartum haemorrhage, preeclampsia

1. Introduction

Anaesthetists are true multitaskers and, in addition to their routine duties, must possess profound knowledge of the physiology and pathology of various medical conditions.

For any anaesthetist working in the delivery room, a solid understanding of physiological particularities in pregnant women is essential. Besides the anatomical changes, hormonal adjustments lead to physiological peculiarities that prepare the body as best as possible for childbirth. For example, increased sensitivity to centrally acting substances and local anaesthetics is normal, as is reduced functional residual capacity and enhanced oxygen consumption. This leads to a decreased apnoea tolerance and a reduced minimum alveolar concentration (MAC) value for inhalational anaesthetics. An increased stroke volume and a rise in heart rate by up to 25% lead to an increased cardiac output. From the 20th week of pregnancy onwards, the uterus can reduce cardiac output depending on position due to the vena cava compression syndrome. In the event of circulatory instability, attention must be paid to placing the pregnant on the left side. These bodily changes are necessary to ensure the increased oxygen and nutrient demands throughout pregnancy. These particularities must be carefully considered when inducing general anaesthesia or performing regional

 IntechOpen

anaesthesia. The anaesthetist must be prepared for a difficult airway, as the tendency for oedema, including the airway, increases the incidence of difficult intubations [1].

Pregnancy is divided into three trimesters. Most emergencies occur around the time of delivery, but incidents can also happen in the second trimester and in the postpartum period. Complications of obstetrics can quickly turn into life-threatening emergencies, which is why the obstetrician must be able to rely anytime on interdisciplinary collaboration. The anaesthetist plays a crucial role in critically ill pregnant women, ensuring not only analgesia but also circulatory stabilisation and, if necessary, airway management. In addition to caring for the mother, the well-being of the unborn child must also be kept in mind, as foetal oxygenation depends directly on maternal hemodynamic until the cord is clamped. Interdisciplinary emergencies in the delivery room present a particular challenge, as multiple disciplines are required simultaneously to protect the lives of both mother and child.

This chapter aims to outline the most prevalent emergencies and their management.

2. Hypertensive pregnancy disorders

Hypertensive pregnancy disorders include various conditions such as gestational hypertension, preeclampsia, eclampsia, and haemolysis, elevated liver enzyme levels, and low platelet count (HELLP) syndrome. With a frequency of 6–8% of all pregnancies, these disorders account for 20–25% of maternal deaths across Europe [2].

The underlying pathophysiology common to all these conditions is inadequate placentation and the insufficient development of the placental vascular system. Although the pathophysiology is not yet fully understood, reduced vascularisation of the placenta leads to increased uteroplacental vascular resistance, resulting in relative hypoperfusion and, thus, placental insufficiency. This can cause foetal growth restriction, and due to generalised endothelial dysfunction, other maternal organ systems may also be affected [3].

The risk factors include a body mass index (BMI) ≥ 25 kg/m^2, pre-existing diabetes or arterial hypertension, as well as primiparity and advanced maternal age. Aside from that, there is an 11–27% risk of recurrent preeclampsia in subsequent pregnancies [2].

The main symptom underlying all these conditions is an elevated blood pressure. The definition of gestational hypertension, also called pregnancy-induced hypertension, is new-onset blood pressure values above 140/90 mmHg during gestation, which are often not associated with complications. However, it is essential to identify serious conditions like preeclampsia early and perform risk stratification. During prenatal check-ups, blood pressure measurement, a detailed medical history, weight monitoring, and urine tests should be included. In recent years, biomarkers such as the ratio of placental growth factor (PlGF) to soluble fms-like tyrosine kinase-1 (sFlt-1) have become significant. Whilst they have a strong negative predictive value for preeclampsia, they are not suitable for diagnosis on their own and do not replace clinical examination [4].

Preeclampsia is categorised as early or late-onset, depending on the onset of symptoms before or after 34 weeks of pregnancy. In addition to elevated blood pressure, preeclampsia is defined by the presence of at least one new-onset organ complication. Acute kidney injury with oedema and proteinuria is typical, but symptoms can vary widely. New-onset dyspnoea must be seen as a warning sign, as well as upper abdominal pain, which could indicate liver involvement. Central nervous symptoms such as headaches, visual disturbances, and dizziness may also occur.

For pregnant women at high risk of preeclampsia, the only effective prevention currently available is the intake of 150 mg of acetylsalicylic acid daily until the 36th week of gestation. There has been evidence that the incidence of preeclampsia can be reduced by approximately 63% [5, 6].

The only causal treatment is the termination of the pregnancy [7]. Delivery should be considered after 34 weeks of pregnancy, after weighing the maternal and foetal risks, but it should take place no later than after 37 weeks [2]. If the condition of the mother and child is stable, vaginal delivery can be attempted. Between the 24th and 34th week of gestation, a conservative approach is preferred, if possible, as neonatal complications are significantly increased at this stage.

High levels of blood pressure are associated with complications for the mother and poor outcomes for the baby. Hospitalisation and antihypertensive medication should be initiated if systolic blood pressure exceeds ≥160 mmHg or diastolic blood pressure ≥ 110 mmHg. The aim of antihypertensive therapy is the prevention of cardiovascular and cerebral complications in the mother [8].

Eclampsia is a rare but severe complication of major preeclampsia, occurring in 2–3% of preeclampsia patients. Eclampsia or an eclamptic seizure is distinguished by the occurrence of tonic-clonic seizures during pregnancy that cannot be attributed to another neurological cause. The foetal circulation is often compromised during a seizure, leading to severe bradycardia, which may necessitate immediate delivery [7]. If prodromal symptoms such as double vision, severe headaches, or other CNS symptoms occur, first-line therapy and prophylaxis is intravenous magnesium sulphate. The initial dose is 4–6 g of magnesium, afterwards ca. 1 g per hour. This can reduce the incidence of eclampsia by half [9].

Ten to twenty percent of all pregnant women with preeclampsia have a HELLP syndrome [2]. The typical laboratory findings—haemolysis, elevated liver enzyme levels, and low platelet count—give the condition its name. A common symptom in the early stages is right upper quadrant pain caused by liver capsule distention. Other symptoms can include nausea, anaemia, proteinuria, and hypertension, similar to preeclampsia, making it difficult to distinguish between these two. Here, as well, termination of pregnancy is the definitive treatment.

The complications of the aforementioned hypertensive pregnancy disease can be severe and require interdisciplinary care. The dysfunction of various organ systems poses a particular challenge for the anaesthetist. For caesarean deliveries, after ruling out contraindications—especially with attention to coagulation disorders—neuraxial techniques are the preferred method [10, 11]. In the context of HELLP syndrome, in addition to the absolute platelet count, the trend of this value is also important. If platelet levels fall rapidly below 80 gpt/l, general anaesthesia should be preferred. The daily intake of 150 mg of acetylsalicylic acid for preeclampsia prophylaxis, after assessing the risk-benefit ratio, does not contraindicate regional anaesthesia [12]. The primary focus, regardless of the chosen anaesthetic technique, is on hemodynamic stabilisation. Blood pressure spikes and hypotension must be avoided at all costs.

Hypertensive pregnancy disorders can also exacerbate up to 7 days postpartum, usually with blood pressure normalising within a few days postpartum in 29–57% of cases. HELLP syndrome can occur postpartum in up to 30% of cases [13, 14]. In order to ensure the best care for both, childbirth should take place at specialised centres familiar with the complications and treatment of pregnancy-related diseases, as well as with the postnatal care of mother and child.

3. Caesarean section

In Europe, an average of 25.2% of babies are born by caesarean section (C-section), and the amount of caesarean birth is increasing globally [15]. The indications for performing a caesarean section are diverse and have been more liberal in the past years. In the case of an uncomplicated pregnancy, the obstetrician decides the mode of delivery together with the pregnant woman as an "informed choice", the wish of the mother is paramount [16]. In emergency situations, the maternal and child's well-being is the top priority. Anaesthetists support obstetricians in many situations, as surgical delivery is not possible without anaesthesia or analgesia. Good consultation within the team should be the priority here.

A primary caesarean section or category 4 C-section is an elective delivery after the 39th week of gestation, aimed before the onset of labour, with the amniotic sac still closed. In addition to maternal request, the most common indications are women who have had previous caesarean sections and a pathological cardiotocography (CTG). The absolute indications for primary caesarean section include malpresentation of the child, prematurity or a placental implantation disorder [17]. In a secondary caesarean section, the decision is made after the onset of labour. This is often not an acute emergency, but there is a certain urgency depending on the indication. Common indications include a pathological CTG, a hypertensive pregnancy disorder or prolonged labour. The timing of the procedure is divided into a standardised scheme according to different levels of urgency, for example, according to the classification scheme of the National Institute for Health and Clinical Excellence [18]. The least urgent category is a category three caesarean section, where mother and child are not compromised, but a fast delivery should be aimed for. An example of this could be an early onset of labour in the case of a planned caesarean birth.

In the event of an urgent caesarean section or category 2 caesarean section, there is a risk to the mother and/or the child that is not immediately life-threatening. The caesarean section must therefore be performed immediately and without delay. A time interval from decision to delivery under 30 minutes should be aimed for.

An emergency caesarean section is also referred to as a category 1 caesarean section or crash C-section, which means that there is a directly life-threatening danger to the pregnant and/or the child. This can be triggered by therapy-resistant foetal bradycardia or severe bleeding, for example, due to uterine rupture or premature placental abruption. As the delivery must take place immediately, the usual preparations such as a detailed enlightenment must be dispensed with. A time interval of less than 20 minutes between the decision and the delivery of the child should be realised in order to improve the outcome. Internationally, a maximum decision-delivery time of 30 minutes is recommended; in Germany, a maximum time of 20 minutes is standard [18, 19]. Apart from Category 1 sections, patients should be offered regional anaesthesia as the first choice [18]. If the coagulation history is unremarkable and the pregnancy is progressing without problems, routine monitoring of coagulation parameters can be dispensed with, especially in urgent situations. The risk of spinal haemorrhage complications is lower in pregnant women due to hypercoagulation [19, 20]. General anaesthesia is routinely used for emergency caesareans from the 20th week of pregnancy in the form of rapid sequence induction (RSI) with subsequent mostly balanced anaesthesia. The incidence of a difficult airway is significantly higher in pregnant women, at around 1 in 250 intubations [21].

An emergency caesarean section is a frequent obstetric emergency. Close consultation and regular training in the interdisciplinary team are essential to optimise the procedure and communication and to keep the time until delivery as short as possible. Particularly in time-critical situations, the roles of each team member must be clearly allocated from the alert of the emergency team to postoperative care.

Perimortem caesarean section is a special case and an absolute rarity. If a parturient suffers a cardiac arrest, every second counts for mother and foetus. In addition to the standard resuscitation of the patient according to the ERC guidelines, the well-being of the child is also paramount. According to current recommendations, if there is no immediate return of spontaneous circulation (ROSC) within 4 minutes, a perimortem caesarean section should be carried out in the 20th week of pregnancy at the latest. Although foetal survival is only possible from the 22nd-24th week of pregnancy, delivery improves maternal haemodynamic and allows adequate chest compressions [22]. Before the 20th week of pregnancy, the focus should be on caring for the mother. Another characteristic is the manual displacement of the abdomen and, thus, the uterus to the left to counteract a vena cava compression syndrome. The possibility of extracorporeal life support should also be considered at an early stage after delivery. This rare incident is another example of how important it is to create structures to ensure a frictionless process and to provide the best possible care for mother and child.

4. Peripartum haemorrhage

Peripartum haemorrhage (PPH) accounts for the majority of interdisciplinary emergencies, with an incidence of 1–3% of all deliveries worldwide. At the same time, the mortality rate for these emergencies is high and constantly increasing. In industrial countries at 13%, and even higher in the countries of the Global South at around 30% [23, 24]. Many of these deaths are demonstrably preventable, and blood loss is often not quantified or initially underestimated [25]. This makes structured action algorithms and a trained interdisciplinary team even more important. Several specialist societies have therefore jointly defined a guideline for the management of haemorrhage emergencies to provide the best possible care for these frequent emergencies. There are also minimum requirements that must be met by the hospitals providing obstetrics.

The term peripartum haemorrhage includes intra- and postpartum haemorrhage and therefore all bleeding before, during and after birth. From a blood loss of ≥500 ml after delivery, independent of the mode of delivery, the WHO speaks of peripartum haemorrhage from ≥1000 ml of severe haemorrhage. If there are clinical signs of haemorrhagic shock, peripartum haemorrhage can be assumed regardless of the estimated extent of blood loss. The causes of haemorrhage are divided into the so-called "4 Ts": Tonus, Trauma, Tissue and Thrombin. Tonus stands for uterine atony, Trauma for any birth injury, Tissue for placental haemorrhage, and placenta accreta spectrum (PAS) and lastly, thrombin for coagulopathies such as disseminated intravascular coagulation (DIC) or HELLP syndrome [23].

The assessment of the bleeding risk includes the evaluation of various factors. On the maternal side, for example, a previous caesarean section or other operations on the uterus, multiparity or a known coagulation disorder. A macrosomia or any type of placental retention disorder as well as hypertensive pregnancy disorders also increase the risk of postpartum haemorrhage. Finally, there are also risk factors during labour, such as prolonged labour or the use of large amounts of oxytocin. At over 95%, most of these incidents occur in the first 24 hours after birth as primary haemorrhage, the main reason being uterine atony (>80%). Secondary haemorrhages are a rarity but are not less dangerous as they usually occur after the patient has been discharged [26, 27].

Uterine atony leads to a contraction weakness of the uterus and thus to a reduced contraction of the myometrial vessels. This is followed by increased bleeding, which can occur after or during placental expulsion. The drugs of first choice are therefore uterotonics such as oxytocin or external compression or stimulation of the uterus. If the placenta is expelled incompletely or delayed, the first step is to manually or surgically remove the remains. Severe bleeding can be tamponaded with a balloon catheter such as the Bakri balloon; the last option in a life-threatening emergency is hysterectomy, in addition to suturing techniques for uterine compression. Uterine atony has a high risk of recurrence. Multiple pregnancies, multiparity, rapid birth order and macrosomic children are also risk factors.

The PAS includes all placental abnormalities, in particular invasive placentation. The placenta grows into the deep wall layers of the myometrium and is categorised as placenta accreta, increta or percreta. The mildest form is placenta accreta, which is also the most common form at around 60%, whilst placenta increta and percreta have a significantly higher complication rate. Due to the worldwide increase in the caesarean section rate, the number of PAS is also increasing, as one of the main risk factors for placental abruption is parturients who have previously given birth by caesarean section. Other risk factors include nicotine abuse, previous curettage and *in vitro* fertilisation [28]. An unrecognised PAS can lead to serious and life-threatening bleeding, which is why early birth planning should take place in a maternity clinic with a multidisciplinary team. Even with early diagnosis, the risk of severe PPH is high depending on the degree of adhesions and the delivery must be performed as a caesarean section. Placenta praevia may be present alongside or at the same time as a PAS. In this case, the inner cervix is partially or completely covered by the placenta. In the case of a deep-seated placenta, the placenta is classified sonographically in the second trimester according to its localisation as placenta praevia marginalis, partialis or totalis. Risk factors here are analogical to the PAS [29]. Depending on the extent of the adhesion, a primary caesarean section should be performed to prevent haemorrhage in the event of a vaginal delivery.

In addition to the uterine atony and PAS, which are mentioned first and occur more frequently in comparison, there are other clinical pictures that can cause intra- and postpartum haemorrhage. The category "trauma" includes, for example, injuries to the birth canal and uterine rupture, which is an absolute emergency for mother and foetus. In the case of a complete rupture, there is a connection from the foetus to the abdominal cavity, which is related to a high rate of mortality for the child; a covered rupture can be subacute. It typically occurs during an attempted vaginal delivery after a previous C-section, but in rare cases, a rupture can also occur spontaneously [30]. In addition to the common disorders of placental abruption already mentioned, the term "tissue" also includes premature placental abruption, which poses a vital threat. With only 0.3–1% of all pregnancies, this complication is rare, but due to placental insufficiency and foetal hypoxia, it poses a vital threat to the unborn child. The infant mortality rate is 12% [31]. On the maternal side, severe haemorrhage and even haemorrhagic shock can occur.

In addition to anaesthesia and analgesia, the interdisciplinary task of the anaesthetist in PPH is to stabilise the circulation and maintain haemostasis. In addition to the provision of blood reserves and availability of coagulation factors, cell salvage and mechanical autotransfusion also play a role in preparation for patient blood management in PPH [23]. In addition, sufficient staff with expertise on the side of the obstetricians and anaesthetists who are familiar with the hospital's internal treatment protocol should be available at an early stage. The hormonal changes during pregnancy also have an influence on haemostasis, which is why there are special features to consider when treating a haemorrhage that must be dealt with in accordance with the PPH guideline. In addition to stabilising the general conditions, such as normothermia, normocalcaemia and a balanced pH, volume therapy should be provided as required and, if necessary, substitution of blood reserves. In addition to surgical measures, uterotonics such as oxytocin or prostaglandins are used if atony is the cause of PPH. As local fibrinolysis is physiologically limited, possible hyperfibrinolysis should always be treated at an early stage by administering tranexamic acid. Point of care procedures such as viscoelastic tests can help to recognise and treat a coagulation disorder at an early stage on the bedside. As, in addition to primary haemostasis, special attention must also be paid to the final stage of coagulation; fibrinogen should be substituted if necessary. In haemorrhagic shock, patients can benefit from early administration and a high ratio of clotting factors or fresh frozen plasma (FFP) to avert dilutional coagulopathy. The substitution of platelet concentrates may be necessary, as the increased plasma volume leads to relative thrombocytopenia. The administration of prothrombin complex concentrate (PCC) may also be indicated, as well as a so-called thrombin burst with the administration of recombinant factor

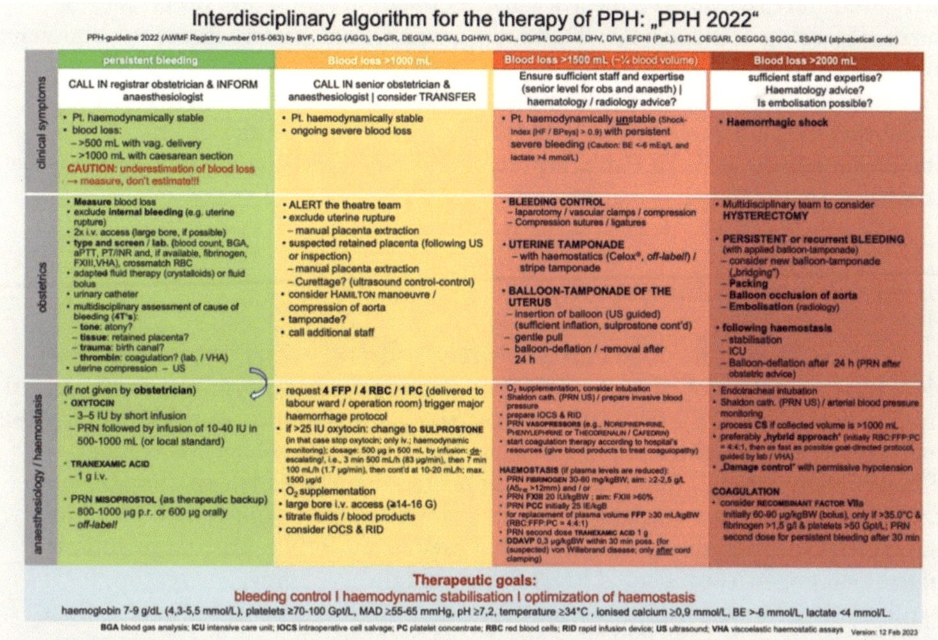

Figure 1.
Interdisciplinary algorithm for the therapy of PPH, based on PPH Guideline 2022, AWMF Registry No. 015/063 [23].

VIIa (rFVIIa) in individual cases [23]. If the bleeding is uncontrolled and the patient cannot be stabilised, the only option is a hysterectomy.

The scheme below must be familiar to every anaesthetist working in the delivery room (**Figure 1**).

5. Amniotic fluid embolism and thromboembolic complications

Thromboembolic events such as pulmonary artery embolism are the main reason for motherly mortality in the United Kingdom, with a prevalence of 1.45 per 100,000 pregnant women [19]. Pregnancy itself poses a risk for thromboembolic complications like pulmonary artery embolism, as increased factor activity during pregnancy leads to a procoagulatory state [32]. Differential diagnosis must include a potentially fatal complication that is often underestimated: Amniotic fluid embolism. Accounting for 5–15% of all worldwide deaths of parturients, it is a major cause of direct maternal deaths [33]. During labour, amniotic fluid leaks into the maternal venous circulation, most likely leading to an anaphylactoid reaction due to the mediator-rich amniotic fluid. The complete pathogenesis is not fully explained. In addition to circulatory depression caused by peripheral vasodilation, pulmonary vasoconstriction, similar to that seen in pulmonary embolism, leads to acute right heart strain, resulting in hypoxia and hypotension. Clinically, this manifests as a compromised circulatory system, potentially progressing to cardiac arrest and multi-organ failure. Differentiating between these diagnoses is challenging. Viscoelastic tests play a major role, as amniotic fluid embolism leads to an immediate coagulopathy. Already in the early stages, hyperfibrinolysis and fibrinogen deficiency can be detected. Coagulation activation and disseminated intravascular coagulation (DIC) may occur, causing further bleeding or thrombosis. These symptoms are completely absent in pulmonary artery embolism.

Symptoms appear acutely and immediately around the time of delivery, and the amniotic fluid embolism is a diagnosis of exclusion. Therapeutically, circulatory stabilisation is the priority. Extracorporeal membrane oxygenation (ECMO) may be considered in individual cases [34].

6. Peripartum cardiomyopathy

Pregnant women are often mistakenly regarded as a healthy and young population, but the number of patients with a pre-existing cardiac risk profile has increased in recent years. From the 24th week of pregnancy, the risk of cardiac decompensation increases in women with a pre-existing cardiac risk profile, which is why interdisciplinary collaboration is important in early pregnancy. These high-risk pregnancies should be planned in a specialised hospital. However, even women with a healthy heart can develop cardiac problems during pregnancy. Besides the aforementioned high blood pressure, congenital heart defects are the most prevalent reasons for cardiac emergencies during gestation. Cardiomyopathies are rare but severe diseases with a high mortality rate [35]. The aetiology is not fully understood. Peripartum cardiomyopathy presents as idiopathic heart failure due to left ventricular systolic dysfunction. The ejection fraction is typically reduced, and the left ventricle is dilated, but the diagnosis remains a diagnosis of exclusion. It is particularly difficult to recognise warning signs such as oedema, dyspnoea and reduced exercise tolerance in a pregnant woman, and the symptoms are often dismissed as normal. The rapid progression with the risk of decompensation necessitates quick diagnosis and treatment. This condition usually occurs towards the end of pregnancy but can also cause problems postpartum [36]. Early cardiology consultation with echocardiography and medication management should be performed promptly and before delivery. Treatment is similar to that of heart failure. In cardiologically stable patients, vaginal delivery is possible, with continuous monitoring of blood pressure and heart rate. If a C-section or epidural anaesthesia is desired, the anaesthetist must proceed cautiously and strictly avoid hypotension to prevent ischaemia, particularly in cases of stenotic heart defects. Outside of emergency situations, anaesthesia for elective caesarean sections can be provided via an epidural catheter, as circulatory depression from epidural administration is usually less pronounced [21].

7. Shoulder dystocia

Shoulder dystocia is a foetal emergency. During labour, even after a normal progression, an abnormal foetal position can occur due to a high shoulder gradient or deep transverse shoulder position. This mechanical obstruction results in a sudden halt of labour during the expulsion phase. The baby has already descended deeply into the birth canal, with the head already delivered, posing a risk of hypoxia due to umbilical cord compression. Approximately 80% of shoulder dystocia can be resolved using the McRoberts manoeuvre, where the obstetrician attempts to enlarge the diameter of the pelvic inlet by repositioning the mother's legs [37]. If this manoeuvre is insufficient to deliver the baby, clear interdisciplinary communication and cooperation are necessary to avoid a fatal outcome. Rapid induction of general anaesthesia in the mother for full relaxation of the pelvic floor is often the only way to deliver the baby. Alternatives include performing a caesarean section, also under general anaesthesia.

8. Conclusion

The spectrum of emergencies in the delivery room is diverse. The MBRRACE (Mothers and Babies: Reducing Risk through Audits and Confidential Enquiries) report investigates maternal mortality and morbidity in the United Kingdom and analyses factors that can lead to a reduction in these deaths. The report shows that anaesthetists are involved in managing a significant portion of obstetric emergencies, as many of the described cases require the baby to be delivered via (emergency) caesarean section or an emergency treatment for the mother [38]. The report highlights the importance of having a clinic-specific interdisciplinary emergency plan in place before a critical situation arises, tailored to the internal structures and conditions of the clinic. This concept should then be regularly practised with all involved disciplines through simulations, training sessions, and case reviews. Equally important is professional debriefing. A study comparing trained and untrained teams showed a significantly reduced decision-to-delivery time in the trained group, with simulation-based training achieving the highest success rate [39]. The teams are prepared for emergency scenarios under realistic conditions to improve reaction times in critical situations. With targeted preparation, effective communication, and a well-trained interdisciplinary team, it should be the goal of every anaesthesiologist and gynaecology department to further reduce maternal mortality worldwide.

Conflict of interest

The authors declare no conflict of interest.

Author details

Kim K. Kutun* and Mark Ulrich Gerbershagen
Department of Anesthesiology, Kliniken der Stadt Köln gGmbH, Cologne, Germany

*Address all correspondence to: gerbershagenm@kliniken-koeln.de

References

[1] Girard T, Palanisamy A. The obstetric difficult airway: If we can't predict it, can we prevent it? Anaesthesia. 2017;**72**:143-147

[2] Hypertensive Pregnancy Disorders: Diagnosis and Therapy. Guideline of the German Society of Gynaecology and Obsterics (S2k-Level, AWMF-Registry No. 015/018, March 2019). pp. 7; 51-52; 67-68. Available from: http://www.awmf.org/leitlinien/detail/II/015-018.html

[3] Hofmeyr R, Matjila M, Dyer R. Preeclampsia in 2017: Obstetric and Anaesthesia Management. Best Practice & Research Clinical Anaesthesiology. Mar 2017;**31**(1):125-138. DOI: 10.1016/j.bpa.2016.12.002. Epub 2016 Dec 18. PMID: 28625300

[4] Tsiakkas A, Saiid Y, Wright A, Wright D, Nicolaides KH. Competing risks model in screening for preeclampsia by maternal factors and biomarkers at 30-34 weeks' gestation. American Journal of Obstetrics and Gynecology. 2016;**215**(1):87.e1-87.e17. DOI: 10.1016/j.ajog.2016.02.016. Epub 2016 Feb 12

[5] Rolnik DL, Wright D, Poon LC, O'Gorman N, Syngelaki A, de Paco MC, et al. Aspirin versus placebo in pregnancies at high risk for preterm preeclampsia. The New England Journal of Medicine. 2017;**377**(7):613-622. DOI: 10.1056/NEJMoa1704559. Epub 2017 Jun 28

[6] Richards EM, Giorgione V, Stevens O, Thilaganathan B. Low-dose aspirin for the prevention of superimposed preeclampsia in women with chronic hypertension: A systematic review and meta-analysis. American Journal of Obstetrics and Gynecology. 2022

[7] Koopmans CM, Bijlenga D, Groen H, Vijgen SM, Aarnoudse JG, Bekedam DJ, et al. Induction of labour versus expectant monitoring for gestational hypertension or mild pre-eclampsia after 36 weeks' gestation (HYPITAT): A multicentre, open-label randomised controlled trial. Lancet. 2009;**374**(9694):979-988. DOI: 10.1016/S0140-6736(09)60736-4. Epub 2009 Aug 3

[8] Abalos E, Duley L, Steyn DW, Gialdini C. Antihypertensive drug therapy for mild to moderate hypertension during pregnancy. Cochrane Database of Systematic Reviews. 2018;**10**(10):2-9. DOI: 10.1002/14651858.CD002252.pub4

[9] Altman D, Carroli G, Duley L, Farrell B, Moodley J, Neilson J, et al. Do women with pre-eclampsia, and their babies, benefit from magnesium sulphate? The Magpie Trial: A randomised placebo-controlled trial. Lancet. 2002;**359**(9321):1877-1890. DOI: 10.1016/s0140-6736(02)08778-0

[10] Lee S, Bang E, Yang E, Lee H, Kang Y, Cho K, et al. Retrospective analysis of anesthesia for cesarean section of the patients with hypertensive disorders in pregnancy for 15 years. The Ewha Medical Journal. 2014;**37**:36. DOI: 10.12771/emj.2014.37.1.36

[11] Palit S, Palit G, Vercauteren M, Jacquemyn Y. Regional anaesthesia for primary caesarean section in patients with preterm HELLP syndrome: A review of 102 cases. Clinical and Experimental Obstetrics & Gynecology. 2009;**36**(4):230-234

[12] Vela Vásquez RS, Peláez RR. Aspirin and spinal haematoma after

neuraxial anaesthesia: Myth or reality? British Journal of Anaesthesia. 2015 Nov;**115**(5):688-698. DOI: 10.1093/bja/aev348

[13] Sharma KJ, Kilpatrick SJ. Postpartum hypertension: Etiology, diagnosis, and management. Obstetrical & Gynecological Survey. 2017;**72**(4):248-252. DOI: 10.1097/OGX.0000000000000424

[14] Magee LA, Smith GN, Bloch C, et al. Guideline No. 426: Hypertensive disorders of pregnancy: Diagnosis, prediction, prevention, and management. Journal of Obstetrics and Gynaecology Canada. 2022;**44**:547-571.e1. DOI: 10.1016/j.jogc.2022.03.002

[15] WHO statement on caesarean section rates: World Health Organization human reproduction programme [WHO/RHR/15.02]. Reproductive Health Matters. 2015;**23**(45):149-150

[16] Gerbershagen MU, Baagil H. Caesarean delivery: A narrative review on the choice of neuroaxially administered opioid and its implications for the multimodal peripartum pain concept. Medicina. 2024;**60**:358. DOI: 10.3390/medicina60030358

[17] Singh N, Pradeep Y, Jauhari S. Indications and determinants of cesarean section: A cross-sectional study. International Journal of Applied and Basic Medical Research. 2020;**10**(4):280-285. DOI: 10.4103/ijabmr.IJABMR_3_20

[18] NICE Guideline. Caesarean Section. Clinical guideline [NG192] [Internet]. 2021.Available from: https://www.nice.org.uk/guidance/ng192 [Accessed: 8 July 2024]

[19] Louwen F, Wagner U, Abou-Dakn M, Dötsch J, Lawrenz B, Ehm D, et al. Caesarean Section. Guideline of the DGGG, OEGGG and SGGG (S3-Level, AWMF Registry No. 015/084. June 2020) [Internet]. Available from: http://www.awmf.org/leitlinien/detail/II/015084.html [Accessed: 20 June 2024]

[20] Moen V, Dahlgren N, Irestedt L. Severe neurological complications after central neuraxial blockades in Sweden 1990-1999. Anesthesiology. 2004;**101**(4):950-959

[21] Bremerich D, Annecke T, Chappell D, Hanß R, Kaufner L, Kehl F, et al. The new S1 guideline "Obsteric analgesia and anesthesia". Anasthesiologie, Intensivmedizin, Notfallmedizin, Schmerztherapie. 2020;**55**:674-685

[22] Jeejeebhoy FM, Zelop CM, Lipman S, Carvalho B, Joglar J, Mhyre JM, et al. Cardiac arrest in pregnancy: A scientific statement from the American Heart Association. Circulation. 2015;**132**:1747-1773

[23] Schlembach D, Annecke T, Girard T, et al. Peripartal haemorrhage: Diagnosis and therapy. Guideline of the German Society of Gynaecology and Obstetrics (S2k-Level, AWMF Registry No. 015/063, June 2022)

[24] Reale SC, Easter SR, Xu X, et al. Trends in postpartum hemorrhage in the United States from 2010 to 2014. Anesthesia and Analgesia. 2020;**130**:e119-e122

[25] Haeri S, Dildy GA 3rd. Maternal mortality from hemorrhage. Seminars in Perinatology. 2012;**36**(1):48-55

[26] Schwendemann WD, Watson WJ. Postpartum hemorrhage. In: Winn HN, Chervenak FA, Romero R, editors. Clinical Maternal-Fetal Medicine. 2nd ed. London: CRC Press; 2021. pp. 10-11

[27] Alonso-Burgos A, Díaz-Lorenzo I, Muñoz-Saá L, et al. Primary and

secondary postpartum haemorrhage: A review for a rationale endovascular approach. CVIR Endovascular. 2024;7:17. DOI: 10.1186/s42155-024-00429-7

[28] Jauniaux E, Alfirevic Z, Bhide AG, Belfort MA, Burton GJ, Collins SL, et al. Placenta praevia and placenta accreta: Diagnosis and management: Green-top Guideline No. 27a. BJOG. 2019;**126**(1)

[29] Downes KL, Hinkle SN, Sjaarda LA, Albert PS, Grantz KL. Previous prelabor or intrapartum cesarean delivery and risk of placenta previa. American Journal of Obstetrics and Gynecology. 2015;**212**(5):669.e1-6669e6

[30] Savukyne E, Bykovaite-Stankeviciene R, Machtejeviene E, Nadisauskiene R, Maciuleviciene R. Symptomatic uterine rupture: A fifteen year review. Medicina. 2020;**56**(11):574. DOI: 10.3390/medicina56110574

[31] Pecks U, Bauerschlag DO. Emergencies in gynaecology and obstetrics. Frauenheilkunde up2date. 2017;**11**(2):139-153. DOI: 10.1055/s-0043-100744

[32] Tan EK, Tan EL. Alterations in physiology and anatomy during pregnancy. Best Practice & Research. Clinical Obstetrics & Gynaecology. 2013;**27**:791-802

[33] Rossi AC, Mulin P. The etiology of maternal mortality in developed countries: A systematic review of the literature. Archives of Gynecology and Obstetrics. 2012;**285**:1499-1503

[34] Tschöp J, Lier H, Annecke T. Anaesthesiological management of amniotic fluid embolism. AINS. 2020;**55**:674-685

[35] Regitz-Zagrosek V, Roos-Hesselink JW, Bauersachs J, Blomström-Lundqvist C, Cifkova R, De Bonis M, et al. ESC guidelines for the management of cardiovascular diseases during pregnancy. European Heart Journal. 2018;**39**:3165-3241

[36] Regitz-Zagrosek V et al. ESC guidelines on the management of cardiovascular diseases during pregnancy. European Heart Journal. 2011;**32**:3147-3197

[37] Shoulderdystocia. Guideline of the DGGG,OEGGG and SGG G (S2k-Level, AWMF Registry No. 015/098, October 2024). pp. 39-41; 59-71. Available from: http://register.awmf.org/de/leitlinien/detail/015-098

[38] Knight M, Bunch K, Patel R, Shakespeare J, Kotnis R, Kenyon S, Kurinczuk JJ. Saving lives, improving mothers' care core report—Lessons learned to inform the future. 2022

[39] Scholz T, Schedlbauer A, Reissig D, Schuster T. Emergency training in the delivery room. The Gynaecologist. 2016;**49**(8):623-627. DOI: 10.1007/s00129-016-3924-z

Chapter 5

Solutions for Insufficient Epidural Analgesia for Planned Vaginal Birth

Lukas Hartmann and Mark Ulrich Gerbershagen

Abstract

Background: Epidural analgesia (EDA) plays an important role in the pain relief and comfort of women during childbirth. Despite its benefits, in some cases, epidural analgesia can fail, or no adequate alternative can be offered if there are contraindications. There is currently no standardized solution for this situation, and it is not uncommon for women in labor to be left alone in this situation. A clear recommendation for an alternative to neuroaxial options for vaginal birth is needed to achieve the goal of alleviating pain, promoting a positive birth experience and avoiding postpartum problems. Based on the literature, this chapter provides a good solution to the problem of inadequate epidural analgesia or contraindications to epidural analgesia.

Keywords: epidural analgesia, pain relief, vaginal birth, inadequate analgesia, failed epidural, alternative pain management, analgesia in labor

1. Introduction

Analgesia during childbirth, particularly epidural analgesia, plays a crucial role in relieving pain and comfort for expectant mothers during the birth process. The importance of this pain relief option lies not only in reducing the sensation of pain but also in promoting a positive birth experience and improving the health of mother and child. Choosing an analgesic method such as epidural analgesia can help to reduce the physical and emotional stress during labor. This allows the expectant mother to relax better, which in turn can make the labor process easier. In addition, effective pain relief can reduce oxygen consumption and catecholamine levels, which is beneficial for both the mother and the newborn. Increased catecholamine levels can lead to hyperglycemia, as well as increased release of fatty acids and increased lactate levels, which can cause acidosis in the mother but also in the fetus. In view of the possibilities of ensuring effective analgesia, the responsibility lies solely with medical care [1].

However, there are situations where the epidural analgesia does not work as expected or cannot be recommended. In such cases, it is important to be able to offer alternative methods of pain relief to support the expectant mother's needs during labor. One option is, of course, reattachment or combined spinal-epidural anesthesia (CSE); however, there are numerous situations where even this is not possible. Technical problems or complications can occur during the first attempt to place the epidural analgesia, which can make re-placement difficult or problematic. This can be caused, for example, by anatomical features of the spine. In some cases, the time between the first attempt and the need for a repeat epidural analgesia may be too short, as the birth may already be too far advanced. Also, after an unsuccessful first attempt, a second attempt may be rejected by the mother and alternative pain relief may be desired. The safe use of neuroaxial analgesia requires developed units with sufficient resources and experienced staff, which are not available in large parts of the world, especially in developing countries [2, 3].

The importance of having a backup option if the epidural anesthesia does not work as planned is to ensure the woman's comfort during the birth process. It is crucial that the medical team is well prepared and agrees on the procedure to be able to react to unexpected situations and offer suitable alternatives. The aim is to alleviate pain and make the birth as comfortable as possible to promote a positive birth experience and support the health of mother and child throughout the birth process. A painful birth can result in postpartum depression or even post-traumatic stress disorder. Careful planning, communication and a willingness to offer a range of options will ensure that the expectant mother's needs are best met during this momentous event. Today's medicine has the means to help in this situation. However, it requires accurate communication and assessment of the right measures. This chapter describes epidural anesthesia and aims to facilitate the choice of alternative options when neuroaxial options fail [4].

2. Epidural analgesia (EDA)

The advantage of neural techniques is that the woman in labor continues to feel contractions and can therefore actively participate in the birth. In epidural analgesia, a local anesthetic with an opioid is injected into the epidural space. The substances gradually diffuse through the dura mater into the subarachnoid space, where they act primarily on the spinal nerve roots and, to a lesser extent, on the spinal cord and paravertebral nerves. Successful epidural analgesia leads to a segmental blockade of the sympathetic and sensory nerves and a decrease in endogenous catecholamine release with the onset of pain relief. Hypotension, or normalization of blood pressure to pre-birth levels, may result from vasodilation resulting from the blockade of the sympathetic nervous system and a decrease in circulating catecholamines [5].

2.1 Indications for an epidural analgesia

The epidural anesthesia offers the woman in labor the possibility of pain relief during birth and is also used for this purpose. It also offers the possibility of longer-term pain relief. The most common indication is therefore the expectant mother's wish. However, there are also maternal illnesses that represent an indication. These are diseases in which pain-related stress causes an intolerable increase in oxygen demand. This can occur in the context of certain heart and lung diseases. Twin deliveries or breech presentation can also be medical indications [4].

2.2 Complications of epidural analgesia

An unnoticed puncture of the dura mater can lead to headaches later on. This is often due to a lack of technique or experience. If an spinal puncture is suspected, fluid can be aspirated *via* the needle. There are various tests for the detection of cerebrospinal fluid. If the aspirated fluid streaks in the syringe filled with saline solution, it is most likely cerebrospinal fluid. If the aspirated fluid is warm, it is probably cerebrospinal fluid. If it is cold, it was injected only a short time ago. A drop on the back of the hand in the glove can already give an indication of the temperature. Testing for glucose using test strips can detect cerebrospinal fluid here.

The physiological blockade of the preganglionic sympathetic fibers can lead to hypotension [2, 3]. These hypotensions occur particularly in cases of unrecognized or untreated hypovolemia. The extent and frequency of hypotension are directly related to the circulating blood volume [6]. Late complications that can occur with epidural analgesia occur hours to days after the procedure. These include bladder dysfunction, headaches or neurological complications up to paraplegic symptoms. Spinal-peridural hematoma, which occurs in patients undergoing anticoagulant therapy or with undetected coagulation disorders, is also a feared complication of epidural analgesia. Neuralgia-like pain in the back, as well as sensory deficits and motor disorders up to a feeling of weakness or paralysis in the legs, which occur within 16 hours, are indications of a spinal-peridural hematoma. In this case, immediate surgical intervention is required to avoid consequential damage. Another complication is cauda equina syndrome. This involves damage to spinal cord fibers from L4 to S3 at the level of the cauda equina, which also results in a paraplegic syndrome. Inflammatory changes such as purulent meningitis or a peridural abscess are also late complications [2, 3].

2.3 Challenges of an epidural analgesia

Absolute contraindications for an epidural analgesia are, of course, refusal by the patient, blood clotting disorders, increased intracranial pressure, infection in the puncture area, septic events and various forms of shock. As the cooperation of the patient is necessary for epidural anesthesia, patients who have allowed themselves to be coerced into this method against their wishes are difficult to manage or are non-compliant. Patients with a tendency to bleed who are being treated with heparin, phenprocoumon, warfarin or combined antiplatelet therapy must not receive an epidural catheter, as there is a risk of bleeding with compression of the spinal cord. Complications include infections, allergic reactions, bleeding, hypotension and bladder emptying disorders. The latter are caused by sympathicolysis. Perforation of the dura mater can lead to post-puncture headache and, in worse cases, to a high level of spinal anesthesia due to ascending analgesics [7]. With an incidence of 10%, catheter malpositions or malfunctions occur, which include disconnections or catheter occlusions and result in the removal of the catheter. Intravascular and intrathecal malpositions occur much less frequently [8].

2.4 Risk factors

Risk factors for an unsuccessful epidural analgesia can be divided into patient-related and procedure-related risk factors. Patient-related factors include obesity. Women with a BMI over 30 kg/m^2 should adopt the sitting position for the epidural analgesia placement. The position of the fetal head also influences the success rate of epidural analgesia. The risk of insufficient epidural analgesia is higher the further away the head is from the ischial spine [9]. Two studies have shown a correlation between the use of oxytocin drops during labor and an increased risk of a failed epidural analgesia [9, 10]. According to the literature, procedural risk factors include a lack of anesthesiology experience [9, 10]. Catheter migration is also a known risk factor for inadequate epidural analgesia. However, the risk is lower if the catheter is inserted 5–6 cm into the epidural space [11].

2.5 Definition of failed epidural analgesia

It is important that a definition is concise and easy to use and that staff are familiar with the pain scale used. The VAS score is a simple and well-known tool that midwives, anesthesiologists and obstetricians are familiar with. Bucstain et al. define failed epidural analgesia as a VAS score ≥ 5 at 30 minutes after insertion of the epidural catheter. Sisman recommends using the Bucstain et al. definition as it allows time to assess the effect of the epidural block [9, 12].

3. Alternative procedures to epidural analgesia

3.1 Spinal anesthesia

Neuroaxial procedures are among the most effective methods of relieving labor pain. Especially in the late stages of vaginal birth, unpredictable moments, instrumental or special gynecological actions require fast and sufficient analgesia. This refers to situations with sudden, often unexpected and particularly pronounced pain intensity. This is where the advantages of spinal analgesia over the gold standard of obstetric epidural anesthesia can dominate. Spinal analgesia is characterized by a rapid onset of pain relief, a profound blockade and less technical feasibility and, like other neuroaxial procedures, is comparatively uncomplicated in pregnant women. There is no possibility of repetition without a new puncture, so the limited duration of effect is a significant disadvantage. Combined spinal and epidural anesthesia offers a solution to the latter [13].

In contrast to peridural analgesia, the local anesthetic is applied lumbarly in the subarachnoid space, the spinal canal, in spinal anesthesia. This directly blocks nerve conduction and creates a reversible sensory, motor and sympathetic blockade. The blockade of the sympathetic fibers often results in a sympathetic blockade and an undesired drop in blood pressure in various forms. In rarer cases, bradycardia/asystole, total spinal anesthesia, post-spinal headaches, hearing loss, spinal hematomas and nerve damage may occur. A systemic toxic effect triggered by the local anesthetic is generally not to be expected. While the epidural space is accessed during epidural analgesia and the substance is injected into this space in front of the dura mater, the dura mater is punctured during an spinal anesthesia and the local anesthetic is injected into the spinal canal. To ensure that no spinal cord fibers are injured, spinal punctures must not be performed higher than L2/3, but preferably below L3/L4. Below this point, the outlets of the spinal cord, the cauda equina, can be touched with the needle, but this does not usually lead to injury. The subarachnoid space contains about 75 ml of cerebrospinal fluid, while the total volume of cerebrospinal fluid is about 130 ml. The cerebrospinal fluid is a transparent liquid that is continuously produced by the choroid plexuses in the ventricles of the brain. Its specific gravity is about 1003 g/cm^3, which plays an important role in the classification of local anesthetics for spinal anesthesia. There are isobaric local anesthetics, which have a similar weight to the cerebrospinal fluid and therefore remain mainly at the injection site. There are also hyperbaric local anesthetics, which have a greater density than the cerebrospinal fluid and can therefore sink into the subarachnoid space. And there are hypobaric local anesthetics, which have a lower density than cerebrospinal fluid and can therefore rise in the subarachnoid space toward the brain. They are no longer commonly used today. Apart from the property of how the local anesthetic is distributed, the cerebrospinal fluid also has a helpful function. The leakage of cerebrospinal fluid from the needle is a clear indication that the subarachnoid space has been successfully accessed. When the cerebrospinal fluid is aspirated, it draws streaks in the saline solution of the syringe.

The nerve fibers are blocked in a specific sequence. The autonomic preganglionic fibers are the first to be affected, which is noticeable by a warming of the skin due to dilatation of the blood vessels. Next, the temperature fibers are blocked, which is why the sensation of cold is eliminated earlier than the sensation of heat. In the further course, fibers are blocked, which now transfer intense pain as needlesticks. The sensation of touch and depth sensitivity is only now switched off and finally the motor function, vibrations and the sensation of position are blocked. In addition to the specific temporal sequence, there is also a spatial sequence of propagation. Looking at the spinal column, the sympathetic blockade is the highest. The sensory blockade takes place two to four segments deeper and the motor deactivation another two segments deeper. There is also a sequence when the effect subsides. The motor functions return first and autonomic functions last, which is why there is a risk of a drop in blood pressure until the end of the spinal anesthesia. The effect is reversed as the local anesthetics are transported away *via* capillaries and lymph. Depending on the type of local anesthetic, degradation takes place in the plasma (amino esters) or in the liver (aminoamides) but not in the subarachnoid space. The following local anesthetics are used for spinal anesthesia, sorted according to their spreading properties and effectiveness. Bupivacaine, levobupivacaine 0.5%, as hyperbaric or isobaric, and ropivacaine 0.5% have a longer duration of action of 160 minutes. Prilocaine 1% isobaric or 2% hyperbaric has a shorter duration of action of 60–120 minutes. Chloroprocaine 1% also has a shorter duration of action of 80–100 minutes. Absolute contraindications are refusal by the patient, blood clotting disorders or anticoagulant therapy, neurological diseases with increased intracranial pressure, sepsis, shock and specific cardiovascular diseases, such as congenital or acquired heart defects [2, 3].

3.2 Combined spinal and epidural analgesia (CSE)

Combined spinal-epidural analgesia combines an initial subarachnoid injection with opioids and a local anesthetic and the placement of an epidural catheter in the epidural space. Spinal analgesia allows a quick onset of action and a lower dose can be used as the catheter provides a safety margin if the dose is too low. It also offers greater hemodynamic stability and less likelihood of motor blockade. Confirmation by a spinal component ensures the correct position of the needle, which also increases the success rate of the epidural catheter [14].

3.3 Intravenous or intramuscular analgesia

Opioids are suitable for intravenous and intramuscular analgesia, but all have similar, dose-dependent, relevant side effects. In addition to nausea, vomiting and sedation, respiratory depression in both mother and child is a feared complication. Possible substances are pethidine, fentanyl and remifentanil as PCA.

3.3.1 Pethidine

Pethidine has long been used in obstetrics as an intramuscular injection. It is an agonist for the μ1 and μ2 receptors in the central nervous system and has approximately 0.125 times the potency of morphine. However, pethidine is metabolized into the active norpethidine, which is only eliminated very slowly and can trigger epileptic convulsions due to its high neurotoxicity. Its half-life in the newborn is also 18–23 hours. The analgesic effect of alternative agents is significantly more potent, and the side effects of nausea and vomiting, as well as the effects on the newborn, make it necessary to seek alternative treatments [15]. Although it is no longer used in postoperative care and traumatology, it was still the most commonly used opioid for labor in Norway in 2009, with 77% [16]. However, this has changed considerably in the last 10 years. It is now only indicated if there are contraindications for epidural analgesia. Problems include the difficulty of control, the widely varying intensity of pain during labor, placental patency and the associated reduced cardiac activity, reduced fetal movement and risk of respiratory depression [17]. None of the studies reviewed here provide a rationale for the use of pethidine either. Pethidine is less analgesic than remifentanil [18]. Pethidine causes more nausea than remifentanil and has more side effects than remifentanil [19]. Overall, taking into account the German S1 guideline, there is therefore no reason to use pethidine when remifentanil is available. It can therefore be definitively stated that pethidine is not a first-choice alternative in cases of insufficient EDA or contraindications to EDA [20].

3.3.2 Remifentanil

In the search for an opiod for the combination of total intravenous anesthesia (TIVA) with propofol, remifentanil came onto the market in the United States in 1991. Remifentanil offers a decisive advantage over other opioids. Due to the propionic acid methyl ester side chain, it allows access for esterases. Non-specific esterases thus ensure rapid metabolization and provide the decisive advantage of a very short half-life. The remifentanilic acid GR90291 produced by cleavage of the side chain is 1000 times less effective and is excreted *via* the kidneys. The short half-life ensures good controllability. For this reason, remifentanil is used in a PCA pump (patient-controlled analgesia). An overdose should be avoided. This is possible with the correct pump setting. During the period of use, there may be a greater decrease in effect than with other opioids. It should also be used *via* an additional intravenous access used solely for PCA. Potential sources of error here are incorrect programming of the PCA pump, too rapid application or incorrect concentration, which can quickly lead to respiratory depression. For this reason, continuous monitoring of oxygen saturation, the possibility of oxygen administration and ventilation and permanent supervision by a midwife are prerequisites for use. Compared to pethidine, remifentanil offers better analgesia and fewer effects on the newborn. The analgesic effect is comparable to fentanyl, but less than an epidural analgesia. It offers a good alternative to pethidine. Due to the high requirements, such as intensive 1-to-1 care by a midwife, it is mainly used when there are contraindications to other variants [15, 21]. The advantages of remifentanil are clear. Although it provides similar pain relief to fentanyl, it is easily controllable due to its short half-life and long-term side effects on the mother or child are significantly less common. Even after administration over 10 hours, the context-sensitive half-life is 3–4 minutes. However, even with remifentanil, a bolus of 1.5 μg/kg bodyweight results in respiratory depression of up to 10 minutes in newborns, which is why the number of ventilations after birth with remifentanil should not be neglected. A study by Marwah et al. mentions a rate of 25% of newborns who had to be ventilated after birth. Another study by Wilson et al. says 10% of newborns required reanimation. Both figures should be viewed with caution, as the term resuscitation is not defined in Wilson's study. In Marwah's study, 25% of the newborns had to be ventilated, but there was no resuscitation. From this, one could conclude that the 10% resuscitations in Wilson's study were also ventilation. Even the term ventilation is ambiguous. In the European Resuscitation Council 2021 Newborn Resuscitation Guidelines of June 2, 2021, one reads of 5% of newborns who need ventilation and 1% who need extensive intubation. A distinction is made here between mask ventilation and intubation. Less than 0.3% require cardiac resuscitation. Various prepartum and intrapartum factors are given as reasons for ventilation and resuscitation in these guidelines; drug analgesia during childbirth is not mentioned here as a possible factor [22]. It can be assumed that 5% of newborns need to be ventilated. As opioids have an effect on breathing, resuscitation probably refers to purely pulmonary resuscitation. In addition, clearing the airway or mask-assisted ventilation is often sufficient in a resuscitation case, as bradycardia in newborns is usually a sign of hypoventilation [23–25]. This means that remifentanil has a respiratory depressant effect, but this is less pronounced if the true starting level is taken. And that is even in uncomplicated births, without opioids, ventilation of the newborn is required in 5% of cases. The advantage of remifentanil is clearly its effective analgesic effect, which is greater than that of pethidine and also superior to that of nitrous oxide. The analgesic effect is not the same as with epidural analgesia in terms of analgesic effect, but it is quite comparable [26–28]. Remifentanil causes less sedation and allows focus and concentration on the birth process [28]. Remifentanil also has a lower risk of intrapartum maternal fever compared to epidural [27]. Disadvantages are a higher respiratory depression compared to epidural analgesia. Respiratory monitoring and oxygen supply options are essential. An anesthetist is also required for induction and the initial titration phase. However, this is also necessary for an epidural. Close monitoring and the presence of trained medical professionals are required throughout the application [27, 29–31]. The advantage over nitrous oxide is that remifentanil is easily available, and patients can control their own requirements to a certain extent *via* PCA using intravenous access.

3.3.3 Fentanyl

Fentanyl is a highly lipid-soluble and protein-bound synthetic opioid, chemically belongs to the anilinoperidines and was synthesized in 1959. With an analgesic potency 100 times higher than that of morphine, the potency is 800 times higher than that of pethidine. The time to reach the maximum effect of fentanyl is 3–4 minutes after iv. administration. It has a shorter half-life than pethidine, but after repeated administration the context-sensitive half-life increases. Several studies have shown that intravenously administered fentanyl is superior to pethidine in the treatment of labor pain, but it may have a dose-dependent adverse effect on infant feeding after birth. In one study, 37% of newborns required the use of the antagonist naloxone after PCA with fentanyl [32, 33]. The literature research also comes to the conclusion that the analgesic effect of fentanyl is comparable to that of remifentanil. However, significantly more newborns had to be ventilated under fentanyl [24]. Other adverse effects such as nausea, vomiting and sedation were also more frequent with fentanyl. These clear disadvantages and the fact that overall there is little evidence on the use of fentanyl in obstetrics speak clearly against fentanyl. The consideration of the German S1 guideline, which favors remifentanyl over fentanyl, also clearly speaks against fentanyl. The use of fentanyl as a first-choice alternative to spinal procedures in obstetrics cannot be recommended [20].

3.4 Nitrous oxide

Nitrous oxide with the molecular formula N_2O, which has a long history in anesthesia, has lost much of its popularity in the last 15 years. It is still used in pediatric anesthesia. In the United Kingdom, Australia and Scandinavia, nitrous oxide has a long tradition as an analgesic in obstetrics. It has the undesirable side effect of nausea and vomiting but has the advantage that when mixed with oxygen, the woman giving birth can inhale it herself relatively safely. Gas mixtures of 50–70% nitrous oxide with 50–30% oxygen are produced, which do not switch off the protective reflexes. Prolonged exposure to nitrous oxide is potentially harmful, but brief use, such as during childbirth, is safe for mother, child and medical personnel [15]. Nitrous oxide provides a similar level of pain relief as paracervical blockade and opioids but does not have the side effects on the newborn that occur with injected opioids. Although mothers report that nitrous oxide is less effective than epidural analgesia, women who have used nitrous oxide report a similar level of satisfaction compared to those who have had an epidural analgesia and would use nitrous oxide again if offered in future pregnancies. Nitrous oxide is easy to administer, inexpensive, does not interfere with uterine contractions, and has no adverse effects on normal physiology and labor progression. Because of its poor tissue solubility, it does not diffuse into the tissues and quickly floods. Therefore, pain relief with nitrous oxide begins within one minute, which is less time than the onset of pain relief with epidural analgesia. It is also less invasive than a peridural anesthetic or opioid injection. By choosing when to put on and take off the mask, the patient can control the level of pain relief. This can increase the feeling of control and reduce the perception of pain. In contrast to epidural analgesia, nitrous oxide allows motor function and freedom of movement to be maintained. It can also induce a feeling of pleasure, relaxation and anxiety relief, so that the woman giving birth is not so worried about her pain. It also requires the birthing woman to concentrate on breathing when using nitrous oxide, which may explain some of the positive effects.

The main disadvantage of nitrous oxide is that it is less effective than other forms of pain management, including neuroaxial analgesia. It also requires repeated self-dosing, so the mask must be held over the face to ensure effective pain management. This could be cumbersome for the birthing woman who is exhausted or tired and does not want to hold the mask. Reported side effects of nitrous oxide include excessive drowsiness (0–24%), nausea (5–36%), vomiting (15%), lightheadedness or dizziness (6–23%), a feeling of detachment and claustrophobia from the mask. Nitrous oxide is also a very potent greenhouse gas and its use is therefore not climate-friendly [34]. Nitrous oxide, a colorless gas with a slightly sweet smell, can be safely ingested when mixed with oxygen. Mixtures with 50% are considered safe, but a mixture ratio of 70% nitrous oxide can also be used without any evidence of unfavorable effects on the newborn. Prolonged exposure to nitrous oxide for more than 15 minutes can lead to neonatal depression [23]. Nitrous oxide is easy to administer, inexpensive, does not interfere with uterine contractions, and has no adverse effects on normal physiology and progression of labor or oxytocin levels [23]. Nitrous oxide has been shown not to be as potent in analgesia as the epidural analgesia, but roughly comparable to pethidine [26, 35]. Consequently, nitrous oxide is less analgesic than remifentanil. Nevertheless, maternal satisfaction with the pain relief of nitrous oxide is seen as positive [36, 37]. Chantrasiri and Sheyklo were unable to demonstrate any effects of nitrous oxide on the newborn [26, 36]. The perception of pain relief correlates more strongly with the euphoric effect and less with the actual analgesic effect of the substance. Agah et al. further describe that the euphoric and anxiolytic effect is caused by an increased release of endogenous opioids [38, 39]. The overall experience with nitrous oxide is rated as positive and 68% of women would choose it again [26, 37, 40]. The side effects described are dizziness, nausea, dry throat, vomiting and drowsiness. However, 65% also state that they have had no side effects [40]. Overall, nitrous oxide leads to a positive birth experience. It meets the needs of those giving birth and leads to satisfaction, even if the pain relief is less severe. The ability to put the mask on and take it off yourself leads to a feeling of self-determination and ensures that the option of continuing to hold the mask in front of the face is lost during sedation. Nitrous oxide is less invasive than remifentanil. The focus on breathing during nitrous oxide intake has a positive effect on individual birth control. However, nitrous oxide is a powerful greenhouse gas. When used in the delivery room, it is inexorably released into the room air. Exposure of staff, other people in the room and the environment must be taken into account. Gas extraction and ventilation should be provided in the room [34].

4. Discussion

The epidural analgesia is an effective and convincing method of providing adequate pain relief for women giving birth during spontaneous vaginal birth. Why do we need another option for peripartum analgesia?

In the United States, around 60% of pregnant women receive an epidural for labor analgesia. In the United Kingdom, only 30% of pregnant women receive an epidural for labor analgesia. In Germany, it was only 24% in 2014 [19, 41]. This shows that even in countries where the healthcare system can provide the resources, not all women can or want to recourse to epidural analgesia. In addition, there are numerous contraindications and other reasons why epidural analgesia is not used and a less invasive alternative is desired. Unfortunately, the number of studies is not sufficient to make a clear statement that can be transferred to the majority of pregnant women. Also, some studies do not have the desired evidence and have very different numbers of cases. With different study designs, different methods and very different numbers of cases, it is not easy to compare the findings of the various studies. Nevertheless, this chapter attempts to list the core statements on individual drugs and to put their significance into context. The main factors investigated were the strength of analgesia, patient satisfaction, the safety of the method used and ultimately, the associated adverse effects [42]. The chapter shows that the opioids pethidine and fentanyl have become less important for the analgesia of vaginal delivery over the last 12 years. In the S1 guideline of the German Society for Anesthesia and Intensive Care Medicine from 2020, a total of 653 experts were asked for their opinions on opioid administration. The participants voted overwhelmingly in favor of remifentanil PCA over other opioids for obstetric analgesia [20]. The following section explains further why pethidine and fentanyl are not considered as alternatives to epidural analgesia.

5. Conclusion

When it comes to relieving labor pain, the epidural analgesia is the first choice worldwide. Direct blockade of the transmission of the pain stimulus is the most effective form of analgesia [1]. If the epidural analgesia does not have the desired effect, it must first be defined what an insufficient effect looks like. The exact definition of failure is unclear. Some define it as a need for general anesthesia, and others say it is when other analgesia medication is necessary. The definition by Bucstain et al., which defines failed EDA as a VAS score ≥ 5 after 30 minutes is clear and easy to implement [9, 43]. In the absence of analgesia 30 minutes after the initial administration, the peridural catheter should be reinserted, or a CSE should be performed directly. In the event of breakthrough pain occurring after a period of 30 minutes during which pain relief has been observed, the administration of an injection into the catheter is indicated. In the event of a further failure after a further 30 minutes, CSE is indicated [43]. Primary options for an insufficient epidural analgesia are available, but limited. It may quickly become impossible to perform another puncture, or it may no longer be desired. As described above, pethidine and fentanyl, although used for this purpose in the past, do not offer a suitable alternative. The most potent analgesia after neuraxial procedures is provided by remifentanil in the form of PCA. However, the use of nitrous oxide prevails in almost all other respects. In terms of pain relief, nitrous oxide is less analgesic but very satisfactory overall. It is easy for patients to administer themselves and does not necessarily require the presence of a doctor. A high level of care by trained specialist staff such as a midwife or physician assistant is sufficient. The side effect profile is not close to zero, but it is low and the side effects are less risky, such as respiratory depression with fentanyl. The application is less invasive. In some of the studies examined, no serious effects on the newborn were observed and the APGAR values are no worse than with other forms of analgesia [26, 36]. However, nitrous oxide can potentiate the respiratory depressant effects of other drugs such as opioids. The idea of whether remifentanil can be used if the effect of nitrous oxide is insufficient has not yet been investigated [44]. There is also evidence of neurotoxicity with nitrous oxide exposure [45]. The data for the previous statements on safety for mother and child are not large enough to be able to reliably assess risks. Even if all previous findings speak in favor of the use of nitrous oxide and nitrous oxide has performed very well in the past and continues to do so in dentistry, it cannot be readily recommended in the specific situation of obstetrics. This approach needs to be investigated further. The impact on staff, which has not been sufficiently investigated, and the harmful effect on the climate are also arguments against the use of nitrous oxide (**Figure 1**).

	Remifentanil	Nitrous oxide
Pain relief	+	-
side effects	-	+
satisfaction	?	+
application	-	+
Doctor necessary	-	+
Newborn UAWs	-	+
Environment/environment	+	-

Figure 1.
Distribution of points. Which therapy is more convincing in which category. The table shows the advantages of the individual medications. + stands for the advantage in the corresponding category. - stands for disadvantage.? stands for no data.

If an effective analgesic option for an epidural analgesia is sought, only remifentanil PCA can be recommended so far. Remifentanil has a proven analgesic effect. The analgesic effect is comparable to that of EDA [27]. Although the side effect profile of remifentanil is more severe than that of nitrous oxide, it has been sufficiently studied and the effects are understood and can be treated. It can be safely assumed that remifentanil is broken down in the maternal and fetal body after 10 minutes and it has no long-term effects on the newborn [23, 24]. However, one must assume an increased number of ventilations in newborns from 5% to >10%. Unfortunately, the data on this is not valid enough. More research is needed here [18, 24]. Although the application is more extensive and invasive than that of nitrous oxide, it effectively fulfills its purpose and provides effective pain relief during childbirth. In order to further investigate and improve the use of remifentanil PCA during childbirth and to revise dosing regimes, the RemiPCA SAFE Network was established in 2008 as a private

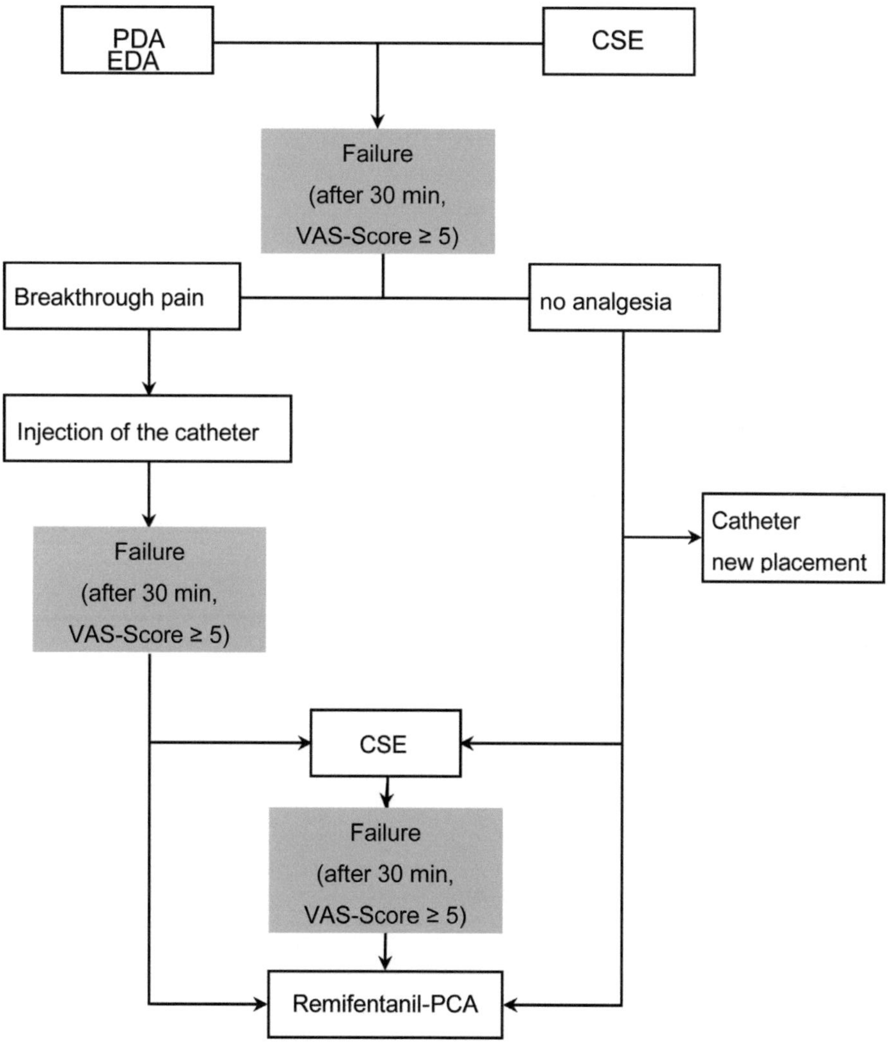

Figure 2.
Algorithm for failure of the epidural analgesia during vaginal birth. Modified algorithm by [43].

initiative. It serves as a register to document applications, improve processes and for quality assurance. By December 31, 2023, 13,933 applications had been registered. This can help with implementation. The following diagram, based on Guasch 2017, shows the steps of first choice for analgesia in vaginal birth (**Figure 2**).

If pain of at least five on the visual analog scale is registered 30 minutes after placement of the epidural analgesia or CSE catheter, the epidural analgesia or CSE is considered insufficient. The reasons may be breakthrough pain, previous pain relief or no analgesia from the outset. Breakthrough pain is primarily treated by injecting the catheter. If no analgesia has been achieved so far, a new catheter is indicated or, in the case of a previous EDA, a CSE. The direct step to remifentanil PCA should also be considered. If there is still no adequate analgesia 30 minutes after the catheter has been injected in the event of breakthrough pain, CSE is indicated. It may also be necessary to switch directly to RPCA. If the CSE is also insufficient, the PCA pump with remifentanil should be selected at this point at the latest. In order to avoid the worst-case scenario of having to assess the efficacy three times for 30 minutes, the use of remifentanil PCA should be considered sooner. The additional use of nitrous oxide for labor analgesia, for example, should be considered with caution, as interactions between nitrous oxide and remifentanil have not yet been adequately investigated [43, 44].

Author details

Lukas Hartmann* and Mark Ulrich Gerbershagen
Hospital Cologne-Holweide, Germany

*Address all correspondence to: hartmann517@web.de

References

[1] Kranke P, Greve S. Anästhesie und Analgesie in der Geburtshilfe. Die Geburtshilfe: Springer Berlin Heidelberg Verlag; 2023

[2] Larsen R. Periduralanästhesie. Anästhesie und Intensivmedizin für die Fachpflege. German. 2016a:218-231. Available from: https://www.lehmanns.de/shop/medizin-pharmazie/37355560-9783662504444-anaesthesie-und-intensivmedizin-fuer-die-fachpflege. DOI: 10.1007/978-3-662-50444-4_14

[3] Larsen R. Spinalanästhesie. Anästhesie und Intensivmedizin für die Fachpflege. 2016b:197-217. German. DOI: 10.1007/978-3-662-50444-4_13

[4] Stefan J, Ortner C, Klein UK. Schmerztherapie während der Geburt. Wien (Vienna): Springer-Verlag Wien; 2017

[5] Hawkins JL. Epidural analgesia for labor and delivery. The New England Journal of Medicine. 2010;**326**(16):1503-1510

[6] Ahnefeld FW, Bergmann H, Burri C, Dick W, Halmágyi M, Hossli G, et al. Lokalanästhesie. Berlin Heidelberg: Springer-Verlang; 1978

[7] Giesler AC. Beurteilung der Aufklärungsqualität einer mediengestützten Aufklärung für die Periduralanalgesie in der Geburtshilfe: Vergleich zwischen einer textorientierten Aufklärung (Flyer) vs. Videoaufklärung. Inaugural-Dissertation. Kiel; 2021

[8] Kessler P. Update rückenmarknahe Regionalanästhesie – weniger Nutzen, mehr Gefahren? 2010. Available from: www.ai-online.info

[9] Bucstain C, Garmi G, Zafran N. Risk factors and peripartum outcomes of failed epidural: A prospective cohort study. Archives of Gynecology and Obstetrics. May 2017;**295**(5): 1119-1125

[10] Agaram R, Douglas MJ, McTaggart RA. Inadequate pain relief with labor epidurals: A multivariate analysis of associated factors. International Journal of Obstetric Anesthesia. Jan 2009;**18**(1):10-4

[11] Hess PE, Pratt SD, Lucas TP. Predictors of Breakthrough Pain during Labor Epidural Analgesia. Boston: Anesth Analog; 2001

[12] Sisman Y, Ekelund K, Strandbygaard J. Failed epidural analgesia during birth. Ugeskrift for Laeger. 2019;**181**(16):V09180650

[13] Töpel L, Wenk M. Spinalanalgesie—Clever nutzen zur vaginalen Geburt [Spinal analgesia—cleverly used for vaginal delivery]. Anasthesiol Intensivmed Notfallmed Schmerzther. Thieme. 2021;**56**(3):210-218. DOI: 10.1055/a-1101-8522. Epub 2021 Mar 16. German

[14] Bajwa SJS, Kulshrestha A. Anaesthesia for laparoscopic surgery: General vs regional anaesthesia. Journal of Minimal Access Surgery. 2016;**12**(1):4-9. DOI: 10.4103/0972-9941.169952

[15] Girard T, Engmann C. Modernes peripartales Schmerzmanagement. PDA oder kurz wirksame Opiate? Gynäkologie. 2012;**2**:24-29

[16] Kranke P, Girard T, Lavand'homme, P., et al. Must we press on until a young mother dies? Remifentanil patient

controlled analgesia in labour may not be suited as a "poor man's epidural". BMC Pregnancy and Childbirth. 2013;**13**:139. DOI: 10.1186/1471-2393-13-139

[17] Ohnesorg H. Systemische Analgesie mit Opioiden zur vaginalen Entbindung. Referenz Geburtshilfe und Perinatalmedizin: Georg Thieme Verlag KG; 2022

[18] Wilson M, MacArthur C, Gao Smith F, Homer L, Handley K, Daniels J. The RESPITE trial: Remifentanil intravenously administered patient-controlled analgesia (PCA) versus pethidine intramuscular injection for pain relief in labour: Study protocol for a randomised controlled trial. European Journal of Anaesthesiology. Elsevier Ltd; 2012;**29**(4):177-185. DOI: 10.1016/S0140-6736(18)31613-1

[19] Mora A. Hilfestellungen für Gebärende mit PDA. Die Hebamme: Georg Thieme Verlag KG; 2014

[20] Bremerich D, Annecke T, Chappell D, Hanß R, Kaufner L, Kehl F, et al. S1-Leitlinie: Die geburtshilfliche Analgesie und Anästhesie. Anästh Intensivmed. 2020;**61**:S300-S339. DOI: 10.19224/ai2020.S300

[21] Bushuven S, Kreuer S, Kranke P. Remifentanil Up2date - Part 1. Anästhesiologie Intensivmedizin Notfallmedizin Schmerztherapie. 2017;**52**:543-553

[22] Madar J, Roehr CC, Ainsworth S, Ersda H, Morley C, Rüdiger M, et al. Versorgung und reanimation des Neugeborenen nach der Geburt: Leitlinien des European resuscitation council 2021 [newborn resuscitation and support of transition of infants at birth]. Notf Rett Med. 2021;**24**(4):603-649. DOI: 10.1007/s10049-021-00894-w. German. Epub 2021 Jun 2

[23] Larsen R. Anästhesie. Deutschland: Elsevier Health Sciences; 2022

[24] Marwah R, Hassan S, Carvalho JC, Balki M. Remifentanil versus fentanyl for intravenous patient-controlled labour analgesia: An observational study. Canadian Journal of Anaesthesia. 2012;**59**(3):246-254. DOI: 10.1007/s12630-011-9625-0. Epub 2011 Nov 5

[25] Spieß C. SOPs in Intensivmedizin und Notfallmedizin. Neugeborenen Erstversorgung: Georg Thieme Verlag Stuttgart; 2013. DOI: 10.1055/b-002-57162

[26] Chantrasiri R, Wanapirak C, Tongsong T. Entonox® versus pethidine in labor pain relief: A randomized controlled trial. International Journal of Environmental Research and Public Health. 2021;**18**(23):12571. DOI: 10.3390/ijerph182312571

[27] Lei X, Yu Y, Li M, Fang P, Gan S, Yao Y, et al. The efficacy and safety of remifentanil patient-controlled versus epidural analgesia in labor: A meta-analysis and systematic review. PLoS One. 2022;**17**(12):e0275716. DOI: 10.1371/journal.pone.0275716

[28] Moran VH, Thomson G, Cook J, et al. Qualitative exploration of women's experiences of intramuscular pethidine or remifentanil patient-controlled analgesia for labour pain. BMJ Open. 2019;**9**:e032203. DOI: 10.1136/bmjopen-2019-032203

[29] Karadjova D, Shosholcheva M, Ivanov E, Sivevski A, Kjaev I, Kartalov A, et al. Side effects of intravenous patient-controlled analgesia with remifentanil compared with intermittent epidural bolus for labour analgesia—A randomized controlled trial. Prilozi. 2019;**40**(3):99-108

[30] Logtenberg SLM, Vink ML, Godfried MB, Beenakkers ICM, Schellevis FG, Mol BW, et al. Serious adverse events attributed to remifentanil patient-controlled analgesia during labour in the Netherlands. International Journal of Obstetric Anesthesia. Elsevier Ltd; Aug 2019;**39**:22-28. DOI: 10.1016/j.ijoa.2018.10.013

[31] Schnabel A, Hahn N, Muellenbach R, Frambach T, Hoenig A, Roewer N, et al. Geburtshilfliche Analgesie in deutschen Kliniken. Remifentanil als Alternative zur Regionalanalgesie. Anaesthesist. 2011;**60**(11):995-1001. DOI: 10.1007/s00101-011-1933-9. German. Epub 2011 Sep 16

[32] Evron S, Ezri T. Options for systemic labor analgesia. Current Opinion in Anaesthesiology. 2007;**20**:181-185

[33] Schäfer M, Zöllner C. Opioide in der Anästhesiologie. In: Rossaint R, Werner C, Zwißler B, editors. Die Anästhesiologie. Berlin: Springer; 2019. pp. 291-314

[34] Vallejo MC, Zakowski MI. Pro-con debate: Nitrous oxide for labor analgesia. BioMed Research International. 2019;**2019**(2019):4618798. DOI: 10.1155/2019/4618798

[35] Czech I, Fuchs P, Fuchs A, Lorek M, Tobolska-Lorek D, Drosdzol-Cop A, et al. Pharmacological and non-pharmacological methods of labour pain relief-establishment of effectiveness and comparison. International Journal of Environmental Research and Public Health. 2018;**15**(12):2792. DOI: 10.3390/ijerph15122792

[36] Sheyklo SG, Hajebrahimi S, Moosavi A, Pournaghi-Azar F, Azami-Aghdash S, Ghojazadeh M. Effect of Entonox for pain management in labor: A systematic review and meta-analysis of randomized controlled trials. Electronic Physician. 2017;**9**(12):6002-6009. DOI: 10.19082/6002

[37] Zanardo V, Volpe F, Parotto M, Giiberti L, Selmin A, Straface G. Nitrous oxide labor analgesia and pain relief memory in breastfeeding women. The Journal of Maternal-Fetal & Neonatal Medicine. 2018;**31**(24):3243-3248. DOI: 10.1080/14767058.2017.1368077

[38] Agah J, Baghani R, Safiabadi Tali SH, Tabarraei Y. Effects of continuous use of Entonox in comparison with intermittent method on obstetric outcomes: A randomized clinical trial. Journal of Pregnancy. Hindawi Publishing Corporation; 2014;**2024**:1-5, Article ID 245907. DOI: 10.1155/2014/245907. Available from: https://pmc.ncbi.nlm.nih.gov/articles/PMC4267458/pdf/JP2014-245907.pdf

[39] Mändle C, Opitz-Kreuter S. Das Hebammenbuch: Lehrbuch der praktischen Geburtshilfe. Stuttgart, Deutschland: Schattauer; 2015

[40] Dammer U, Weiss C, Raabe E, Heimrich J, Koch MC, Winkler M, et al. Introduction of inhaled nitrous oxide and oxygen for pain management during labour—Evaluation of Patients' and Midwives' satisfaction. Geburtshilfe und Frauenheilkunde. 2014;**74**(7):656-660. DOI: 10.1055/s-0034-1368606

[41] Halliday L. Epidural analgesia in labor: A narrative review. International Journal of Gynecology & Obstetrics. Nov 2022;**159**(2):356-364

[42] Marchand K, Oviedo-Joekes E, Guh D. Client satisfaction among participants in a randomized trial comparing oral methadone and injectable diacetylmorphine for long-term opioid-dependency. BMC Health Services Research. 2011;**11**:174

[43] Guasch E, Iannuccelli F, Brogly N, Gilsanz F. Failed epidural for labor: What now? Minerva Anestesiologica. 2017;**83**(11):1207-1213. DOI: 10.23736/S0375-9393.17.12082-1. Epub 2017 Jun 12

[44] Manuel W, Hugo Van A, Dorothee B, Karin Becke, Paul K, Frank L, et al. Deutschen Gesellschaft für Anästhesiologie und Intensivmedizin (DGAI) der Deutschen Gesellschaft für Gynäkologie und Geburtshilfe (DGGG). Einsatz von Lachgas zur Schmerztherapie unter der Geburt. Gemeinsame Stellungnahme. Nuernberg & Berlin; 2014

[45] Zhen Y, Dong Y, Wu X, Xu Z, Lu Y, Zhang Y, et al. Nitrous oxide plus isoflurane induces apoptosis and increases beta-amyloid protein levels. Anesthesiology. Oct 2009;**111**(4):741-52

Section 4

Anesthesia in Dentistry

Chapter 6

Considerations and New Perspectives of Locoregional Anesthesia in Dentistry

Ciprian Ioan Roi, Alexandra Roi and Mircea Riviș

Abstract

The locoregional anesthesia has been administrated in dentistry for more than 100 years, being essential for pain management. Almost every dental procedure requires a temporary sensory loss of hard or soft tissues of the oral cavity. The aim of this chapter is to emphasize the most relevant aspects of locoregional anesthesia in dentistry, specifically related to anesthesia evolution over the decades, clinical anatomy, differences between plexus and peripheric troncular anesthesia techniques, risk patients for local anesthesia administration, complications, trypanophobia, problems in achieving local anesthesia and new perspectives. This complex chapter presents up-to-date information in a clear and concise manner, that can be useful for students, dentists, for oral and maxillofacial surgeons. The detailed knowledge presented in the next pages along with the schematic figures can be used for a better understanding of the local anesthesia and help the practitioner to obtain a complete anesthesia of the territory of interest.

Keywords: dental anesthesia, applied anatomy, anesthesia techniques, accidents and complications, trypanophobia, locoregional anesthesia

1. Introduction

Local anesthesia is essential for pain management in dentistry. Dental treatments can be associated with mechanical, thermal, or chemical stimuli, eliciting a painful response. Such dental treatments may include oral surgery, periodontal, endodontic, prosthetic and restorative treatments. Local anesthesia is used to provide temporary sensory loss to allow for the delivery of dental treatment.

The oral cavity is innervated by branches of the trigeminal nerve. The maxillary and mandibular nerves provide nerve fibers for the maxillary bones, gingiva, dental pulp and periodontal ligaments, ensuring sensory innervation to these structures. It is essential for the practitioner to have knowledge about the clinical anatomy, anesthesia landmarks and the territory of innervation in order to perform dental treatment without pain.

The local anesthesia in dentistry can be delivered topic or by infiltration. The topic anesthesia is used mainly for superficial procedures, before infiltration anesthesia, in children or adults with anxiety. The infiltration can be local or troncular/block anesthesia. The local infiltration is used mainly where the cortical bone is thinner as in the maxillary bone. In the mandible, this technique can be used only anterior to the mental foramen. The troncular anesthesia is used when dental or surgical procedures are indicated on a wider anatomical area or where the cortical bone is thicker, preventing the anesthetic substance from diffusing.

The doctor who is performing the locoregional anesthesia must keep in mind that the anesthetic substance is not an unharmful drug deposited in a lively organism. Each patient must be carefully evaluated prior to local anesthesia administration and establish the accidents and complications that can occur. Patient comorbidities, such as hepatic, renal, or blood diseases among the patient's medication can interfere with the metabolization or excretion of the local anesthetic substances. All these aspects must be taken into account when choosing the type of anesthetic substance, the anesthesia technique and the dosage of the anesthetic. The fundamental principle that should be adhered to is a minimum dose of local anesthetic with maximum results.

Regarding the accidents and complications that can occur during or after the local anesthesia administration, the dentist or the specialist performing the local anesthesia must be aware of the clinical signs and patient symptoms and take emergency measures to reduce the local or general implications and stopping the progression.

2. Brief history

2.1 Before 1840

Since ancient times, mankind tried to resolve one of the biggest problems: tooth pain. The tomb of Hesy-Re, an Egyptian who lived 4600 years ago and was referred to as "the best among those who treat teeth," has the earliest known written record of a dentist [1]. 2250 BC: The cure for tooth cavity discomfort is discovered on a clay tablet from Babylonia. Gum mastic and henbane seed were combined to create the cement that was utilized [2]. The Papyrus of Eber, an Egyptian manuscript, describes dental conditions and several ways to treat oral discomfort as early as 1700 BC. Hippocrates and Aristotle wrote about dentistry later, around the year 500–300 A.C., showing different techniques for anesthesia of dental pain [3]. Most of the anesthesia techniques consisted of natural (herbal) and pharmaceutical methods to mitigate tooth discomfort.

Dental pain was treated with a variety of methods, including herbal medicine, injections, inhalations and the use of chemicals that were eaten, administered topically, prayed for, and anointed saints like St. Appollonia. Before Decius persecuted the Christians, there was a small revolt in Alexandria that resulted in the suffering of several virgin martyrs, including Apollonia. Legend has it that throughout her ordeal, all her teeth were forcibly extracted or smashed. St. Apollonia became the specific intercessor for those with tooth disorders and, naturally, the patron saint of dentists and anyone suffering from toothaches or other dental problems because of the nature of the torment she underwent rather than betray her faith [4].

Greek army surgeon Dioscorides proposed for dental pain a mouthwash made of a concoction of therapeutic ingredients cooked in vinegar, including henbane roots (hyoscyamine), marshmallow, pellitory, nutmeg-flower, plantain, and capers, among other ingredients. He wrote a 5-volume "Materia medica" that included thorough descriptions of 1000 medications with plant, animal and mineral origins [4, 5].

In the Middle Ages, dentistry was not yet acknowledged as a separate profession, thus barbers and blacksmiths frequently provided dental care. Patients endured agonizing agony during extractions and other treatments since dental pain control techniques were still somewhat archaic. Significant progress was made during the Renaissance in a number of disciplines, including dentistry and medicine [6, 7]. Doctors, dentists and patients were able to do almost anything to reduce pain during surgery. Chinese and Indian doctors used marijuana and hashish. In various parts of the world, both opium and alcohol were often used.

Before 1840, patients did not enter terrified in the operating room for oral procedures. Why? Because there is no anesthesia. In his book "We Have Conquered Pain", Dennis Fradin states: "Surgeons were known to enter the operating room with a bottle of whiskey in each hand: one for the patient and the other for the doctor to be able to bear the cries of the patient" [8].

Every anesthesia technique employed failed to provide enough pain alleviation. Surgeons and dentists thus worked as fast as they could. However, even the most rapid physician might inflict great pain. As a result, rather than endure the pain of surgery or tooth extraction, people typically opt to suffer from a variety of oral illnesses, such as tumors, oral or cervical odontogenic infections, or complete tooth extraction.

2.2 After 1840

2.2.1 Modern general anesthesia beginnings

The born of modern anesthesia is stated around the year 1844 when using nitrous oxide and diethyl ether, respectively, dentists Horace Wells in 1844 and William T. G. Morton in 1846 made the initial discoveries of the miracle of anesthesia for painless surgery [9].

Horace Wells made an effort to prove that breathing nitrous gas was a reliable method of surgical anesthetic. Unfortunately, at the last minute, the booked patient decided not to have the treatment done. A young student who was there consented to have his wisdom teeth removed, but he moaned and moved while it was being done. It was not until much later that the young kid claimed to have "actually did not feel any real pain," despite the apparent failure. Regretfully, the degraded Dr. Wells withdrew from more public demonstrations of nitrous gas efficacy [10].

The agent that many other dentists were using, nitrous oxide, was not working well for Dr. Morton, a young dentist from Boston. Though it was extremely uncomfortable, few patients would put up with his innovative method of fitting dentures. He knew that if he could create a painkiller that worked better, his business would expand rapidly [11, 12]. William Morton extracted a tooth without any pain on September 30, 1846, from a patient who consented to breathe ether—the same substance that long had employed in 1842. Morton used a patient having surgery to demonstrate in public the anesthetic effects of ether. On October 16, 1846, Morton gave the patient anesthesia in Boston, Massachusetts. The procedure, which involved extracting a tumor from the patient's lower jaw, was then carried out by the surgeon, Dr. Warren [9].

Oliver Wendell Holmes first used the term "anesthesia" in a November 21, 1846, private letter to Dr. Morton. As the ether-induced shift was physiologic, Holmes also considered the terms antineurotic, aneuric, neroleptic, neurolepsia and neurostasis. However, he dismissed these terms as "too anatomical" [13].

2.2.2 Local anesthesia in dentistry

The local anesthesia in dentistry had a 40-year delay after the general anesthesia discovery. The invention of the modern hypodermic needle by American physician Zophar Jayne in 1841 marked a significant advancement in the field of local anesthetic [14].

2.2.3 Cocaine first usage

In Göttingen, Germany, Albert Niemann, a pharmacology graduate student, was extracting cocaine from coca leaves. Twenty more years later, while still a graduate student in Vienna, Sigmund Freud started testing the effects of coca leaves on himself. He was surprised to feel how deeply numbing it made his tongue feel. Cocaine was not initially accepted by surgeons as a safe anesthetic. However, for tooth extractions, dentists started using it subcutaneously. Although a very good anesthetic was obtained, the nonstandard dosage resulted in several undesirable systemic side effects, including tachycardia, giddiness and excitement. Dentists were already limiting their subcutaneous cocaine use 6 years later [15, 16].

2.2.4 Vasoconstrictors

German physician Heinrich Braun made a pioneering contribution to the development of a safer local anesthetic in 1903. Braun introduced adrenaline to a cocaine solution because he was aware of the hormone's effects on vasoconstriction. He then gave himself long-lasting anesthesia by injecting the new solution into his arm.

William Stewart Halsted and William John Hall first presented the idea of conduction anesthesia in writing around the same period. More effective and pleasant anesthesia was made possible by the idea of numbing tissues farther away from the injection site by anesthetizing the nerve by depositing the anesthetic substance close to the nerve. This allowed for a more focused and targeted anesthetic technique and decreased the number of injections required [13, 17].

2.2.5 Procaine

After years of research and development, German scientist Alfred Einhorn finally synthesized procaine in 1904 and filed a patent for it under the brand name Novocaine. Dentists began using this anesthetic because they found it to be quite helpful. Novocaine turned out to be the safest and most efficient substitute for cocaine, although having less potent anesthetic properties than cocaine [18].

2.2.6 Lidocaine

The pivotal discovery was made in 1943 in Stockholm, Sweden by Nils Löfgren and Bengt Lundqvist. This new molecule, designated LL30, would eventually become lidocaine, the first amide local anesthetic. Lidocaine has an extended duration of action, superior potency, less tissue irritation and less allergenicity than Novocaine. The Food and Drug Administration authorized the use of lidocaine, or Xylocaine (Astra), in the United States in November 1948 [19].

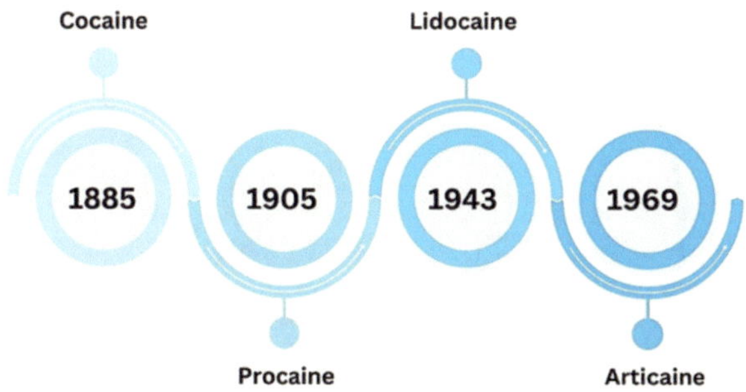

Figure 1.
Timeline of local anesthetic sintetization (personal design and propriety of the authors).

2.2.7 Other anesthetic substances

Several other amide local anesthetics were created after lidocaine was successfully used in dentistry, including mepivacaine in 1957, bupivacaine in 1957, prilocaine in 1969, articaine in 1969 and etidocaine in 1972 (**Figure 1**) [19].

3. Clinical anatomy

Trigeminal nerve is the fifth pair of cranial nerves, being a mixt nerve, providing both sensory and motor innervation. It presents three branches, which originate at the level of the Gasser ganglion OPHTHALMIC - V1 division; MAXILLARY- V2 division and 3. MANDIBULAR- V3 division, as shown in **Figure 2**.

- ensures SENSITIVE innervation of:

  1. facial soft *tissues*

  2. oral mucous membranes apart from the pharyngeal mucosa and the base of the tongue

- ensures MOTOR innervation of mandible muscles:

  - masticatory muscles:

  - masseter

  - temporal

  - medial pterygoid

  - lateral pterygoid

- mylohyoid muscle

- the anterior belly of the digastric muscle

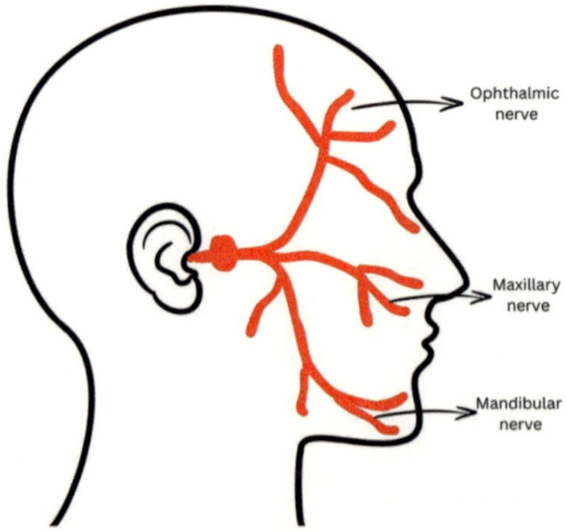

Figure 2.
Trigeminal nerve representation (personal design and propriety of the authors).

- tensor veli palatini
- tensor tympani muscle

3.1 Ophthalmic nerve - V1

The ophthalmic nerve is the smallest of the three divisions of the trigeminal nerve. The nerve splits into its three major branches when it leaves the skull through the superior orbital fissure:

- Frontal nerve
- Lacrimal nerve
- Nasociliary nerve

It provides sensory innervation to the following structures:

- forehead and scalp
- frontal, ethmoid and sphenoid sinuses
- upper eyelid and its conjunctiva
- cornea
- dorsum of the nose
- lacrimal gland
- parts of the meninges and tentorium cerebelli (recurrent tentorial branch)

Due to the no implication in dentistry, this branch will be not extensively presented.

3.2 Maxillary nerve - V2

Is the second branch of the trigeminal nerve with the origin at the level of Gasser's ganglion (**Figure 3**).

3.3 Mandibular nerve - V3

Is the largest branch of the trigeminal nerve with the origin also at the level of Gasser's ganglion (**Figures 4** and **5**).

The mandibular nerve and its branches ensure the skin sensitivity of the temporal region, ear, cheek, lower lip and chin. Regarding the innervation of the mucosa, the mandibular nerve provides sensitive innervation of the cheek mucosa, ⅔ anterior parts of the tongue mucosa, the lower lip and the buccal side of the mandibular alveolar ridge from the mental foramen to the midline. The mandibular nerve, ensures the sensitivity of the mandibular teeth and the mandible bone. Is the only branch with motor fibers for masticatory musculature.

The inferior alveolar nerve block has the highest failure rate of all anesthesia techniques used in the mandible, due to the inherent anatomical conditions. The inferior alveolar nerve, artery and vein are located in the mandible canal, as

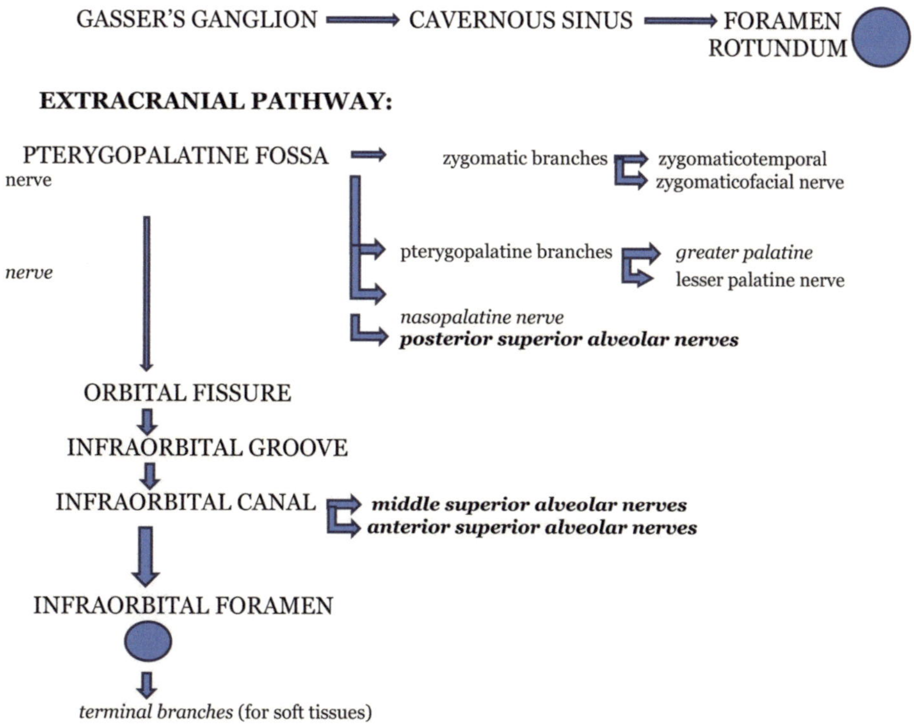

Figure 3.
The pathway of the maxillary nerve. (personal design and propriety of the authors).

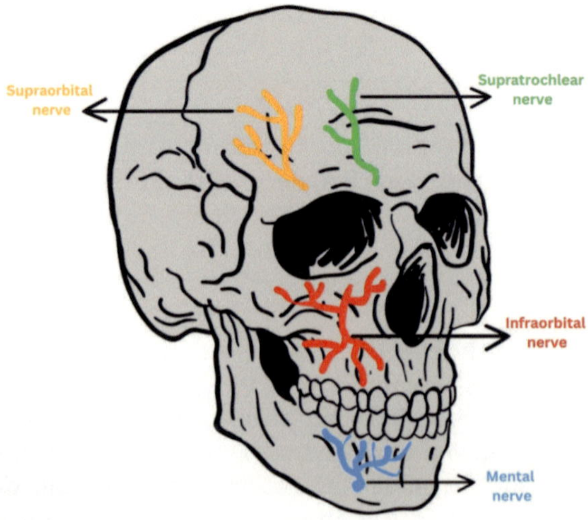

Figure 4.
Oftalmic and maxillary nerve representation (personal design and propriety of the authors).

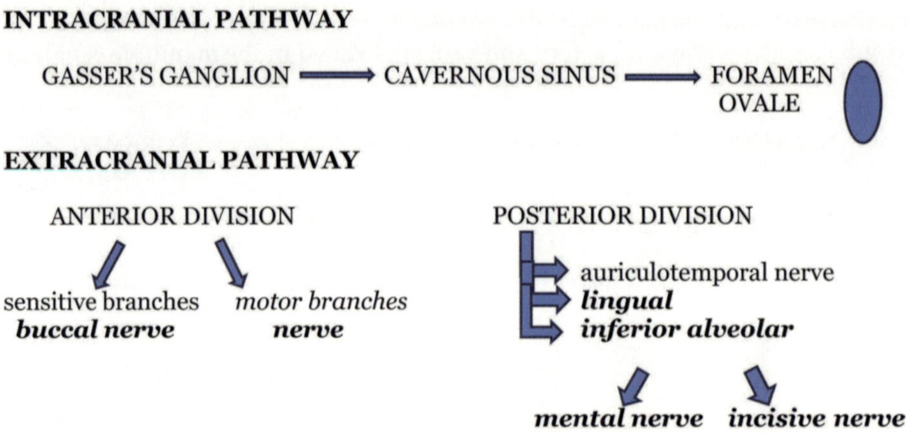

Figure 5.
Mandibular nerve pathway. (personal design and propriety of the authors).

known as the mandibular canal, which is 2–4 mm in diameter and is patterned in an S shape. The mandibular canal approximates the lingual plate in the first molar area and is most laterally positioned in the third molar region, closest to the buccal cortical bone. The canal route ends at the mental foramen. The mental foramen is located between the first and second premolars, roughly 7.5 mm from the inferior border of the jaw, in its lowest position. This is where the incisive and mental nerves split off from the inferior alveolar nerve. The mental nerve emerges from the foramen and provides sensory innervation for the lip, chin and buccal mucosa anterior from the foramen and the incisive nerve remains in the bone and provides sensory innervation for the anterior teeth. There are many common anatomical variants of the mandibular canal, including a bifid canal, trifid canal and enlarged canal (**Figure 6**) [20, 21].

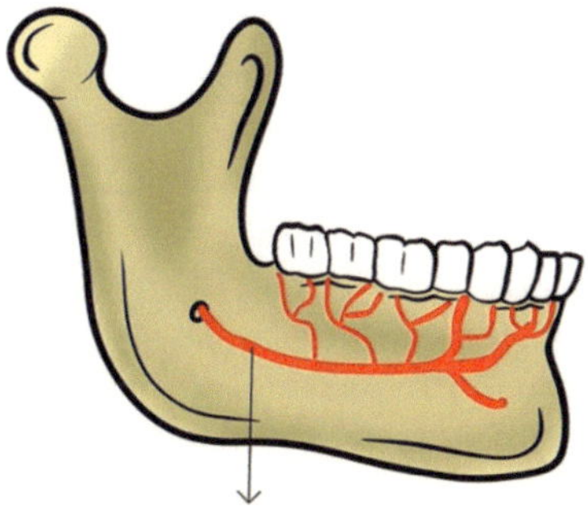

Figure 6.
Inferior alveolar nerve representation (personal design and propriety of the authors).

4. Local anesthesia techniques in dentistry: Plexus vs. troncular

4.1 Plexus anesthesia

This type of local anesthesia technique is widely used in dentistry due to its advantages: atraumatic anesthesia, simple technique and minimal risks of accidents and complications. The anesthetic substance is deposited under the mucosa and upper from the periosteum.

The local conditions that are necessary to exist for performing this anesthesia are: bone cortical as thin as possible and the bone spongy very well represented so that the anesthetic substance can reach the nerve plexus.

In the maxilla, these conditions are met in all teeth, except for the first molar, due to the vestibular presence of the zygomatic-alveolar crest, made of compact, thick bone, which does not allow the anesthetic substance to diffuse through it. The posterior superior alveolar nerve, the middle superior alveolar nerve, and the anterior superior alveolar nerves form the superior dental plexus. The plexus is located in the alveolar process of the maxilla and gives rise to both dental and gingival branches. It innervates the teeth of the upper jaw [22, 23].

At the level of the mandible bone, plexus anesthesia can be performed only on the front teeth, where the vestibular bone plate is thinner. The lateral teeth, premolars and molars, no longer benefit from plexus anesthesia due to the thick vestibular bone, formed by the external oblique line at this level.

Plexus anesthesia can be used for endodontic treatments, cavity preparation, periodontal procedures, oral surgery and implantology.

4.2 Troncular anesthesia

Troncular anesthesia is also a regional anesthesia type. This technique is based on injecting the local anesthetic substance in the immediate vicinity of a major nerve trunk, so that the local anesthesia occurs in the area of distribution of this nerve, distal to the injection site of the anesthetic solution. In dentistry, troncular anesthesia is used in the maxilla for the posterior superior alveolar nerve at the tuberosity, the anterior superior alveolar nerves and the terminal branches of the infraorbital nerve at the suborbital foramen, the anterior palatine nerve, the nasopalatine nerve. In the mandible, it is used for the inferior alveolar nerve and its terminal branches-incisive and metal nerves, the lingual nerve and the buccal nerve.

Peripheral troncular anesthesia follows anesthetic infiltration along the peripheral branches of the mandibular and maxillary nerve branches of the trigeminal nerve.

Troncular anesthesia techniques are indicated whenever anesthesia through infiltration is not good enough, the patient accuses pain or technically it cannot be performed. This situation occurs when the bone layer around the tooth is very compact and therefore, the local anesthetic cannot diffuse to the dental apex in sufficient concentrations for obtaining adequate anesthesia.

As a deep tissue anesthesia, it offers several advantages, including comprehensive anesthesia of both soft and hard tissues, prolonged duration of action, and the utilization of low doses of local anesthetic. The disadvantages are represented by the long duration of anesthesia, which can be a cause of accidental injury of soft tissues such as lips, and cheeks traumatized by biting. Also, nerve injury can be obtained because the main scope of this type of anesthesia is injecting the local anesthetic, closer to the nerve, which cannot be precisely located in the soft tissues. There is a risk of puncturing the blood vessels located in the proximity of the nerve trunks, this is the main reason that this type of anesthesia is not recommended for patients with blood disorders or anticoagulant treatment.

5. Risk patients for local anesthesia administration

5.1 Anticoagulant treatments

Traditionally, the proper anticoagulation therapy for patients receiving oral anticoagulant medication was determined by assigning them to one of three categories: for low-risk treatments, the anticoagulant medication did not need to be changed; for moderate-risk procedures, coumarin withdrawal was advised 2 days prior to the surgery, and the INR was verified the day of the procedure; and for high-risk dental procedures, a heparin regimen was highly advised [24].

Before administering local anesthesia, it is vital to ensure that the patient is prepared regarding the INR values that must be within therapeutic ranges (2.0–4.0). Values that surpass the top limit may result in protracted bleeding, even when just local anesthesia is administered. Prolonged bleeding may occur due to tissue damage, or injury of blood vessels by the needle, resulting in the forming of hematomas and other serious complications like obstruction of superior airways [25]. For this reason, the Spix technique for inferior alveolar nerve anesthesia, and the tuberosity technique for superior and posterior alveolar nerve anesthesia is not recommended.

5.2 Elderly patients

A decline in patient capacity for physiological, physical, or psychological functioning is the hallmark of frailty, a multifaceted condition. Over the past 10 years, there has been a significant growth in the usage of local anesthesia among the fragile population. Due to their increased susceptibility to local anesthetics, older individuals should not get more local anesthetic than what is recommended for their weak condition. Furthermore, it makes sense to advise lowering the amount and concentration of LA given to elderly patients in order to lessen resorption.

To lower the danger of systemic toxicity in this situation, it is recommended to lower the local anesthesia administrated and the doses of local anesthetics used. For example, for lidocaine, the optimal concentration indicated is 10 $mg.mL^{-1}$ without exceeding the dose of 4–5 $mg.kg^{-1}$ [26].

5.3 Pregnancy

The dentist is concerned about the use of systemically absorbed anesthetics in women patients who are pregnant or nursing. Therefore, the consequences of any anesthetic given to a pregnant woman must be taken into account for both the mother and the fetus.

Because most medications as well as local anesthetics used simply diffuse over the placenta, the potential teratogenic effects must be considered. Despite being in the 2–4 weeks pre-differentiation phase, the embryo is resistant to teratogenic effects. The 4–10 weeks that follow the previous menstrual cycle are the riskiest after this time when organogenesis occurs [27]. In the second trimester of pregnancy, the danger of teratogenicity is becoming less significant due to the fact that significant organogenesis has taken place. Elective dental treatment under locoregional anesthesia is frequently recommended to be completed during the second trimester to prevent labor, supine hypotensive syndrome and overall discomfort.

The amount of free anesthetic molecules that reach the fetus determines the prenatal harm from the local anesthetic. The anesthetic dosage, type of anesthesia administration, the presence of vasoconstrictors, the maternal metabolism and excretion, the pH levels of the mother and the fetus, the anesthetic's pKa, and the extent of protein binding between the mother and the fetus, all can affect the fetal exposure. Head and neck local anesthetic administration offers a risk of greater plasma levels and, consequently, a higher drug concentration reaching the fetus due to increased vascularity [28].

The United States Food and Drug Administration categorized local anesthetics used in dentistry based on their level of risk to the fetus when injected during pregnancy. It is stated that there are no harmful effects on the fetus for Categories A and B. There is insufficient evidence to conclude that local anesthetics in category C are teratogenic in humans, but they have been demonstrated to be so in animal fetuses. Currently, the anesthetic agent that best combines safety and efficacy for expectant mothers is thought to be 2% lidocaine with 1:200,000 epinephrine [29].

Both articaine—for which there are no controlled trials in pregnant women—and bupivacaine and mepivacaine are categorized into category C because of the possibility of fetal bradycardia resulting from their usage. Pregnant women can get up to five cartridges of 1:100,000 epinephrine (or ten cartridges of anesthesia with a 1:200,000 epinephrine concentration) in a single dental appointment [30].

5.4 Cardiovascular disease

The dentist should be aware when administrating local anesthesia for dental procedures on this category of patients that nowadays are numerous. Both in healthy patients and cardiovascular affected, the patients experience stress and discomfort as a result of inadequate local anesthesia, which causes the body to generate more endogenous catecholamine. Remember that the quantity of epinephrine secreted endogenously is higher than the amount used for dental anesthesia [31]. Thus, even in patients with cardiovascular illness, a local anesthetic containing epinephrine may be chosen to provide sufficient amounts of anesthesia and hemostasis.

The cardiovascular pathologies that can interfere with local anesthesia administration are represented by arterial hypertension, ischemic heart disease, myocardial infarction, arrhythmias and endocarditis. Before any administration of anesthesia for dental procedures, a previous consultation with the patient by a cardiologist must be performed [32].

In the administration of local anesthesia, we must take into account the general and locoregional effects of anesthetic substances on the cardiovascular system through the vasodilator effect of all anesthetic substances, and the action of the associated vasoconstrictors: peripheral vasoconstriction, tachycardia, hypertension.

In recent (less than 6 months) or repeated myocardic infarction: due to the increased risk of reinfarction, any intervention under local or general anesthesia is performed only on the indication of the cardiologist. In previous heart attacks (more than 6 months), local anesthesia can be performed with a normal amount of vasoconstrictor.

In the case of patients presenting with cardiovascular disease, the recommended dosage of adrenaline is 0.04 mg, in contrast to the 0.2 mg dosage typically administered to a healthy adult [33]. Additionally, because adrenaline-containing anesthetics reach the general circulation quickly by intraligamental and intraosseous injection, these techniques are not recommended for patients with cardiovascular diseases [34].

5.5 Hepatic implications

Particular attention should be paid to patients with liver diseases (chronic hepatitis, cirrhosis, malignant tumors), due to the hepatic metabolism of local anesthetic substances from the amide group, which is disturbed, and leads to the accumulation of anesthetic substance or metabolites in the general circulation that can trigger the intoxication reactions. Among all the anesthetic substances, from the amide group, articaine is preferred due to its predominantly plasmatic and only partially hepatic metabolism. In severe forms of liver function impairment, it is recommended to use anesthetics from the esters group (Procaine, Chlorprocaine) with plasma metabolism.

5.6 Renal disease

Anesthetic substances and their metabolites are eliminated by the kidneys. Alteration of renal function causes the accumulation of anesthetic substances at the blood serum level, with the risk of overdose. Limited amounts of Al will be used for patients with altered function of the kidneys.

5.7 Diabetes mellitus

In the case of patients with diabetes mellitus, performing local anesthesia presents some risks related to the effect of inhibiting insulin action and increasing blood sugar given by catecholamines used as vasoconstrictor adjuvants and increased susceptibility to infectious complications. These risks are minimal in the compensated phase of the disease. The recommendation is to administer anesthetics associated with adrenaline in a maximum dose of 1:200,000.

6. Complications

6.1 Allergic reactions

It is not recommended to use a local anesthetic if the patient has a known allergy to it or any of its constituents. The only absolute contraindication to local anesthesia administration is allergy reaction. True allergic responses to local anesthetics are actually very uncommon. Roughly 1% of all responses that happen during local anesthetic are thought to be allergic in nature [35].

Allergic complications can be prevented by questioning the patient about known allergies and, in the case of the presence of known allergies, by avoiding the administration of the specific substance. When there is a suspicion of a possible allergy, the patient will be referred to an allergology specialized service to carry out specific tests.

Allergy to local anesthetic substances from the ester group is more common than to those from the amide group. Allergies to the agents with a preservative role in the anesthetic substances have been demonstrated: methylparaben added for the bacteriostatic role and preservative of anesthetics, and sodium disulfite- an antioxidant agent of the associated vasoconstrictor agents.

There are two recognized forms of allergic responses to local anesthetics: type I reactions mediated by immunoglobulin E (IgE) and type IV reactions mediated by T cells. On the other hand, delayed type IV responses are mostly brought on by topical anesthetics and are distinguished by localized edema. Allergic reactions can range from aphthous ulceration to anaphylaxis [36, 37].

6.2 Intravascular injection

Apart from allergic reactions, another unfavorable consequence of local anesthetics is toxic reactions. These complications arise due to the administration of anesthesia being unsuccessful, resulting in the aspiration not being performed correctly. In such cases, the local anesthetic is injected intravascularly, leading to adverse effects on the central nervous system and cardiovascular system. The clinical signs that can appear as a toxic response are represented by convulsions, hypotension, bradycardia, and in rare instances, cardiovascular collapse, coma and even death [38].

The amount of the anesthetic that is injected into the systemic circulation determines the general toxicity of the local anesthetic. This condition, known as dose-dependent local anesthetic systemic toxicity (LAST), primarily affects children as opposed to adults. When the local anesthesia is administered correctly, most of the time there are no significant adverse effects. However, some organs that are highly vascularized as the brain and heart, may suffer adverse effects if repeated local anesthesia is performed or if an intravascular injection is made by mistake [39].

When the intravascular levels of the local anesthetic are not excessive, the inhibitory neurons in the central nervous system are often blocked initially, resulting in the onset of excitatory symptoms, including diplopia, seizures and involuntary muscular fasciculations. Subsequently, when the anesthetic's plasma concentration rises, depression symptoms, such as commas, respiratory arrests and unconsciousness, may manifest.

The cardiovascular system is the second most vulnerable to adverse effects, after the nervous system. When increasing concentrations of the local anesthetic impede the function of sodium channels in the heart muscle, bradycardia frequently occurs first. In the end, prolonged systemic absorption of local anesthetics may result in complete cardiac arrest, ventricular dysrhythmias and atrioventricular blocks [40].

6.3 Ocular complications

Consequences from an intravascular injection of local anesthetic when performing troncular or plexal anesthesia into the maxillary artery might cause ocular complications. The oculomotor, trochlear and abducens nerves may become anesthetized as a result of the anesthetic solution flowing retrogradely through the lacrimal and optic arteries.

The most frequently observed adverse effect is transient diplopia, which is attributable to the firm deposition of the anesthetic substance within the orbit with the elevation of the eyeball. It vanished after 15 minutes to 24 hours. Other ocular complications that can appear are represented by transient uniocular blindness, strabismus and complete or partial visual loss. After the administration of anesthesia of the inferior alveolar nerve block technique, anesthesia may cause permanent visual loss in one eye. Following the administration of prilocaine and the extraction of multiple teeth, complete loss of one eye's vision was reported. Two months later, the loss of eyesight remained [41].

6.4 Nerves injury

The frequency of temporary or permanent nerve damage associated with local anesthetic in dental practice is estimated to range substantially from 1:750,000 to 1:42 disruptions per injection [42].

Diverse and often not supported by evidence opinions have been expressed on the cause of injection-related nerve damage. Three mechanisms are proposed [43]:

- Direct mechanical injury may occur as a result of the needle penetrating the nerve during the anesthetic procedure.
- Indirect mechanical injury manifests as a consequence of intraneural hemorrhage, which in turn gives rise to the formation of a hematoma and granulation tissue. This is followed by the development of constrictive scarring and hypoxia.
- Local anesthetic-induced neurotoxicity involving axon or myelin with cellular structural degradation, or both.

6.4.1 Direct mechanical injury

This complication arises when there is an interruption to the continuity of the nerve, either partially or entirely, during the administration of local anesthetic. The nerves most frequently affected are the inferior alveolar nerve, lingual nerve, mental nerve and infraorbital nerve. This can be attributed to the variable position in the soft tissues of the IAN on the medial surface of the ramus before entering in the mandibular canal. The same situation is also encountered at the lingual nerve. In contrast, the mental and infraorbital nerves are located in the osseous foramen where the needle is inserted.

6.4.2 Indirect mechanical injury

Nerve compression can result in complete crushing with axonal disruption (axonotmesis) or localized demyelination with ischemia. If nerve compression is severe enough, it can also create blockages in nerve conductivity and neuropeptide synthesis (neuropraxia).

Concomitant vascular alterations and nerve damage can result in ischemia episodes, artery occlusion from the vasa nervorum and hemorrhage inside the nerve sheaths. Despite the protective effect of the collagen coating on nerve vascular plexuses, sufficiently aggressive traumas may result in changes in the permeability of the epidermis and, in more severe cases, lesions in the endoneurial vessels with the occurrence of edema and intrafascicular hemorrhages secondary to nerve injury. In addition to creating a hypoxic environment that exacerbates neuropathic pain symptoms, these alterations can also lead to axonal compression and crushing due to hemorrhage and edema [44].

6.4.3 Local anesthetic-induced neurotoxicity

All local anesthetics used in dentistry have varying degrees of neurotoxicity. The degree of local and systemic neurotoxicity is directly proportional to the injected dose. Of the anesthetics most frequently linked to a greater incidence of neurotoxicity, articaine and prilocaine are the most commonly used. The higher the concentration and dose of the local anesthetic substance, the greater the neurotoxicity. The development of paresthesia is more strongly correlated with 4% anesthetic solutions (prilocaine and articaine) than with lower concentrations [45].

The clinical manifestations are diverse, encompassing paresthesia, dysesthesia and allodynia, as well as permanent anesthesia.

6.5 Transient facial nerve palsy

This complication may occur either during or after the inferior alveolar block, when the anesthetic agent is deposited too deeply in the Spix technique, directly in the parotid gland. Facial paralysis develops within minutes of the injection and remits within a few hours. To avoid this adverse effect, it is essential to perform an accurate evaluation of the anesthetic landmarks. The hemi-face is paralyzed, the patient cannot do facial expressions, such as closing an eye or smiling. Drooping skin around the brow, eye, cheek and mouth.

The transient facial nerve palsy that occurs several hours or even days after the administration of local anesthetics has a number of potential causes [46, 47]:

- the anesthetic substance or the needle's mechanical damage, which causes ischemic neuritis and a sympathetic vascular reflex
- mechanical injury that awakens a dormant varicella or herpes simplex-zoster virus
- inflammation of the neural sheath
- damage to the nerves as a result of the local anesthetic's breakdown products
- opening the mouth for a lengthy time and straining the facial nerve
- intravascular injection

No specific treatment is necessary.

6.6 Needle breakage

The fracture of a needle during the administration of local anesthetic is an extremely rare occurrence. The advent of standardized disposable cannulas composed of robust stainless steel may have almost eliminated the most prevalent cause in the past, namely fatigue fracture of sterilized reusable dental needles [48].

The potential causes of this complication are as follows:

- needle fabrication defects
- choosing the wrong type of needle
- suddenly, the needle changes in direction
- patient movement
- violent contraction of pterygomandibular muscles
- inappropriate injection techniques
- multiple injections with the same needle

This complication is most frequently observed in the inferior alveolar block-spix technique, performed on adults with needles of a small diameter. In the case of mandibular blocks, the use of a needle with a gauge of 27 or less is advised. In order to facilitate retrieval in the event of breakage, a long needle with a minimum of 5 mm of exposed tip is recommended. In addition to this, the following measures should be employed in order to prevent this complication: the needle should not be bent and the needle shank should not be inserted into any tissues, as fractures are more prevalent in the most vulnerable areas, which is the union between the stem and cap [49, 50].

The management of this accident must be prompt and accurate, with the objective of locating the broken needle before it migrates into the oral or cervical soft tissues. The needle fragment may move and cause serious complications, including potentially fatal bleeding from the major cervical blood arteries. In the event of a needle breakage and visible fragment, hemostatic forceps or Pean forceps should be promptly employed to grasp the fragment. It is important to note that the fragment may disappear as soon as the patient moves, swallows, or the dentist uses digital manipulation to relax the soft tissues.

7. Fear of dental anesthesia

Fear of receiving dental care is one of the main reasons patients postpone visiting the dentist. The dread of local anesthetic needles is a significant aspect of this phobia complex, and many patients avoid dental treatments because of this anxiety [51]. The needle phobia is called trypanophobia and it is included in the medical aspect of the fears, unlike aichmophobia, belonephobia and enetophobia which are concerned with the fear of pins, needles and sharp objects respectively [52]. Phobia is defined as a type of anxiety disorder when an individual has an excessive level of fear toward a specific situation or object, which affects their daily functioning and quality of life.

Unfortunately, this fear manifests even in children, and an anxious child will become an anxious adult with a fear of dental anesthesia.

Symptoms:

- increased anxiety
- avoidance of needles
- increased blood pressure
- restlessness
- tremor
- dizziness
- profuse sweating
- muscle weakness
- dry mouth
- suffocation sensations
- psychomotor agitation
- even vasovagal syncope

The management of trypanophobia is a highly complex process that employs a range of techniques. These include the use of anxiolytic premedication and melotherapy, which is a method of suppressing the sympathetic nervous system and reducing adrenergic and neuromuscular activity. Virtual Reality Exposure Therapy (VRET) is another effective approach that helps to relax and distract the patient, thereby reducing anxiety, improving compliance and achieving non-disruptive behavior during dental anesthesia. Topical anesthesia can also be used to reduce pain on needle insertion.

Aromatherapy is the most effective non-pharmacological technique for anxiolysis and relaxation because it can influence pain perception and anxiety relief using orange, chamomile, lavender and lemongrass oils.

Acupuncture is a minimally invasive technique that has been demonstrated to reduce general and pre-anesthetic anxiety. Auricular acupuncture has been shown to relieve anxiety by modulating the autonomic nervous system, suppressing the sympathetic nervous system, stimulating the parasympathetic nervous system, inhibiting noradrenaline and reducing sympathetic hyperactivity.

Canine-assisted therapy is also a therapeutic relief method that improves the physical condition and mental health of patients who suffer from trypanophobia [53].

Patients with trypanophobia may find relief from their fear by using coping methods such as deep breathing, muscular relaxation and lying down while receiving an injection [54].

The tripartite components of the pathological fear response, namely physiology, behavior and cognition, along with the general subjective experience of dread, represent the primary targets of psychological therapies for trypanophobia. Distraction, visual and auditory examples have been identified as particularly effective in improving the condition. A three-step methodology has been established to assist patients in overcoming their trypanophobia, comprising relaxation, control and progressive exposure [55].

8. Failures in achieving local anesthesia

In order to facilitate analysis, the success criteria for anesthesia should be separated into two distinct groups: those pertaining to the success of the anesthesia technique itself and those pertaining to the success of pulp anesthesia. The majority of anesthetic procedures have historically relied on the assessment of soft tissue numbness as a primary indicator of anesthetic efficacy. For instance, in the majority of cases following maxillary molar anesthesia infiltration, soft tissue numbness may not be discernible, leading the patient to conclude that the anesthesia was ineffective. In such a scenario, the anesthetic's effectiveness would be more reliably indicated by the presence of pain upon access cavity preparation or a lack of reaction to thermic tests than by the absence of soft tissue numbness [56].

Failures of dental anesthesia procedures may result in an unpleasant treatment session for both the patient and the dentist. Patients may choose to postpone dental treatments, which could result in a decline in oral health. If the frequency of dental anesthesia errors increases, dentists may feel inept and regret their time spent in the field [57].

The typical range for molar anesthesia failures is 15% in pulps that are not inflamed and 44–81% in pulpitis [58].

8.1 Etiologic factors

Anesthesia failures may be attributed to a multitude of factors, including those pertaining to the patient's anatomy, pathology, or psychological state, as well as the dentist's selection of an anesthetic approach. It is reasonable to consider anesthetic failure if anesthesia symptoms are not promptly identified within a reasonable time frame of 10 to 15 minutes following the administration of anesthesia [59]. The etiologic factors can be [60]:

- *Anatomical:* accessory nerve supply (inferior alveolar nerve can have anastomosis with mylohyoid nerve, branch from cervical cutaneous nerves C1, C2 or auriculotemporal nerve), variable anatomic course of nerves, variations in infraorbital or mental foramen position, bifid alveolar nerve or bifid mandibular canal), anastomosis nerve branches on midline;

- *Pathological:* local inflammation with acid environment, trismus, infections, previous surgery with scars where the anesthetic diffusion is weak;

- *Inadequate technique*: This is the most significant factor that contributes to the failure of anesthesia in dentistry. The anesthetic substance must be deposited in close proximity to the nerve. Additionally, the inappropriate selection of instruments and equipment may also be a contributing factor;

- *Pharmacological*: patient's vices such as chronic alcohol abuse, narcotics or deficiencies in metabolization or excretion of anesthetic substances;

- *Psychological*: anxiety, trypanophobia.

8.2 Measures

It is possible to avoid anesthesia failures by undertaking a comprehensive anamnesis of the patient, assessing the relevant anesthesia landmarks and respecting them, selecting the most appropriate technique in accordance with local conditions (avoiding the deposition of local anesthetics in inflamed tissues with hyperaemia and vasodilatation), adjusting the vasoconstrictor dosage, and using the minimum amount of anesthetic substances with the highest potential. In the event that all of the aforementioned measures are duly observed and yet the anesthesia in question fails to provide painless dental treatment, it is necessary to resort to a complementary anesthesia technique, such as intrapulpal, intraosseous or intraligamentary [61].

9. New perspectives in local anesthesia

The field of local anesthesia in dentistry is one that is subject to constant development. Researchers are engaged in the pursuit of new methods and anesthetic substances that will enable dental treatment to be delivered to patients without the discomfort that is typically associated with such procedures. In the majority of cases, patients recall the anesthetic pain rather than the discomfort associated with dental procedures. The factors that may contribute to anesthetic pain can be attributed to local anesthetic properties, damage to the oral mucosa caused by the anesthetic's penetration, subperiosteal injection, high pressure from the anesthetic's spread, low or high temperature and low pH.

9.1 Alternative delivery methods

Computer-controlled local anesthetic delivery (CCLAD) refers to electronic injection tools that can be set to a variety of speed settings, thereby enabling the administration rate of a local anesthetic to be regulated without the production of painful anesthesia. A plethora of systems are currently available on the market, including: Examples of such systems include Morpheus, QuickSleeper anesthesia, No Pain III™ Computer-controlled local analgesic delivery, CDS-IOA, CDS-ILA using Wand STA device, Dentapen, Calajet, Computer-controlled local analgesic delivery, Calajec, SleeperOne®, I Ject device and SleeperOne5 [62]. A few systems have the advantage of not using a needle for injecting the anesthetic substances, instead utilizing a high-pressure system.

9.2 Advances in topical oral anesthesia

Commercially available gels, ointments, solutions, and adhesive patches for oral usage contain dental topical anesthetic compositions. The most often utilized anesthetic ingredients in topical formulations include tetracaine hydrochloride, lidocaine, benzocaine, and benzocaine with butamben [63]. The goal of innovative drug delivery systems is to reduce the toxicity of local anesthetics when administered in dentistry while extending their anesthetic efficacy. These systems are based on technologies like hydrogels, patches, cyclodextrins, liposomes, and biopolymers [64].

9.3 Light controlled anesthesia

One of the most promising methods to regulate the effects of medications, apart from exposure to ultrasonic, magnetic, or electrical fields, is through the use of light.

This method's main idea is to create agents that can switch back and forth between two different forms, one of which has biological activity and the other does not. As of right now, a number of photo-switchable substances have been identified as having the ability to inhibit the transmission of nerve impulses. These substances include azo-propofol, azo derivatives of fentanyl, photo-switchable modulators of metabotropic glutamate receptors 4 (mGlu4) and 5 (mGlu5), a photo-switchable inhibitor of glycine transporter 2, and azo derivatives of capsaicin. QAQ and fotocaine are the most promising photo-switchable voltage-gated sodium channel blockers available at this time [65].

9.4 Reversal agents for local anesthesia

Local anesthetics are often categorized into three groups based on their onset of action and duration of action. The first group comprises low-potency, short-duration anesthetics, the second intermediate-potency and duration anesthetics, and the third high-potency, long-duration anesthetics. Given that a typical dental procedure lasts approximately 47 minutes, a local anesthetic with intermediate strength and duration can be employed for these procedures.

The first nonselective α-adrenergic blocking medication, phentolamine mesylate, was commercially available for the reversal of soft tissue anesthesia and the accompanying functional impairments caused by intraoral anesthesia with a local anesthetic that also contained a vasoconstrictor. The same amount and technique used for local anesthesia administration must be used for efficacy [66].

10. Conclusions

Local anesthesia in dentistry is a vast and multifaceted subject, encompassing a range of disciplines including anatomy, pharmacology, physiology and related fields. For patients, the key figure in this field is the professional dentist, who is equipped with the knowledge and expertise to deliver painless dental treatment. In order to maintain the highest standards of care, continuous education and training are essential.

Acknowledgements

The authors would like to acknowledge "Victor Babeș" University of Medicine and Pharmacy Timișoara for their support in covering the costs of publication for this book chapter.

Author details

Ciprian Ioan Roi[1], Alexandra Roi[2]* and Mircea Riviș[1]

1 Department of Anesthesiology and Oral Surgery, "Victor Babeș" University of Medicine and Pharmacy, Eftimie Murgu, Timișoara, Romania

2 Department of Oral Pathology, "Victor Babeș" University of Medicine and Pharmacy, Eftimie Murgu, Timișoara, Romania

*Address all correspondence to: alexandra.moga@umft.ro

References

[1] Cervino G. Milestones of dentistry: Advent of anesthetics in oral surgery. Dentistry Journal (Basel). 2019;**7**(4):112. DOI: 10.3390/dj7040112

[2] Prichard D. A brief history of dental anesthesia [Internet]. 2013. Available from: https://www.speareducation.com/spear-review/2013/08/a-brief-history-of-dental-anesthesia

[3] Leclant J. Médecine et art dentaire dans l'ancienne Egypte [Medicine and dentistry in ancient Egypt]. Bulletin de l'Académie Nationale de Chirurgie Dentaire. 1987;**33**(33):153-154

[4] Spielman AI. History of dental Anesthesia. In: Illustrated Encyclopedia of the History of Dentistry. 2023. Available from: https://historyofdentistryandmedicine.com/

[5] Koutroumpas D, Lioumi E, Koutroumpas H. Dioscorides on dental and oral treatments. Dental Historian: Lindsay Club Newsletter. 2022;**67**:17-26

[6] Hasebe A. The evolution of dental anesthesia: From Ancient remedies to modern comfort. Oral Health Case Reports. 2023;**9**:105

[7] Su SY, Chen WT, Chiang CJ, Yang YW, Lee WC. Oral cancer incidence rates from 1997 to 2016 among men in Taiwan: Association between birth cohort trends and betel nut consumption. Oral Oncology. 2020;**107**:104798. DOI: 10.1016/j.oraloncology.2020.104798. Epub 2020 May 17

[8] Chele N, Motelica G. Anestezia Loco-regională în Stomatologie și Chirurgia OMF. 1st ed. Chisinau: EDITURA UNIVERSITĂȚII DE STAT DE MEDICINĂ ȘI FARMACIE „NICOLAE TESTEMIȚANU"; 2020. 4 p

[9] Weaver JM. The history of the specialty of dental anesthesiology. Anesthesia Progress. 2019;**66**(2):61-68. DOI: 10.2344/anpr-66-02-12

[10] Fenster JM. Ether Day: The Strange Tale of America's Greatest Medical Discovery and the Haunted Man Who Made it. New York, NY: HarperCollins; 2001

[11] Knapp RB. The Gift of Surgery to Mankind. A History of Modern Anesthesiology. Springfield, IL: Charles C. Thomas; 1983

[12] Robinson DH, Toledo AH. Historical development of modern anesthesia. Journal of Investigative Surgery. 2012;**25**(3):141-149. DOI: 10.3109/08941939.2012.690328

[13] Miller RD. Miller's Anesthesia. 7th ed. Philadelphia, PA: Churchill Livingstone Elsevier; 2010

[14] Calthorpe N. The history of spinal needles: Getting to the point. Anaesthesia. 2004;**59**:1231-1241. DOI: 10.1111/j.1365-2044.2004.03976.x

[15] Ramírez-Carrasco A, Butrón-Téllez Girón C, Sanchez-Armass O, Pierdant-Pérez M. Effectiveness of hypnosis in combination with conventional techniques of behavior Management in Anxiety/pain reduction during dental Anesthetic infiltration. Pain Research & Management. 2017;**2017**:1434015. DOI: 10.1155/2017/1434015. Epub 2017 Apr 11

[16] Nathan J, Asadourian L, Erlich M. A brief history of local anesthesia. International Journal of Head and Neck Surgery. 2016;**7**:29-32. DOI: 10.5005/jp-journals-10001-1261

[17] Rankin JS. William Stewart Halsted: A lecture by Dr. Peter D. Olch. Annals of Surgery. 2006;**243**(3):418-425. DOI: 10.1097/01.sla.0000201546.94163.00

[18] Grzybowski A. The history of cocaine in medicine and its importance to the discovery of the different forms of anaesthesia. Klinika Oczna. 2007;**109**(1-3):101-105

[19] Donaldson M, Goodchild JH. Lidocaine turns 70: The evolution of dental local anesthesia. General Dentistry. 2018;**66**(3):6-9. Erratum in: Gen Dent. 2018 Jul-Aug;66(4):6

[20] Mortazavi H, Baharvand M, Safi Y, Dalaie K, Behnaz M, Safari F. Common conditions associated with mandibular canal widening: A literature review. Imaging Science in Dentistry. 2019;**49**(2):87-95. DOI: 10.5624/isd.2019.49.2.87. Epub 2019 Jun 24

[21] Ai CJ, Jabar NA, Lan TH, Ramli R. Mandibular canal enlargement: Clinical and radiological characteristics. Journal of Clinical Imaging Science. 2017;7:28. DOI: 10.4103/jcis.JCIS_28_17

[22] Rodella LF, Buffoli B, Labanca M, Rezzani R. A review of the mandibular and maxillary nerve supplies and their clinical relevance. Archives of Oral Biology. 2012;**57**(4):323-334. DOI: 10.1016/j.archoralbio.2011.09.007. Epub 2011 Oct 11

[23] Murakami G, Ohtsuka K, Sato I, Moriyama H, Shimada K, Tomita H. The superior alveolar nerves: Their topographical relationship and distribution to the maxillary sinus in human adults. Okajimas Folia Anatomica Japonica. 1994;**70**(6):319-328. DOI: 10.2535/ofaj1936.70.6_319

[24] Scully C, Wolff A. Oral surgery in patients on anticoagulant therapy. Oral Surgery, Oral Medicine, Oral Pathology, Oral Radiology, and Endodontology. 2002;**94**(1):57-64. DOI: 10.1067/moe.2002.123828

[25] Miladinović M, Duka M, Mladenović D, Mladenović S, Mladenović L, Hadžibeti M. Dental patients on oral anticoagulant therapy. Acta Medica Medianae. 2013;**52**:48-51. DOI: 10.5633/amm.2013.0108

[26] Cuvillon P, Lefrant JY, Gricourt Y. Considerations for the use of local anesthesia in the Frail elderly: Current perspectives. Local and Regional Anesthesia. 2022;**15**:71-75. DOI: 10.2147/LRA.S325877

[27] Fayans EP, Stuart HR, Carsten D, Ly Q, Kim H. Local anesthetic use in the pregnant and postpartum patient. Dental Clinics of North America. 2010;**54**(4):697-713. DOI: 10.1016/j.cden.2010.06.010

[28] Lee JM, Shin TJ. Use of local anesthetics for dental treatment during pregnancy; safety for parturient. Journal of Dental Anesthesia and Pain Medicine. 2017;**17**(2):81-90. DOI: 10.17245/jdapm.2017.17.2.81. Epub 2017 Jun 29

[29] Zhou X, Zhong Y, Pan Z, Zhang J, Pan J. Physiology of pregnancy and oral local anesthesia considerations. PeerJ. 2023;**11**:e15585. DOI: 10.7717/peerj.15585

[30] Favero V, Bacci C, Volpato A, Bandiera M, Favero L, Zanette G. Pregnancy and dentistry: A literature review on risk management during dental surgical procedures. Dentistry Journal. 2021;**9**(4):46. DOI: 10.3390/dj9040046

[31] Niwa H, Sugimura M, Satoh Y, Tanimoto A. Cardiovascular response to epinephrine-containing local anesthesia in patients with cardiovascular

disease. Oral Surgery, Oral Medicine, Oral Pathology, Oral Radiology, and Endodontics. 2001;**92**(6):610-616. DOI: 10.1067/moe.2001.118903

[32] Cruz-Pamplona M, Jimenez Y, Pérez MG. Dental considerations in patients with heart disease. Journal of Clinical and Experimental Dentistry. 2011;**3**:97-105. DOI: 10.4317/jced.3.e97

[33] Kim C, Hwang KG, Park CJ. Local anesthesia for mandibular third molar extraction. Journal of Dental Anesthesia and Pain Medicine. 2018;**18**(5):287-294. DOI: 10.17245/jdapm.2018.18.5.287. Epub 2018 Oct 31

[34] Meechan JG. Supplementary routes to local anaesthesia. International Endodontic Journal. 2002;**35**(11):885-896. DOI: 10.1046/j.1365-2591.2002.00592.x

[35] Wildsmith JA, Mason A, McKinnon RP, Rae SM. Alleged allergy to local anaesthetic drugs. British Dental Journal. 1998;**184**(10):507-510. DOI: 10.1038/sj.bdj.4809676

[36] Mathison M, Pepper T. Local anesthesia techniques in dentistry and oral surgery. In: StatPearls [Internet]. Treasure Island (FL): StatPearls Publishing; 2024. Available from: https://www.ncbi.nlm.nih.gov/books/NBK580480/# [Accessed: June 1, 2023]

[37] Jiseon L, Ju-Young L, Hyun JK, Kwang SS. Dental anesthesia for patients with allergic reactions to lidocaine: Two case reports. Journal of Dental Anesthesia and Pain Medicine. 2016;**16**(3):209-212

[38] Noormalin A, Shahnaz M, Rosmilah M, Mujahid SH, Gendeh BS. Ige-mediated hypersensitivity reaction to lignocaine - A case report. Tropical Biomedicine. 2005;**22**:179-183

[39] Macfarlane AJR, Gitman M, Bornstein KJ, El-Boghdadly K, Weinberg G. Updates in our understanding of local anaesthetic systemic toxicity: A narrative review. Anaesthesia. 2021;**76**(Suppl. 1):27-39. DOI: 10.1111/anae.15282

[40] Janev N, Ouanounou A. Local anesthetics in oral and maxillofacial medicine: Pharmacology, adverse effects, drug interactions and clinical manifestations. Journal of Oral and Maxillofacial Anesthesia. 2024;**3**:2. DOI: 10.21037/joma-23-27

[41] Rishiraj B, Epstein JB, Fine D, Nabi S, Wade NK. Permanent vision loss in one eye following administration of local anesthesia for a dental extraction. International Journal of Oral and Maxillofacial Surgery. 2005;**34**(2):220-223. DOI: 10.1016/j.ijom.2004.04.010

[42] Hillerup S, Jensen RH, Ersbøll BK. Trigeminal nerve injury associated with injection of local anesthetics: Needle lesion or neurotoxicity? Journal of the American Dental Association (1939). 2011;**142**(5):531-539. DOI: 10.14219/jada.archive.2011.0223

[43] Pogrel MA, Bryan J, Regezi J. Nerve damage associated with inferior alveolar nerve blocks. Journal of the American Dental Association (1939). 1995;**126**(8):1150-1155. DOI: 10.14219/jada.archive.1995.0336

[44] Alvites R, Rita Caseiro A, Santos Pedrosa S, Vieira Branquinho M, Ronchi G, Geuna S, et al. Peripheral nerve injury and axonotmesis: State of the art and recent advances. Cogent Medicine. 2018;**5**(1):1-45. DOI: 10.1080/2331205X.2018.1466404

[45] Aquilanti L, Mascitti M, Togni L, Contaldo M, Rappelli G, Santarelli A. A systematic review on nerve-related

adverse effects following mandibular nerve block anesthesia. International Journal of Environmental Research and Public Health. 2022;**19**(3):1627. DOI: 10.3390/ijerph19031627

[46] Jenyon T, Panthagani J, Green D. Transient facial nerve palsy following dental local anaesthesia. BML Case Reports. 2020;**13**(9):e234753. DOI: 10.1136/bcr-2020-234753

[47] Ghafoor H, Haroon S, Atique S, Ul Huda A, Ahmed O, Bel Khair AOM, et al. Neurological complications of local anesthesia in dentistry: A review. Cureus. 2023;**15**(12):e50790. DOI: 10.7759/cureus.50790

[48] Pogrel MA. Broken local anesthetic needles: A case series of 16 patients, with recommendations. Journal of the American Dental Association (1939). 2009;**140**(12):1517-1522. DOI: 10.14219/jada.archive.2009.0103

[49] Ferreira BB, Fernanda BL, Stabile GAV. Needle fracture during local anesthesia: How to proceed? International Journal of Clinical Dentistry. 2013;**6**:331-339

[50] Thompson M, Wright S, Cheng LH, Starr D. Locating broken dental needles. International Journal of Oral and Maxillofacial Surgery. 2003;**32**(6):642-644. DOI: 10.1054/ijom.2003.0430

[51] Armfield J. The avoidance and delaying of dental visits in Australia. Australian Dental Journal. 2012;**57**(2):243-247. DOI: 10.1111/j.1834-7819.2012.01697.x

[52] Abhavya J, Ramesh H, Karthyayani PS, Fathima SK, Priyal G, Sudhanshu J, et al. Trypanophobia among medical students - An overlooked concern. Clinical Epidemiology and Global Health. 2023;**20**:101257. ISSN 2213-3984. DOI: 10.1016/j.cegh.2023.101257

[53] Sreenivasagan S, Pendem S, Ravi P, Krishnakumar VB. To assess the prevalence of dental anxiety and assess the efficacy of vibraject and to assess prevalence of dental phobia. Dentistry. 2018;**5**:08. DOI: 10.4172/2161-1122.1000491

[54] Wong NSM, Yeung AWK, Li KY, McGrath CP, Leung Y. Non-pharmacological interventions for reducing fear and anxiety in patients undergoing third molar extraction under local anesthesia: Systematic review and meta-analysis. International Journal of Environmental Research and Public Health. 2022;**19**:11162. DOI: 10.3390/ijerph191811162

[55] Davis T III, Ollendick T. Empirically supported treatments for specific phobia in children: Do efficacious treatments address the components of a phobic response? Clinical Psychology: Science and Practice. 2005;**12**:144-160. DOI: 10.1093/clipsy/bpi018

[56] Parirokh M, Abbott PV. Present status and future directions—Mechanisms and management of local anaesthetic failures. International Endodontic Journal. 2022;**55**(Suppl. 4):951-994

[57] Gazal G, Omar E, Fareed WM, Alsharif A, Bahabri R. Impact of maxillary teeth morphology on the failure rate of local anesthesia. Saudi Journal of Anaesthesia. 2020;**14**(1):57-62. DOI: 10.4103/sja.SJA_542_19

[58] Bhalla VK, Taneja S, Chockattu SJ. Failure of molar anesthesia in endodontics: A systematic review. Saudi Endodontic Journal. 2021;**11**(3):283-291. DOI: 10.4103/sej.sej_152_20

[59] Boronat-López A, Peñarrocha-Diago M. Failure of locoregional anesthesia in dental practice. Review of the literature. Medicina Oral, Patología Oral y Cirugía Bucal. 2006;**11**:E510-E513

[60] Madan GA, Madan SG, Madan AD. Failure of inferior alveolar nerve block: Exploring the alternatives. Journal of the American Dental Association (1939). 2002;**133**(7):843-846. DOI: 10.14219/jada.archive.2002.0298

[61] Blanton PL, Jeske AH. ADA Council on scientific affairs; ADA division of science. Avoiding complications in local anesthesia induction: Anatomical considerations. Journal of the American Dental Association (1939). 2003;**134**(7):888-893. DOI: 10.14219/jada.archive.2003.0288

[62] Altuhafy M, Sodhi GS, Khan J. Efficacy of computer-controlled local anesthesia delivery system on pain in dental anesthesia: A systematic review of randomized clinical trials. Journal of Dental Anesthesia and Pain Medicine. 2024;**24**(4):245-264. DOI: 10.17245/jdapm.2024.24.4.245

[63] Meechan JG. Intraoral topical anesthesia. Periodontology 2000. 2008;**46**:1

[64] Franz-Montan M, Ribeiro LNM, Volpato MC, Cereda CMS, Groppo FC, Tofoli GR, et al. Recent advances and perspectives in topical oral anesthesia. Expert Opinion on Drug Delivery. 2017;**14**(5):673-684. DOI: 10.1080/17425247.2016.1227784

[65] Noev A, Kuznetsov N, Korenev G, Morozova N, Vasil'ev Y, Suvorov N, et al. A novel photoswitchable azobenzene-containing local anesthetic ethercaine with light-controlled biological activity in vivo. International Journal of Molecular Sciences. 2022;**23**(10):5352

[66] Tavares M, Goodson JM, Studen-Pavlovich D, Yagiela JA, Navalta LA, Rogy S, et al. Soft Tissue Anesthesia Reversal Group. Reversal of soft-tissue local anesthesia with phentolamine mesylate in pediatric patients. Journal of the American Dental Association. Aug 2008;**139**(8):1095-104. DOI: 10.14219/jada.archive.2008.0312. Erratum in: J Am Dent Assoc. 2008 Oct;139(10):1312. PMID: 18682624

Section 5

Thoracic Anesthesia

Chapter 7

Anesthetic Management of Bronchoscopic Lung Volume Reduction

Robert Owen

Abstract

Bronchoscopic lung volume reduction (BLVR) is a new and emerging technique for the symptomatic management of severe chronic obstructive pulmonary disease (COPD) with hyperinflation. Although this procedure carries significantly less morbidity and mortality compared to open lung volume reduction surgery, there are still significant risks, most notably the risk of pneumothorax. A thorough understanding of patient pathophysiology and procedural steps is vital for ensuring both a successful procedure and safe outcome. Careful attention must be paid towards ventilation strategy during Chartis measurement and valve deployment. Limiting absorptive atelectasis and avoiding sudden increases in airway pressures such as from coughing or bucking on extubation are vital steps to prevent pneumothorax. The implementation of a BLVR program requires a multidisciplinary team to prepare patients for the procedure, and carry them through safely to hospital discharge.

Keywords: COPD, bronchoscopic lung volume reduction, endobronchial valves, pneumothorax, Chartis

1. Introduction

Chronic obstructive pulmonary disease (COPD) remains a significant source of morbidity and mortality in the United States and across the world. In 2022, it was the sixth leading cause of death in the United States [1]. Emphysema, a subset of COPD, carries the hallmark of loss of pulmonary elasticity resulting in enlarged airspaces, outflow obstruction, and hyperinflation. Hyperinflation, in turn, leads to poor respiratory mechanics, increased intrathoracic pressure, parenchymal loss, worsening pulmonary hypertension, and ultimately reduced functional capacity and mortality.

2. Lung volume reduction

One management strategy for COPD with hyperinflation is lung volume reductions surgery (LVRS). The National Emphysema Treatment Trial (NETT) established the viability of LVRS in improving functional capacity [2]. Beyond this, however, NETT found a survival benefit in those patients with upper-lobe predominant emphysema and poor baseline exercise tolerance. LVRS, however, is an invasive surgery with significant morbidity and mortality. The 90-day mortality rate in NETTT following LVRS was 7.9%. Pulmonary morbidity was 30% and cardiovascular morbidity 20%. This unfavorable risk profile provided the impetus for innovation and achieving the physiologic conditions of LVRS without the high morbidity and mortality.

3. Bronchoscopic lung volume reduction

Bronchoscopic lung volume reduction (BLVR) is an innovative technique for achieving lung volume reduction without the risks of LVRS. There are three different bronchoscopic procedures performed to achieve lung volume reduction: endobronchial valve (EBV) placement, lung volume reduction coil (LVRC) placement, and bronchoscopic thermal vapor ablation (BTVA). The Global Initiative for Chronic Obstructive Lung Disease (GOLD) 2023 Report states "In select patients with advanced emphysema, bronchoscopic interventions reduce end-expiratory volume and improve exercise tolerance, health status and lung function at 6–12 months following treatment." [2]. EBVs receive a level of evidence A, whereas LVRC and BTVA both receive a level of evidence B. Ultimately, each of these modalities work to reduce hyperinflation. This in turn leads to improved ventilation/perfusion (V/Q) mismatch, decreased work of breathing, and improved quality of life.

3.1 Lung volume reduction coils

Lung volume reduction coils (LVRC) are nitinol coils placed within subsegmental airways. The nitinol material has memory-form properties that allow the coil to assume a pre-determined shape after deployment. The coils not only stent open small airways, thus allowing for exhalation, but also compress nearby lung parenchyma, leading to volume reduction. Currently, in the United States, PneumRx Inc. produces the RePneu® LVRC system (**Figure 1**) [3]. Compared to the thoroughly investigated EBV, LVRC may not only benefit patients with heterogeneous emphysema, but homogenous emphysema as well [4]. Similarly, LVRC may be used in patients with collateral ventilation, whereas EBV cannot. This unique property makes LVRC a viable alternative to patients who would benefit from lung volume reduction, however do not have a morphology or anatomy that lends itself to successful EBV placement.

3.2 Bronchoscopic thermal vapor ablation

Bronchoscopic thermal vapor ablation (BTVA) involves the administration of heated water vapor to airway segments to induce an inflammatory response leading to fibrosis and parenchymal loss. While it is less studied than other forms of BLVR, a 2023 meta-analysis including a combined total of 112 patients demonstrated significant improvements in lung function tests as well as quality of life, particularly in the first three months following BTVA [5]. Similar to EBV, BTVA is most useful in patients with upper-lobe predominant emphysema. Unlike EBV, however, BTVA effectiveness is not limited by the presence of collateral ventilation.

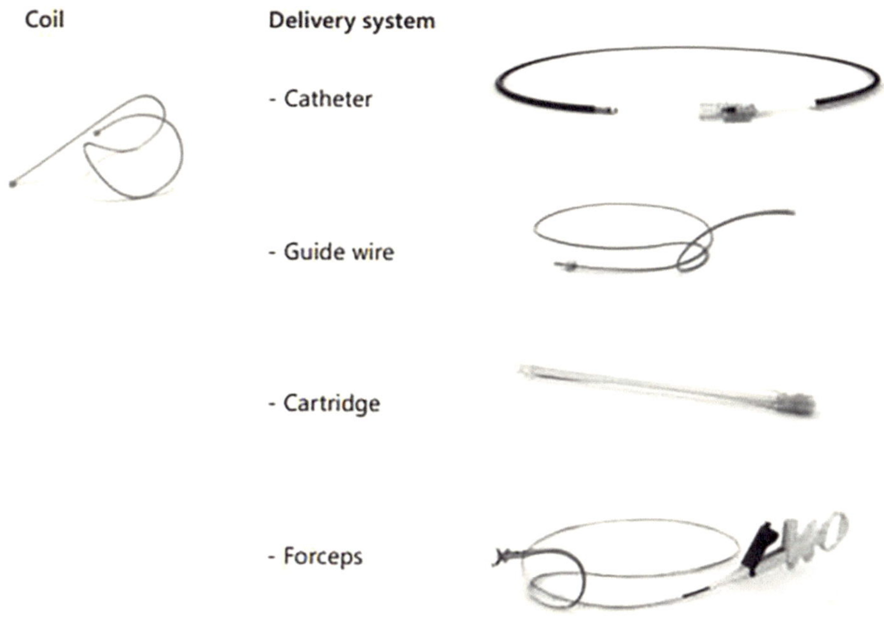

Figure 1.
RePneu® LVRC and delivery system [3].

3.3 Endobronchial valves

Endobronchial valves are one-way valves to allow egress of air from diseased lung segments, however prevent reinflation, leading to atelectasis. In the United States, two EBVs are approved by the FDA for BLVR: the Zephyr® valve by Pulmonx and the Spiration valve by Spiration (**Figure 2**) [6].

EBV, as might be suggested by their GOLD recommendations, seem to be the BLVR modality with the greatest quality of evidence. Indeed, a 2024 meta-analysis from Zhang et al. showed that compared to standard care as well as other BLVR modalities, EBV placement was the most effective at improving 6-minute walking distance (6MWD), forced-expiratory volume in 1 second (FEV1), and residual

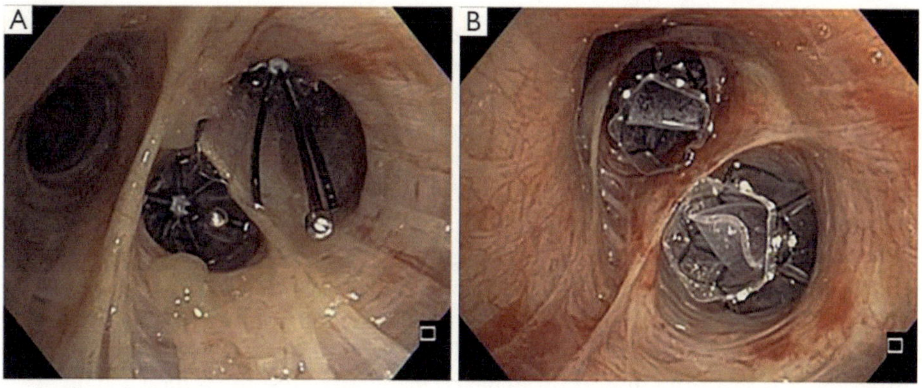

Figure 2.
Spiration valve. (A) and Zephyr® valve, and (B) [6].

volume (RV) at 6 and 12-month follow-up [7]. Given the strength of evidence behind this modality, the remainder of this chapter will focus on the EBV placement, with particular emphasis on anesthetic management.

3.3.1 Patient selection and preprocedural testing

Candidates for EBV placement are those with emphysema with hyperinflation who remain symptomatic despite optimal medical therapy. While no consensus regarding pulmonary function testing exists, Slebos et al. recommends a post-bronchodilator FEV1 15–50% of predicted value, total lung capacity (TLV) > 100% predicted, and RV > 175% predicted value [8]. The patient should demonstrate a reasonable period of reliable smoking cessation and a high resolution commuted tomography (CT) scan should demonstrate an absence of concomitant pulmonary pathology, particularly malignancy. Slebos et al. also recommend the following as exclusion criteria for EBV placement: pulmonary hypertension (pHTN) defined as a pulmonary artery systolic pressure (PASP) > 55 mmHg, hypoxemia defined as an arterial partial pressure of oxygen (PaO2) < 45 mmHg on room air, hypercarbia defined as an arterial partial pressure of carbon dioxide (PaCO2) > 60 mmHg on room air, or unstable cardiovascular disease [8]. It is important to note that clinical judgment still plays an important role in absence of consensus criteria.

The most critical factor in patient selection for EBV placement is the absence of collateral ventilation. Collateral ventilation can happen between adjacent alveoli (pores of Kohn), between bronchioles and alveoli (canals of Lambert) and between bronchioles (channels of Martin). A high resolution CT demonstrate intact pulmonary fissures is highly suggestive of absence of collateral ventilation. Lack of collateral ventilation is so critical to patient selection because EBVs work by precluding air entry into diseased lung segments. This process would be rendered useless in the presence of collateral ventilation.

In addition to the necessary imaging and laboratory testing to ensure a patient is an appropriate candidate, differential perfusion imaging or quantitative single photon emission CT (SPECT) in combination with traditional CT can help quantify blood flow to various lung segments. The goal of EBV placement should be to target the highest volume segments of lung that receive the least blood flow. This is done to optimize V/Q mismatch.

3.3.2 Procedural considerations

The anesthesiologist must be cognizant of the procedural steps to EBV placement as well as the potential complications. The primary complication of EBV placement is pneumothorax. The prevalence of pneumothorax following EBV placement is as high as 34%, with the majority developing within the first 72 hours following valve placement [9, 10]. Many aspects of anesthetic management will be geared towards minimizing the risk of pneumothorax.

The procedural steps are also of paramount importance to the anesthesiologist. The first of these is the exclusion of collateral ventilation using the Chartis measurement system. Despite pre-procedural imaging and testing suggesting a lack of collateral ventilation, some patients will still have prohibitory degrees of collateral ventilation, it is therefore important to perform one final test to exclude it. The Chartis measurement system consists of a catheter with a flow-meter at the tip as well as an occlusive balloon. The catheter is positioned within the bronchus of the target lobe (as determined by preoperative differential perfusion scan and/or SPECT with CT) and the balloon inflated to occlude flow into the target lobe. Expiratory flow is expected to decrease after several breaths. The failure of expiratory flow to decrease by an expected amount is indicative of prohibitive collateral ventilation. The Chartis measurement system is demonstrated in **Figure 3** [11].

Following Chartis measurement and confirmation of lack of collateral ventilation, the bronchus is measured for valve sizing. Subsequently the valve is deployed. Zephyr® valves accommodate bronchioles from 4.0–8.5 mm and have a low-profile option for shorter segment bronchioles. Spiration valves accommodate bronchioles from 4.75–8.75 mm. Following valve deployment, the valve can be observed for proper functioning. An example of a properly functioning valve can be seen in Video 1 (https://www.flexclip.com/share/6908880fa41a85b0b7e8689c6ac6fffcfef856e.html).

Following valve deployment, the risk of pneumothorax dramatically increases. This is due to atelectasis of excluded lung segments, with expansion of non-excluded segments with an accompanying rapid increase in airway pressures. Additionally, rapid expansion of can exceed pulmonary plasticity, resulting in bronchoalveolar fistula and resultant pneumothorax [9]. Any pre-existing pleural adhesions may also present anchoring points for parenchymal rupture when treated lung segments collapse, resulting in pneumothorax [9]. Finally, "trapped lung" or pneumothorax ex vacuo, similar to after thoracentesis, can also be a cause of pneumothorax following valve placement.

3.3.3 Anesthetic considerations

The overarching goals of the anesthesiologist during EBV placement are to allow adequate visualization for the proceduralist, avoid false-negatives on Chartis measurement, minimize the risk of pneumothorax, all while maintaining adequate oxygenation, ventilation, hemodynamics, and anesthetic depth.

To allow adequate visualization and working conditions, general endotracheal anesthesia with a large (8.0–8.5 mm) endotracheal tube should be used which will accommodate the bronchoscope. Induction of anesthesia should be dictated by the

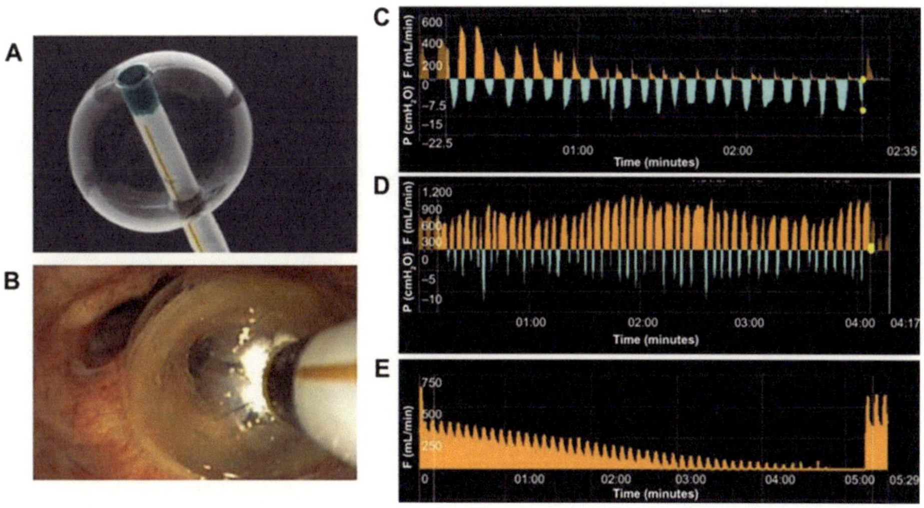

Figure 3.
Chartis measurement system: Panels A and B show the system hardware, while panels C-E show readouts of pressure and flow measurements [11].

patient's underlying cardiovascular comorbidities. In the absence of contraindication, muscle relaxation is useful in avoiding injury from unexpected patient movement or cough. Utilizing total intravenous anesthesia (TIVA) with propofol and remifentanil infusions for maintenance of general offers several benefits. Firstly, as propofol has less of an inhibitory effect on hypoxic pulmonary vasoconstriction (HPV), the hypoxemia that may result from shunt following alveolar collapse can be minimized. Remifentanil allows for adequate control of hemodynamics during a highly stimulating procedure with little to no postoperative pain. Additionally, both agents, but particularly remifentanil can facilitate a smooth and cough-free emergence and extubation. Avoidance of coughing and sudden increases in intrathoracic pressure are vital to the efforts of preventing pneumothorax. Small amounts of dexmedetomidine, intravenous lidocaine, as well as topicalization of the carina with lidocaine can further assist in this effort. Lastly, TIVA ensures continuous delivery of anesthetic agents in a shared airway procedure, while minimizing exposure to anesthetic gasses by procedural and operating room staff. If TIVA is to be utilized, one can consider processed electroencephalogram (EEG) monitoring to observe depth of anesthesia.

Ventilation strategy is a top priority in the formation of an anesthetic plan. Initially, a "lung-protective" ventilation strategy utilizing a tidal volume (TV) of 6–8 ml/kg of ideal body weight, while utilizing positive end-expiratory pressure (PEEP) to avoid atelectasis and minimize driving pressures is appropriate. During Chartis measurement, bronchial collapse can lead to false-negative readings, therefore increasing the PEEP to 10 mmHg is recommended to avoid this. During valve deployment, a lower TV and PEEP should be used to minimize risk of pneumothorax. As such, a TV of 4 ml/kg ideal body weight and a PEEP of 0 mmHg is utilized to mitigate the rapid increases in airway pressure.

Careful management of fraction of inspired oxygen (FiO_2) can also help minimize pneumothorax risk. Lentz et al. performed a small before-and-after cohort study observing the effects of a standard or protocolized minimal FiO_2 to maintain an oxygen saturation (SpO_2) >89%, where they demonstrated a reduction in pneumothorax rate from 31% in the standard FiO_2 group, to 7% in the reduced FiO_2 group [12]. The proposed theory behind this reduction is that the lower FiO_2, slows absorption atelectasis and prevents nitrogen washout in the treated lung, thus slowing the rate of airway pressure rise. Though small, this study provides some justification for a minimized FiO_2 approach particularly immediately before and during valve placement.

As mentioned, a cough-free emergence and extubation should be the goal in order to minimize sudden elevations in airway and intrathoracic pressure. Topicalization of the carina with local anesthetic can facilitate this. As can a slow, titrated emergence using a decreasing remifentanil infusion. Neuromuscular blockade should be completely reversed, utilizing quantitative train of four monitoring to ensure appropriate reversal. Surprisingly, some of these patients may already start to develop therapeutic atelectasis of treated lung segments with decreased hyperinflation by the time they are ready for extubation. Thus, their work of breathing may already be lessened.

3.3.4 Postprocedural considerations

Despite all preventative measures, pneumothoraxes still can occur. As such, equipment for emergent chest tube placement needs to be readily available in the bronchoscopy suite. Some institutions may find it helpful to gather all of these supplies into a "pneumothorax cart". This cart can remain either inside or immediately adjacent to

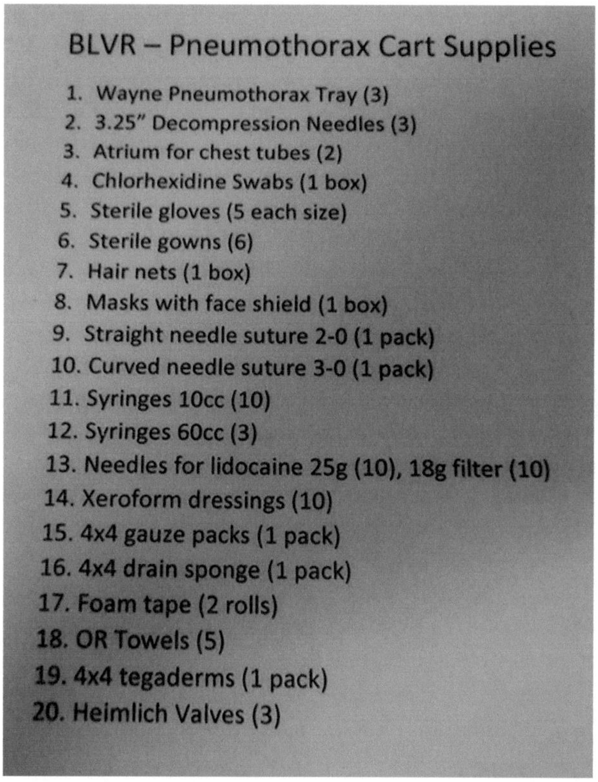
BLVR – Pneumothorax Cart Supplies

1. Wayne Pneumothorax Tray (3)
2. 3.25" Decompression Needles (3)
3. Atrium for chest tubes (2)
4. Chlorhexidine Swabs (1 box)
5. Sterile gloves (5 each size)
6. Sterile gowns (6)
7. Hair nets (1 box)
8. Masks with face shield (1 box)
9. Straight needle suture 2-0 (1 pack)
10. Curved needle suture 3-0 (1 pack)
11. Syringes 10cc (10)
12. Syringes 60cc (3)
13. Needles for lidocaine 25g (10), 18g filter (10)
14. Xeroform dressings (10)
15. 4x4 gauze packs (1 pack)
16. 4x4 drain sponge (1 pack)
17. Foam tape (2 rolls)
18. OR Towels (5)
19. 4x4 tegaderms (1 pack)
20. Heimlich Valves (3)

Figure 4.
Example supply list for BLVR pneumothorax cart.

the bronchoscopy suite. An example of a supply list for a pneumothorax cart can be seen in **Figure 4**. Given that the risk of pneumothorax remains high within the first 72 hours after valve deployment, it is recommended that this cart follow the patient throughout their hospital stay. The hospital stay should be for at least 72 hours after valve deployment, and should be extended if any pneumothorax occurs. Patients should be kept in a monitored setting such as a step-down unit or ICU for the duration of their stay. So that all staff members are aware of the risks for these patients, an identifying "pneumothorax risk" armband can be used, similar to allergy or fall risk armbands. A chest radiograph should be obtained after extubation, prior to leaving the procedural area. Serial radiographs should be obtained during the hospitalization. These films can not only monitor for developing pneumothorax but can also show progression of therapeutic atelectasis in treated lung segments.

Should a pneumothorax occur, its management will depend on its severity. All pneumothoraxes can be dangerous, and those patients who are candidates for EBV placement tend the be the ones who will tolerate a pneumothorax the least. However, small, asymptomatic pneumothoraxes, such as ex vacuo pneumothoraxes, do often occur and can be managed with more frequent radiographs and prolonged hospitalization. Any symptomatic pneumothorax, or small pneumothorax that progresses to become symptomatic should be managed with chest tube placement. In the event of hemodynamic instability suggestive of tension physiology, a chest tube must be immediately placed. If time nor appropriately trained personnel are available, needle decompression can be considered to temporize until definitive chest tube placement. If air leak persists following chest tube placement, additional measures such as a larger bore chest tube, addition of suction, or removal of 1–2 EBVs can be considered [9]. Surgery with pleurodesis remains an option in those patients with persistent air leak despite increasingly aggressive measures. If after successful chest tube placement, the patient experiences symptomatic relief and there is no air leak for >24 hours, with either stable or decreasing pneumothorax size on radiographs, chest tube removal can be considered.

3.4 Creating a BLVR program

When thinking of implementing a BLVR program at an institution, it is imperative to create a multidisciplinary team of stakeholders. In addition to pulmonologists performing the procedure, anesthesiologists, nursing, radiologists, critical care physicians, and thoracic surgeons should be included in the planning process. Protocols for preprocedural testing, procedural performance, anesthesia management, and postoperative care should be created. Particular attention should be paid to educating nursing staff on signs and symptoms of pneumothorax, as well as escalation plan for pneumothorax management. With appropriate team education and engagement from all interested parties, plans can be put in place to safely move patients through these life-changing procedures.

4. Conclusions

BLVR offers a less invasive alternative to traditional LVRS in patients with severe, symptomatic emphysema with hyperinflation. Different bronchoscopic procedures exist for lung volume reduction: EBV, LVRC, and BTVA. Of these, EBV is the most well-studied, but carries a high pneumothorax risk and requires an absence of collateral ventilation. As such, preprocedural testing to ensure patients are appropriate candidates for EBV placement is critical. Preprocedural imaging is also vital for planning anatomical targets for treatment. The anesthesiologist plays an invaluable role in safely moving patients through the procedure. Anesthetic management is geared towards the goals of providing adequate exposure, ensuring lack of false negatives during Chartis measurement, minimizing the risk of pneumothorax, and maintaining homeostasis. A detail-oriented approach to ventilatory management facilitates both in preventing false negatives in Chartis measurement, and in minimizing the risk of pneumothorax. Efforts to ensure smooth emergence and extubation pay huge dividends in minimizing pneumothorax risk. A TIVA utilizing propofol and remifentanil infusions offers several benefits to anesthesiologists. Awareness of pneumothorax risk and steps in management by all staff caring for EBV placement patients helps ensure patient safety. Protocols should be created for pneumothorax prevention and management. When creating a BLVR program, a multidisciplinary team of pulmonologists, anesthesiologists, critical care physicians, thoracic surgeons, radiologists, and nursing can ensure all interested parties are prepared to care for these complex and challenging patients.

Conflict of interest

The author declares no conflict of interest.

Author details

Robert Owen
MetroHealth Medical Center, Cleveland, OH, USA

*Address all correspondence to: rowen1@metrohealth.org

References

[1] Kochanek KD, Murphy SL, Xu JQ, Arias E. Mortality in the United States. In: NCHS Data Brief, no 492. Vol. 2024. Available from: https://www.cdc.gov/nchs/data/databriefs/db492-tables.pdf#4. Hyattsville, MD: National Center for Health Statistics; 2022. DOI: 10.15620/cdc:135850

[2] Fishman A, Martinez F, et al. A randomized control trial comparing lung volume-reduction surgery with medical therapy for severe emphysema. The New England Journal of Medicine. 2003;**348**:2059-2073. DOI: 10.1056/NEJMoa030287

[3] Klooster K, ten Hacken NHT, Franz I, Kerstjens HAM, van Rikxoort EM, Slebos D-J. Lung volume reduction coil treatment in chronic obstructive pulmonary disease patients with homogeneous emphysema: A prospective feasibility trial. Respiration. 2014;**88**(2):116-125. DOI: 10.1159/000362522

[4] Yildiz F. The efficacy of lung volume reduction coil treatment in patients with severe chronic obstructive pulmonary disease (COPD) type II respiratory failure. International Journal of Chronic Obstructive Pulmonary Disease. 2020;**15**:479-486. DOI: 10.2147/COPD.S218785

[5] Zhi L, Liao L, Wu Z, et al. Impact of bronchoscopic thermal vapor ablation on lung volume reduction in patients with emphysema: A meta-analysis. BMC Pulmonary Medicine. 2023;**23**:405. DOI: 10.1186/s12890-023-02689-w

[6] Kurman J, Hogarth D. Bronchoscopic lung volume reduction: Who, what, where, when? Shanghai Chest. 2021;**5**(29):3. DOI: 10.21037/shc-2019-ipab-15

[7] Zhang R, Zheng Z, Bian Y, Deng M, Herth FFJ, Hou G. Efficacy and safety of bronchoscopic lung volume reduction for chronic obstructive pulmonary disease: A systematic review and network meta-analysis. Expert Review of Respiratory Medicine. 2024;**18**(8):631-644. DOI: 10.1080/17476348.2024.2388293

[8] Slebos DJ, Shah PL, Herth FJ, Valipour A. Endobronchial valves for endoscopic lung volume reduction: Best practice recommendations from expert panel on endoscopic lung volume reduction. Respiration. 2017;**93**(2):138-150. DOI: 10.1159/000453588

[9] van Dijk M, Sue R, et al. Expert statement: Pneumothorax associated with one-way valve therapy for emphysema: 2020 update. Respiration. 2021;**100**(10):969-978. DOI: 10.1159/000516326

[10] Criner GJ, Sue R, Wright S, et al. A Multicenter randomized controlled trial of Zephyr endobronchial valve treatment in heterogeneous emphysema (LIBERATE). American Journal of Respiratory and Critical Care Medicine. 2018;**198**:1151-1164

[11] Koster D, Slebos D. The fissure: Interlobar collateral ventilation and implications for endoscopic therapy in emphysema. International Journal of Chronic Obstructive Pulmonary Disease. 2016;**11**:765. DOI: 10.2147/COPD.S103807

[12] Lentz RJ, Low SW, et al. Association between inspired oxygen fraction and pneumothorax after endobronchial valve placement for emphysema. Annals of the American Thoracic Society. 2023;**20**(6):926-929. DOI: 10.1513/AnnalsATS.202208-664RL

Section 6

Anesthesia in Ophthalmology

Chapter 8

Essentials of Ocular Anesthesia: Techniques, Indications, and Complications

Jatinder Bali and Ojasvini Bali

Abstract

Ocular anesthesia provides pain relief and immobilization of the eye while minimizing local and systemic complications in ocular surgery. This review discusses various types of anesthesia techniques including topical, regional (local), and general anesthesia, highlighting their indications, techniques, and potential complications in ocular surgery. Local anesthesia, encompassing topical drops, retrobulbar, peribulbar, and sub-Tenon's blocks, is the preferred choice for most intraocular surgeries due to its safety profile and efficacy. It is indicated where general anesthesia is unnecessary and patient cooperation is achievable, like cataract extraction, glaucoma surgeries, corneal transplantation, and retinal procedures. However, local anesthesia may be contraindicated in cases of known allergies, nystagmus, high myopia, staphyloma, enophthalmos, or when prolonged surgery duration is anticipated. Patient preparation, preoperative education, assessment of bleeding risks, and ocular anatomy is crucial to optimize outcomes and avoid complications like wrong-site surgery. Various anesthetic agents and adjuncts, like lignocaine, bupivacaine, hyaluronidase, epinephrine, and sodium bicarbonate, are utilized to achieve optimal anesthesia. The complications associated with ocular anesthesia range from transient visual impairment to serious events like brainstem anesthesia and retrobulbar hemorrhage. Understanding these risks and proper management strategies is essential for minimizing adverse outcomes. This review underscores the importance of tailored anesthesia choice based on individual patient characteristics and surgical requirements to ensure optimal surgical outcomes.

Keywords: ocular anesthesia, pain relief, topical anesthesia, regional anesthesia, general anesthesia, local anesthesia, intraocular surgery, complications

1. Introduction

Ocular surgery is performed under different types of anesthesia—topical, local, or general anesthesia. Local anesthesia is the most employed technique due to its safety profile and reduced dependence on the patient's general health. It is a simple to perform technique with a rapid onset of action and provides effective analgesia with low intraocular pressure and a dilated pupil even in patients with comorbidities.

This is very useful in resource-constrained developing countries with high volumes of cataract surgeries, such as India as it is more economical and makes daycare surgery possible for developing countries (**Table 1**) [1, 2].

1.1 History of anesthesia

The history of anesthesia dates back before the 1846 demonstration of the first ether anesthetic. There are several ancient texts which mention the use of pain-reducing substances in both the ancient as well as medieval literature. Ancient texts from China, India, and Arabia mention pain-reducing analgesic practices. European monks mentioned herbal drinks for painless healing. In the eighteenth century, a Japanese surgeon Seishu Hanaoka demonstrated a herbal anesthetic for painless surgery made from several alkaloidal substances [3, 4].

On 16 October 1846, William Morton and John Warren at Massachusetts General Hospital gave the first public demonstration of ether anesthesia. This is officially recorded as the beginning of anesthetic practice according to modern literature. The news of the painless removal of the lump under the jaw of Gilbert Abbott spread quickly, ether was used in Dumfries and London by 19 December 1846, and this reduced patient suffering significantly. Before ether, surgery was extremely painful and risky. The famous story of Robert Liston's surgery 1847 for bladder stone when the patient ran away and locked himself in a lavatory only to have the surgeon break

- Topical anaesthesia

Involves using eye drops for surface anesthesia (e.g., proparacaine 0.5%, xylocaine 2–4%). Commonly used for cataract surgery and minor ocular procedures. Benefits include avoiding needles and preserving patient cooperation. The downside is the lack of akinesia (inability to stop voluntary eye movement).

- Retrobulbar block

Involves injecting anesthetic into the muscle cone behind the eye. Indicated for most intraocular surgeries such as cataract extraction, glaucoma surgery, and retinal detachment surgery. Provides profound anesthesia and akinesia, but carries risks like globe perforation and optic nerve injury.

- Peribulbar block

Involves injecting anesthetic around the orbit, outside the muscle cone. Used for similar indications as the retrobulbar block, but with fewer complications. Requires a larger volume of anesthetic, which can increase the risk of brainstem anesthesia. Sub-Tenon's Block

- Anesthetic is injected under Tenon's capsule around the sclera.
- Suitable for surgeries requiring both anesthesia and akinesia. It has lower complication rates than needle-based techniques but requires surgical tools and skills. Subconjunctival hemorrhage is a common complication.
- Intracameral anesthetic mydriatic (ICAM)

Delivery of the anesthetic agent in the anterior chamber. Preservative free drug used. Used mainly as an adjunct for supplementing topical anesthesia and mydriasis. Reduces the intraoperative pain but no effect on postoperative pain and discomfort.

- General anaesthesia

Involves inducing unconsciousness and complete muscle relaxation. Reserved for patients who are uncooperative, children, or those undergoing major surgeries. Offers full anesthesia and akinesia but has increased systemic risks and requires airway management

Table 1.
Common types of ocular anaesthesia.

down the door and complete the surgery after securing the patient once again has been documented. Liston was one of the early users of this innovation. In November 1847, James Simpson introduced chloroform in Edinburgh. Although more potent, chloroform had severe side effects, including sudden death and liver damage, but was easier to use and became popular [4].

Over the next four decades, many anesthetic agents were introduced, but few endured. In 1877, cocaine was introduced for local anesthesia, followed by local infiltration, nerve blocks, and spinal and epidural anesthesia. These methods improved surgical conditions by reducing the depth of anesthesia needed. Newer surgical procedures could be attempted. The 1910s and 1920s were decades of advancements in airway control with tracheal tubes and intravenous induction agents like barbiturates. The 1940s introduced muscle relaxants, starting with curare, first used in Montreal in 1943 and in the UK in 1946. Halothane, introduced in the mid-1950s, improved inhalational anesthesia with easier use.

Today, anesthesia is highly advanced, with less toxic and more effective agents. Anesthetists are involved in preoperative care, intensive care, obstetrics, emergency medicine, and pain management. Anesthesia is very safe in high-income countries, with a mortality rate under 1 in 250,000, and continues to evolve with ongoing advancements (**Figure 1**) [1, 4].

1.2 Ophthalmology and anesthesia

In ophthalmology, the ancient Indian text composed in 800 BC and covering practices dating from 3000 BC when the earliest instruments are uncovered, Susruta Samhita gives reference of anesthesia in ocular surgeries, including some inhalational techniques. Around the same time, the Egyptian surgeons employed carotid compression to temporarily reduce blood flow and minimize pain during eye procedures. Karl Koller pioneered the use of cocaine for ocular surgery in 1884, the same year Herman Knapp utilized it for retrobulbar block. Later, in 1914, van Lint achieved orbicularis akinesia through local injection [4, 5].

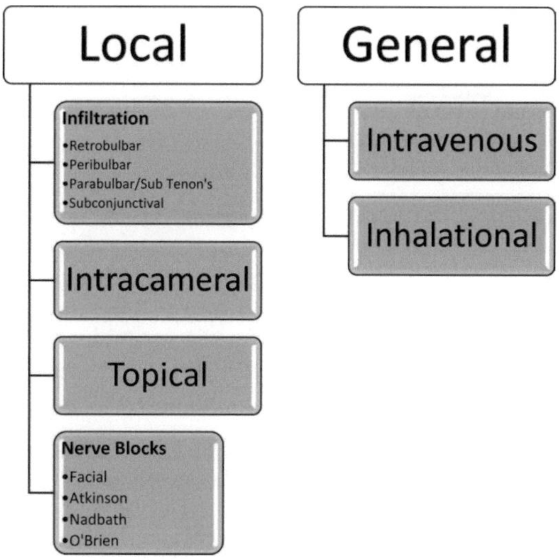

Figure 1.
Types of ocular anesthesia.

2. Regional (local) anesthesia

2.1 Indications

Local anesthesia is suitable for almost all ocular surgeries in adults. These include:

- Cataract extraction
- Glaucoma surgery
- Keratoplasty (corneal transplantation)
- Other corneal surgeries
- Iridectomy
- Squint surgery
- Retinal detachment surgery.

Almost all intraocular surgeries can be performed under regional anesthesia, including cataract extraction, corneal transplantation, glaucoma surgeries, vitreoretinal surgeries, scleral buckling, strabismus repair, and enucleation [5, 6]. Local ocular anesthesia is indicated in surgeries where general anesthesia is not required and where patient cooperation is essential. However, it is not possible if the patient cannot lie still and in paediatric cases where general anesthesia should be preferred (**Table 2**).

2.2 Goals

The primary goals of regional anesthesia for successful ocular surgery are as follows (**Table 3**).

1. Globe and conjunctival anesthesia
2. Orbicularis muscle akinesia
3. Ocular akinesia
4. Low intraocular and intraorbital pressure.

Indications for ocular anaesthesia
Includes cataract surgery, glaucoma surgery, corneal transplantation, retinal detachment surgery, strabismus repair, vitreoretinal surgeries, scleral buckling, and minor ocular procedures (e.g., iridectomy, pterygium surgery).
Absolute contraindications
Confirmed allergy to local anesthetic agents and nystagmus.
Relative contraindications
High myopia (long axial length), staphyloma (weak spot in the eye wall), enophthalmos (deep-set eyes), extended duration of surgery, uncooperative patients, children, and those with uncontrollable neurological movements. General Anesthesia may be considered in these cases

Table 2.
Indications and contraindications for ocular anaesthesia.

- Common anesthetic agent preparations

  Lignocaine (rapid onset, short duration), Bupivacaine (long duration), Hyaluronidase (enhances diffusion), Epinephrine (increases intensity and duration, reduces bleeding).

- Topical anesthesia technique

  Administered through eye drops; suitable for minor surgeries and cataract surgeries. Advantageous as it avoids needles and maintains patient cooperation but does not provide akinesia.

- Retrobulbar block technique

  Involves inserting a needle into the muscle cone; provides profound Anesthesia and akinesia. Risks include globe perforation, optic nerve injury, and retrobulbar hemorrhage.

- Peribulbar Block Technique

  Injection is made outside the muscle cone with a shorter needle; requires a larger volume of anesthetic. Benefits include a reduced risk of globe penetration but risks brainstem Anesthesia due to the larger volume required.

- Subconjunctival Anesthesia Techniques

  Anterior Subconjunctival: 1.5–2 mL,Anterior Subconjunctival, Used for Pterygium and glaucoma Surgery, Supplemented by Intracameral anesthetic and mydriatic (for MSICS) Manual Small Incision Cataract Surgery Advanced Subconjunctival (ASCAN): Up to 10 mL, 2% plain lignocaine or 50/50 mix with 0.5% bupivacaine with hyaluronidase (30 IU/mL), Upper outer quadrant of the eye into sub-Tenon's space

- Sub-Tenon's Block Technique

  Anesthesia delivered under Tenon's capsule; requires surgical tools and skills. Has a lower risk of complications compared to needle-based techniques, though it may cause subconjunctival hemorrhage.

- General Anesthesia Technique

  Suitable for patients who are uncooperative or those undergoing complex or prolonged surgeries. It offers comprehensive Anesthesia but carries higher systemic risks and potential ocular complications from intubation.

Table 3.
Anesthetic agents and techniques.

Transient Decrease in Visual Acuity
Temporary vision loss potentially due to optic nerve blockade or ischemia. Management includes reassuring the patient and providing supportive care.
Globe Penetration
Accidental puncture of the globe during needle-based anesthesia techniques. Immediate management involves stopping the injection and seeking ophthalmologic evaluation.
Optic Nerve Injury
Direct trauma to the optic nerve, particularly associated with retrobulbar blocks. To prevent, avoid deep needle insertion and monitor the patient's vision closely. Prompt ophthalmologic care is essential.
Retrobulbar Hemorrhage
Bleeding behind the eye that can increase intraocular pressure. Management includes monitoring intraocular pressure and, if necessary, surgical decompression to alleviate pressure.
Brainstem Anesthesia
Caused by the spread of anesthesia to the brainstem, leading to respiratory or cardiovascular symptoms. Management involves providing supportive care and stabilizing the patient's respiration and cardiovascular function.
Diplopia
Double vision resulting from injury to the extraocular muscles. It is typically observed postoperatively and may require surgical correction if persistent. Oculocardiac Reflex
Triggered by manipulation of the eye or its structures, leading to bradycardia or arrhythmias. Managed by monitoring the patient's cardiac rhythm and, if necessary, administering anticholinergic medications.
Subconjunctival Hemorrhage
Bleeding under the conjunctiva, commonly occurring with the sub-Tenon's block. Generally self-limiting and does not require specific treatment.

Table 4.
Complications and management of ocular anaesthesia.

These goals can be achieved through various local anesthesia techniques, including surface anesthesia, facial nerve block, and retrobulbar block. A combination of surface anesthesia and peribulbar block is also effective (**Table 4**) [5, 6].

3. Types of local anesthesia techniques

3.1 Surface (topical) anesthesia

Surface anesthesia is achieved by topical instillation of anesthetic solutions such as:

- 2 to 4% xylocaine/lignocaine
- 1% amethocaine
- 0.5% proparacaine (most preferred).

Typically, a drop of anesthetic solution is instilled every 4 minutes, four times, to achieve sufficient conjunctival and corneal anesthesia. Cataract surgery by phacoemulsification can often be performed with topical anesthesia alone. This is used primarily for cataract surgery. It is advantageous because it does not impair vision and avoids the use of needles. However, it does not provide ocular akinesia (immobility of the eye), and patient selection is critical [6, 7].

3.2 Facial nerve block

For intraocular surgery, it is important to block the facial nerve, which supplies the orbicularis oculi muscle. This prevents the patient from squeezing their eyelids during surgery. There are several methods to achieve orbicularis akinesia:

3.2.1 Van lint block

This technique blocks the terminal branches of the facial nerve, resulting in localized akinesia of the orbicularis oculi muscle without facial paralysis. The anesthetic is injected in deeper tissues above the eyebrow and below the inferior orbital margin, through a point about 2 cm behind the lateral orbital margin (**Figure 2**).

3.2.2 O'Brien block

The facial nerve is blocked at the neck of the mandible, near the condyloid process. The needle is inserted until it contacts the periosteum, and then 4 to 6 ml of anesthetic is injected while withdrawing the needle. This method can cause pain and unwanted facial paralysis.

3.2.3 Nadbath block

In this technique, the facial nerve is blocked as it exits the skull through the stylomastoid foramen. This block can also be painful.

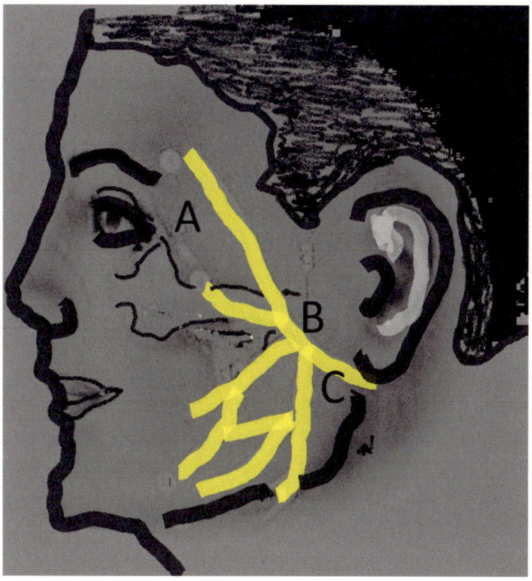

Figure 2.
Facial blocks. A. Van Lint B. Atkinson C. Nadbath.

3.2.4 Atkinson block

This involves blocking the superior branches of the facial nerve by injecting anesthetic at the inferior margin of the zygomatic bone [5, 6, 8].

3.3 Retrobulbar block

The retrobulbar block, introduced by Herman Knapp in 1884, involves injecting 1.5–2 ml of anesthetic solution (2% xylocaine with added hyaluronidase 5 IU/ml, with or without adrenaline) into the muscle cone behind the eye. The injection is administered through the inferior fornix or the skin of the lower eyelid, with the eye in a primary gaze. The needle is directed straight back, then slightly upward, and inward towards the apex of the orbit, to a depth of 2.5 to 3 cm. This block anesthetizes the ciliary nerves, ciliary ganglion, and the third and sixth cranial nerves, providing globe akinesia, anesthesia, and analgesia. The fourth cranial nerve, which is outside the muscle cone, is usually not affected.

Complications of the retrobulbar block can include retrobulbar hemorrhage, globe perforation, optic nerve injury, and extraocular muscle palsies (**Figure 3**) [5, 6, 8].

3.4 Peribulbar block

The peribulbar block, described by Davis and Mandel in 1986, has largely replaced the combination of retrobulbar and facial blocks due to its fewer complications and the absence of a need for a separate facial block. This technique involves injecting 6 to 10 ml of local anesthetic solution into the peripheral space of the orbit, from where it diffuses into the muscle cone and eyelids, providing globe and orbicularis akinesia and anesthesia.

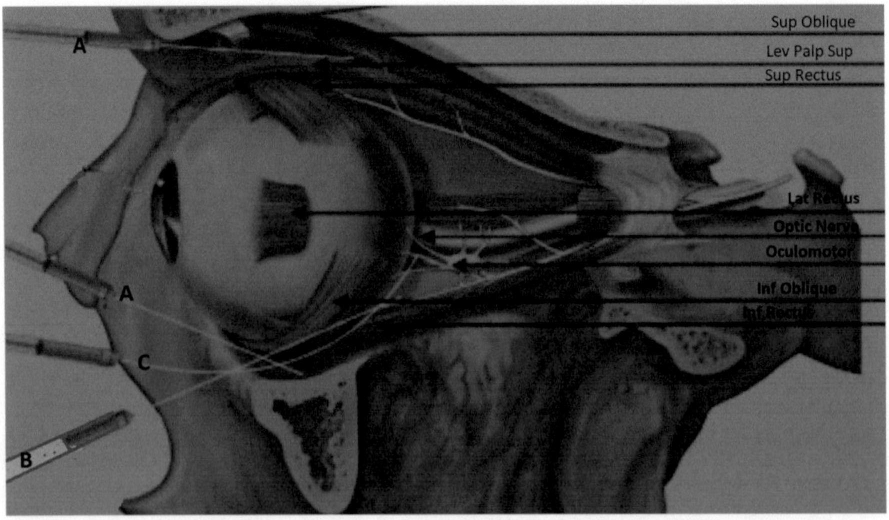

Figure 3.
Infiltration blocks (schematic). Legend: A. Peribulbar B. Parabulbar/Subtenon's C. Retrobulbar.

The block is usually administered via two injections:

1. Through the upper lid (at the junction of the medial one-third and lateral two-thirds)

2. Through the lower lid (at the junction of the lateral one-third and medial two-thirds).

After injection, orbital compression is applied for 10 to 15 minutes. The anesthetic solution used for peribulbar anesthesia consists of a mixture of 2% lignocaine and 0.5 to 0.75% bupivacaine (in a 2:1 ratio), with hyaluronidase 5 IU/ml and adrenaline [5, 6, 8, 9].

3.5 Sub-Tenon's block

Administered by injecting anesthetic under Tenon's capsule using a special blunt cannula, creating a space around the sclera. This technique is associated with fewer complications and provides adequate anesthesia for most ocular surgeries [5, 6, 10].

3.6 Subconjunctival anesthesia

The anterior subconjunctival approach uses a combination of 1.5–2 milliliters of anesthetic mixture given subconjunctivally and supplemented with commercially available intracameral anesthetic and mydriatic for manual small incision cataract surgery and without ICAM for pterygium surgery [11]. Another method called advanced subconjunctival anesthesia (ASCAN) technique involves inserting a 25-gauge, 16 mm needle through the conjunctiva and Tenon's capsule in the upper outer quadrant of the eye. The anesthetic used is either 2% plain lignocaine or a 50/50 mix with 0.5% bupivacaine, combined with hyaluronidase (30 IU/mL). Up to 10 mL of this solution is injected posteriorly into the sub-Tenon's space [12].

3.7 Intracameral anesthesia

Intracameral anesthesia is a technique where anesthetic agents are injected directly into the anterior chamber of the eye. This method is becoming increasingly popular in cataract surgery, and often a mixture of lignocaine (0.5–1.0%) with pupil dilating agents like tropicamide injection 0.02% and phenylephrine 0.31% is used as an adjunct to surface or topical anesthesia. The main advantage of intracameral anesthesia is its ease of application through a preexisting corneal wound. Research comparing various local anesthesia techniques for phacoemulsification shows that combining topical anesthesia with intracameral lidocaine (0.5 to 1%) is generally more effective in reducing intraoperative pain compared to topical anesthesia alone [13, 14]. However, evidence is mixed regarding its impact on postoperative pain. Studies show no significant difference in postoperative pain levels between the two methods [13, 15]. Additionally, there is limited information on how intracameral anesthesia affects participant satisfaction, with one small study indicating no substantial difference [13, 16]. Regarding the need for additional intraoperative anesthesia, data is inconclusive, and no significant difference was found in a meta-analysis [13]. Intracameral lidocaine supplementation did not increase the risk of intraocular toxicity or loss of corneal endothelial cells according to the evidence available [13, 16]. However, the evidence on intraoperative adverse events is limited and needs to be interpreted with caution. The surgeon satisfaction scores improved with the use of intracameral anesthesia [13, 16].

In summary, intracameral anesthesia with lidocaine reduces intraoperative pain during cataract surgery more effectively than topical anesthesia alone, but its impact on postoperative pain and participant satisfaction remains unclear [13, 14]. The method does not seem to affect the risk of complications or toxicity significantly [13, 17].

3.8 Contraindications

3.8.1 Absolute contraindications

- Confirmed allergy to the anesthetic agent.
- Nystagmus (uncontrolled eye movement).
- Contraindications specific to the surgery being performed.

3.8.2 Relative contraindications

- High myopia (long eye in the anterior-posterior axis).
- Staphyloma (protrusion of the eye wall at a weak spot).
- Enophthalmos (deep-set eyes).
- Expected prolonged duration of surgery.
- Patients unable to cooperate, such as children, those with neurological disorders, or uncooperative adults [5, 6, 8].

4. General anesthesia

4.1 Indications

General anesthesia is indicated for:

- Infants and children
- Anxious or uncooperative adults
- Mentally retarded adults
- Cases of perforating ocular injuries
- Major surgeries, such as exenteration
- Patients who prefer or require general anesthesia.

4.2 Considerations

During ocular surgery under general anesthesia, the use of muscle relaxants, endotracheal intubation, and controlled respiration is preferred. Care must be taken to avoid carbon dioxide retention, which can cause choroidal swelling and prolapse of ocular contents when the eye is opened. Agents that do not raise the intraocular pressure should be preferred in perforating eye injuries. This technique is reserved for patients who are unable to cooperate, such as children or those with uncontrollable movements. This carries its own risks and requires careful management, particularly concerning the avoidance of intraocular pressure increases [5, 6, 8].

5. Patient preparation

5.1 Education

"The more you sweat in training, the less you bleed in war," is a famous idiom which holds true even in preparation for surgery. Educating the patient about what to expect during surgery is crucial to reduce anxiety and enhance patient cooperation.

5.2 Preoperative assessment

A thorough preoperative assessment should be performed, including:

- Inquiry about bleeding disorders and medications such as anticoagulants or antiplatelet agents. Anticoagulant therapy can often be continued if within therapeutic ranges.
- Measuring the axial length of the eye to assess the risk for complications, especially when considering retrobulbar anesthesia.

5.3 Avoidance of wrong site surgery

To prevent wrong-site surgery, the operative eye should be clearly marked on the day of surgery [4, 5, 6, 8, 14].

6. Anesthetic agents

The choice of anesthetic agents and their combinations is crucial for effective anesthesia:

- Lidocaine and Bupivacaine: Lidocaine provides rapid onset of action, while bupivacaine offers a longer duration of anesthesia.
- Hyaluronidase: Enhances diffusion of the anesthetic, leading to more rapid and complete anesthesia.
- Epinephrine: Increases the intensity of anesthesia, reduces bleeding, and slows systemic uptake. However, it may cause retinal ischemia and should be avoided in patients with cerebrovascular diseases.
- Sodium Bicarbonate: Adjusts the pH of the anesthetic solution to enhance diffusion of the anesthetic agent [5, 6, 8, 13].

7. Complications and management

7.1 Transient decrease in visual acuity

Due to optic nerve blockade or ischemia, patients should be informed about this potential to reduce anxiety during surgery.

7.2 Permanent vision loss

From globe penetration, optic nerve trauma, or central retinal artery occlusion.

7.3 Brainstem anesthesia

A serious complication characterized by symptoms such as respiratory difficulty, hypertension, and unconsciousness. Such patients should be intubated and given sedation, supportive ventilation, vasoactive support, oxygen, and fluid replacement.

7.4 Diplopia

Caused by injury to extraocular muscles, typically from improper injection technique.

7.5 Oculocardiac reflex

May cause cardiac arrhythmias during ocular surgery. Prophylactic anticholinergics like atropine have been used, although their effectiveness varies.

7.6 Retrobulbar haemorrhage

Rapid orbital swelling due to arterial hemorrhage requires monitoring and may necessitate surgical intervention if intraocular pressure rises significantly [5, 6, 8].

8. Conclusion

Local anesthesia remains the preferred method for most ocular surgeries due to its safety, efficacy, and cost-effectiveness. Proper technique, patient selection, and awareness of potential complications are essential for successful outcomes in ocular anesthesia.

Acknowledgements

We extend our sincere gratitude to Nandan Bali, Dr. Amulya Sahu, Dr. BK Nayak, Dr. Anil Tanwar, and Dr. Naveen Neeraj for their invaluable support and contributions to the development of this chapter. Their expertize and insights have significantly enriched the content and enhanced the quality of this work. We are deeply appreciative of their collaboration throughout the writing process.

Conflict of interest

The authors declare no conflict of interest.

Author details

Jatinder Bali[1]* and Ojasvini Bali[2]

1 NBEMS Course Coordinator, Hindu Rao Hospital and NDMC Medical College, New Delhi, India

2 Department of Pediatrics, All India Institute of Medical Sciences, New Delhi, India

*Address all correspondence to: drbaliacademia@gmail.com

References

[1] Kelly DJ, Farrell SM. Physiology and role of intraocular pressure in contemporary anesthesia. Anesthesia and Analgesia. 2018;**126**(5):1551-1562

[2] Lee LA, Posner KL, Cheney FW, Caplan RA, Domino KB. Complications associated with eye blocks and peripheral nerve blocks: An American society of anaesthesiologists closed claims analysis. Regional Anesthesia and Pain Medicine. 2008;**33**(5):416-422

[3] Matioc AA. An Anesthesiologist's perspective on the history of basic airway management: The "artisanal anesthetic" era: 1846 to 1904. Anesthesiology. 2017;**126**:394-408. DOI: 10.1097/ALN.0000000000001508

[4] Wilkinson D. History of Anaesthesia: A Personal View. World Federation of Societies of Anaesthesiologists. WFSA; 2024. Available from: https://wfsahq.org/about/history/history-of-anaesthesia/

[5] Johnson RW. History of ophthalmic anaesthesia. In: Kumar C, Dodds C, Gayer S, editors. Ophthalmic Anaesthesia, Oxford Specialist Handbooks. 2012; online ed. Oxford: Oxford Academic; 2012. DOI: 10.1093/med/9780199591398.003.0010 [Accessed: August 26, 2024]

[6] Friedman DS, Reeves SW, Bass EB, Lubomski LH, Fleisher LA, Schein OD. Patient preferences for anaesthesia management during cataract surgery. The British Journal of Ophthalmology. 2004;**88**:333-335

[7] Assia EI, Pras E, Yehezkel M, Rotenstreich Y, Jager-Roshu S. Topical anesthesia using lidocaine gel for cataract surgery. Journal of Cataract and Refractive Surgery. 1999;**25**:635-639

[8] Mather SJ, Kong KL, Vohra SB. Loco-regional anaesthesia for ocular surgery. Anticoagulant and antiplatelet drugs. Current Anaesthesia and Critical Care. 2010;**21**:158-163

[9] Davis DB II, Mandel MR. Posterior peribulbar anesthesia: An alternative to retrobulbar anesthesia. Journal of Cataract and Refractive Surgery. 1986;**12**:182-184

[10] Hansen EA, Mein CE, Mazzoli R. Ocular anesthesia for cataract surgery: A direct sub-Tenon's approach. Ophthalmic Surgery. 1990;**21**:696-699

[11] Dev S, Bali J, Narang S, Miglani S, Arneja J. Minimal anesthetic manual small-incision cataract surgery (MSICS): A novel technique in use for anesthesia in MSICS. Indian Journal of Ophthalmology. 2022;**70**(11):4029-4031. DOI: 10.4103/ijo.IJO_1335_22

[12] Wu S, Tang KC. Advanced subconjunctival anesthesia for cataract surgery. Asia-Pacific Journal of Ophthalmology (Philadelphia, PA.). 2018;7(5):296-300. DOI: 10.22608/APO.2018231. Epub 2018 Sep 28

[13] Minakaran N, Ezra DG, Allan BD. Topical anaesthesia plus intracameral lidocaine versus topical anaesthesia alone for phacoemulsification cataract surgery in adults. Cochrane Database of Systematic Reviews. Vol. 2020, Issue 7. London, UK: World Federation of Societies of Anaesthesiologists (WFSA); 2020

[14] Gills JP, Cherchio M, Raanan MG. Unpreserved lidocaine to control discomfort during cataract surgery using topical anesthesia. Journal of Cataract and Refractive Surgery.

1997;**23**(4):545-550. DOI: 10.1016/s0886-3350(97)80211-8

[15] Joshi R. A single drop of 0.5% proparacaine hydrochloride for uncomplicated clear corneal phacoemulsification. Middle East African Journal of Ophthalmology. 2013;**20**(3):221

[16] Carino NS, Slomovic AR, Chung F, Marcovich AL. Topical tetracaine versus topical tetracaine plus intracameral lidocaine for cataract surgery. Journal of Cataract & Refractive Surgery. 1998;**24**(12):1602-1608

[17] Ghai AK, Bali J, Sethi N, Rajaure S, Sarkar S. Cardiovascular effects of diluted intracameral combination of 0.02% tropicamide, 0.31% phenylephrine, and 1% lidocaine during phacoemulsication to manage intraoperative miosis. Taiwan Journal of Ophthalmology. 2024;**14**:242-247

Section 7

Regional Anesthesia

Chapter 9

Fascial Plane Blocks

Mohammed Khamis

Abstract

Fascial plane blocks have been widely introduced as a competitive alternative to paravertebral, epidural, and perineural blocks. They represent a paradigm shift as they do not require visualization of the nerves or injection of local anesthetic close to the nerves. However, there are a number of controversial issues surrounding these new blocks, including their efficacy, evidence, indication, and technique. This has not diminished their popularity or their acceptance into protocols, guidelines, and clinical practice. Although they undoubtedly have a role to play in modern anesthesia, a deeper understanding of fascia is required to improve outcomes.

Keywords: regional anesthesia, local anesthetic drugs, fascial plane block, ultrasound, pain management

1. Introduction

Fascial plane blocks (FPBs) are regional anesthesia techniques that involve injecting local anesthetic into the space ("plane") between two distinct fascial layers. Local anesthetic spread to nerves passing within this plane and adjacent tissues to achieve analgesia. Fascia, in this context, is defined as a sheet of connective tissue that surrounds or separates muscles and surrounding organs. Fascia is mainly composed of collagen fibers filled with a hydrated matrix of glycosaminoglycan and infiltrated by fibroblasts and adipocytes. The interfacial plane contains the fat-glycosaminoglycan complex and provides gliding and cushioning between structures and a pathway for nerves and vessels. These planes are popular targets for ultrasound-guided local anesthetic injection between the muscle layers of the thoracic, abdominal, and paraspinal regions close to the paravertebral space and vertebral canal. The relevant musculofascial anatomy of these regions, together with the nerves involved in visceral and somatic innervation, is a must. This knowledge will assist in sonographic landmark recognition and block performance, as well as knowledge of possible pathways and obstacles for local anesthetic spread. It is also essential for the further development and refinement of FPBs, with a focus on improving their safety, efficacy, and clinical utility [1].

2. Anatomical and physiological considerations

There are two types of fascia: superficial, which is located between the skin and muscle (not the area of our interest), and deep fascia, which – as mentioned above – is a complex fibrous-collagenous connective tissue that surrounds muscles.

Depending on the thickness, deep fascia is subdivided into two types: epimysial and aponeurotic. Epimysial fascia is thinner (150–200 μm), localized to the muscle, and attached to it via tiny fibrous septa and can be identified in pectoralis and latissimus muscles. Conversely, aponeurotic fascia is thicker (600–1400 μm), may enclose more than one muscle, and is less firmly attached to muscles such as thoracolumbar fascia and rectus sheath [2].

3. Sites of the block

Fascial blocks can be performed in the abdominal wall (Transversus abdominis plane (TAP) block-Rectus sheath block-Quadratus lamborum (QL) block – External oblique intercostal block) and thoracic region (Erector spinae block-Pectoral nerve (Pecs) block – serratus block) as well as lower limb (fascial iliaca block).

3.1 TAP block

Since first described by Rafi et al. [3] and McDonnell et al. [4], the TAP block is a widely used block to provide analgesia to the lower and lateral abdominal wall, where local anesthetic is delivered in the neurovascular plane between the internal oblique and transversus abdominis muscles.

Anatomy: The lateral part of the abdominal wall includes the following muscles.

The external oblique muscle takes its origin from the lower eight ribs and runs downwards to be inserted in the iliac crest. The fibers arising from the upper and middle ribs run infero-anteriorly and join a thick aponeurosis, which anteriorly joins the aponeurosis from the transversus abdominis and internal oblique muscles, forming the linea alba.

The internal oblique muscle is deeper and originates from the inguinal ligament and the iliac crest. It is inserted into the linea alba and the lower six costal cartilage.

The transversus abdominis muscle fibers arise from, the iliac crest, the lumbodorsal fascia, and the inner surfaces of lower six costal cartilage and inguinal ligament. It runs transversely across the abdomen and inserts into the linea alba (**Figure 1**).

3.1.1 Sensory innervation of the abdominal wall

Thoracic nerves T6–T11 which passes along their corresponding intercostal space, then crosses under the costal cartilages entering into the fascial plane between transversus abdominis muscle and internal oblique muscle.

Thoracic nerve 12. It runs anteriorly, crossing the lumbocostal arch to run along with the other lower intercostal nerves between the transversus abdominis muscle and the external oblique muscle.

Ilioinguinal and iliohypogastric nerves (T12/L1) both are branches from the lumbar plexus and enter the transverse abdominis plane near to the iliac crest.

3.1.2 Indications for tap block

TAP block is indicated for surgeries at the level of or below umbilicus (uppermost sensory levels around T9/10). This level of the block is supported by findings in a cadaveric study that observed the spread of local anesthetic following a single posterior TAP injection [5]. So, TAP block can be used in cesarean section, abdominal hysterectomy, open appendectomy, and inguinal hernia repair.

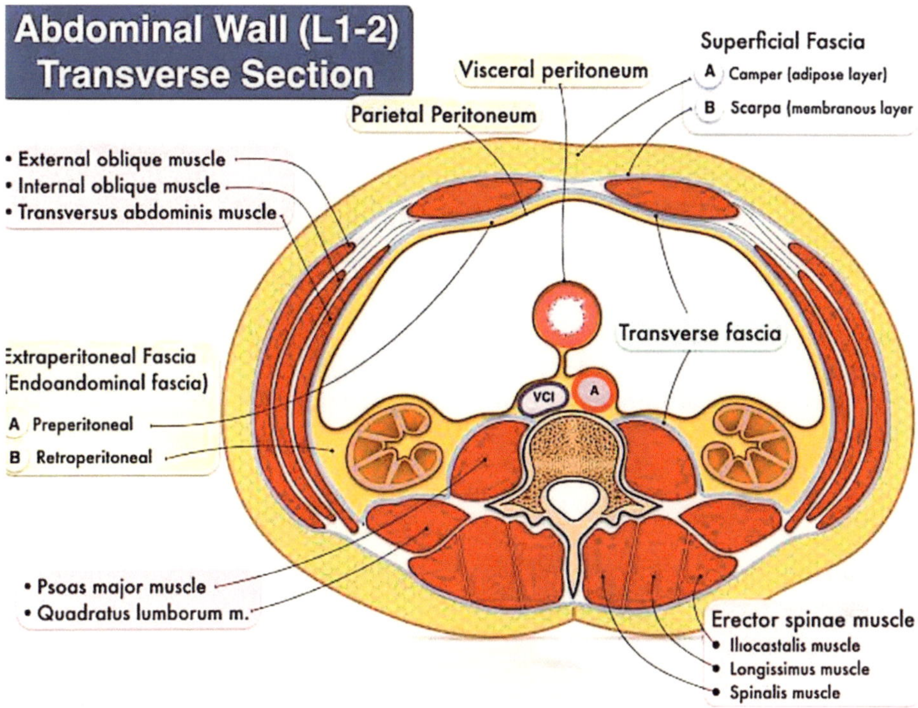

Figure 1.
Cross-section of the abdomen showing three muscles of abdominal wall. Note. Adapted from: Anatomy of the abdominal wall, by O.R. Tarhan, 2024 (https://www.turkcerrahi.com/en/general-surgery-articles/abdominal-wall-and-hernias/abdominal-wall-anatomy/).

3.1.3 Contraindications

As with any regional anesthetic technique, absolute contraindications are patient refusal, local anesthetic allergy, and infection at the injection site. Relative contraindications are abnormal coagulation profile and surgery at the injection site.

3.1.4 Technique

3.1.4.1 Patient preparation

- Intravenous line established.
- Monitoring (ECG – NIBP-Pulse oximetry).
- Complete resuscitation equipment and medications.
- Skin preparation with antiseptic solution (chlorohexidine 0.5%).
- Sterile gloves and mask.
- Ultrasound machine with high frequency linear probe with probe cover and sterile gel.
- Long acting local anesthetic (bupivacaine, ropivacaine, or levobupivacaine) guided by toxic dose calculation.

3.1.4.2 Performing the block (posterior injection)

Patient is placed in supine position. Area of interest is the space between costal margin and iliac crest in the mid-axillary line, where the probe is placed horizontally to visualize three muscle layers: external oblique, internal oblique, and transversus abdominis. The needle entry is 2 to 3 centimeters medial to the probe, then introduced in plane to the fascial plane between internal oblique and transversus abdominus (**Figure 2**).

The local anesthetic solution is slowly injected; a successful block is identified by the separation of the muscles by hypoechoic well-circumscribed fusiform solution (**Figures 3** and **4**). As a rule, fascial plane techniques require large volumes of local anesthetic to block numerous small abdominal wall nerves (in TAP block, usually 30 ml). Maximum local anesthetic doses must be calculated to avoid the effects of systemic toxicity.

3.1.5 Complication of TAP block

Fortunately, TAP blocks have a high safety profile with a low incidence of considerable complication. Complications reported include:

- Block Failure
- Local anesthetic toxicity
- Intraperitoneal injection
- Intestinal injury
- Liver injury

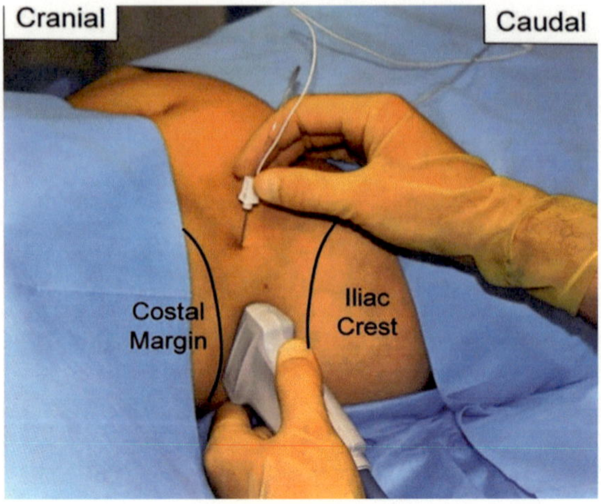

Figure 2.
Transducer position and in-plane needle technique for the posterior TAP block. Note. Image from "Transversus Abdominis Plane Block" Anesthesia tutorial of the week 239, September 2011, P. 7.

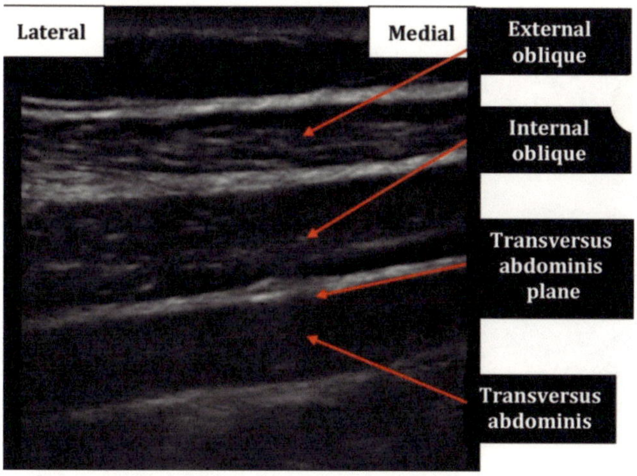

Figure 3.
Ultrasound identification of the three muscle layers. Note. Image from "Transversus Abdominis Plane Block" Anesthesia tutorial of the week 239, September 2011, P. 7.

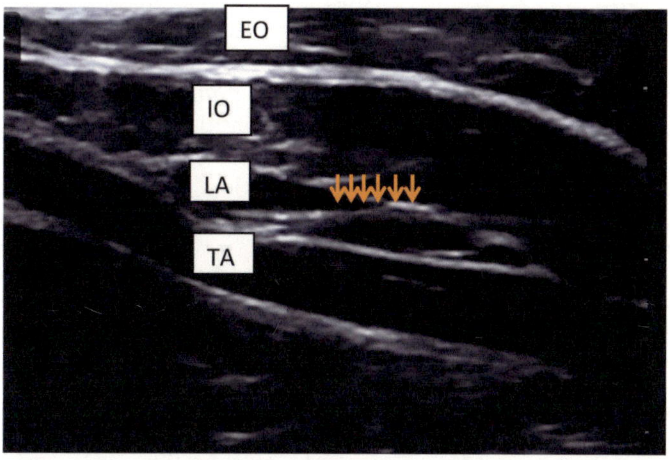

Figure 4.
Ultrasound image showing local anesthetic deposition in the correct plane (EO: external oblique – IO: internal oblique- TO: transversus abdominus – LA: local anesthetic – arrows indicate the needle). Note. Adapted from: Ref. [6].

3.2 Quadratus lumborum block

In 2007, Quadratus lumborum blocks (QLBs) were introduced by Dr. Rafa Blanco as a variant of TAP block known as (no pops TAP). It has been suggested that (QLB) is more reliable than the TAP block for achieving both visceral and somatic analgesia of the abdomen [7].

Anatomy: quadratus lumborum is the deepest muscle of the back. It takes origin from the posteromedial aspect of the iliac crest and inserts into the medial border of the twelfth rib and the transverse processes of the first four lumbar vertebrae. The thoracolumbar fascia surrounds the muscle and is considered a component of the myofascial girdle that surrounds the lower trunk and is crucial for posture, weight bearing, and stabilization of the lumbar spine (**Figure 5**).

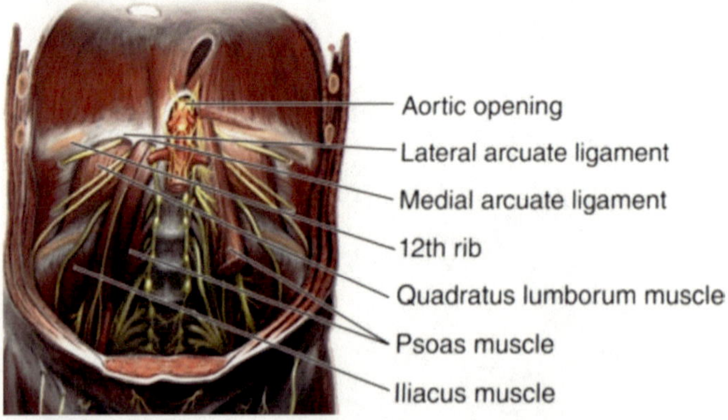

Figure 5.
The anterior aspect of the muscles of posterior abdominal wall and illustrating the relations of QL muscle. Note. Image from: https://www.nysora.com/topics/abdomen/ultrasoundguided-transversus-abdominis-plane-quadratus-lumborum-blocks/

The thoracolumbar fascia is divided into three layers; the most anterior layer is adherent to the anterior surface of both quadratus lumborum and psoas muscles. The middle layer passes between the erector spinae muscles and quadratus lumborum, and the most posterior layer encloses the erector spinae muscle [8].

The middle and posterior layers merge laterally, giving rise to the lateral raphe, which in turn joins with the transversus abdominis and internal oblique muscles. The middle layer is attached to the transverse processes of the vertebra (**Figure 6**) [9].

It is worth noting that the QL muscle is surrounded by vital structures that make these blocks difficult because of the possibility of organ damage; it is important to pay

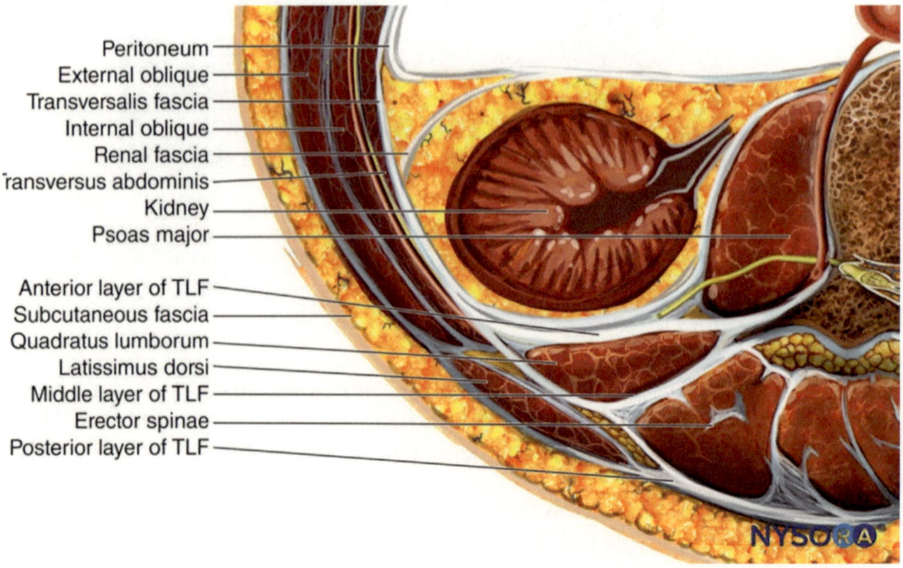

Figure 6.
The three layers of thoracolumbar fascia and their relation to posterior abdominal wall muscles. Note. Image from: https://www.nysora.com/topics/abdomen/ultrasoundguided-transversus-abdominis-plane-quadratus-lumborum-blocks/

sufficient attention to understanding their relative anatomy. The QL muscle is located behind the lower part of the kidney and its surrounding fat. In addition, the ascending and descending colon are anterior to the muscle.

The lumbar arteries arise from the posterior aspect of the aorta at the level of the first four lumbar vertebrae; these blood vessels run posteriorly behind the sympathetic chain and behind the quadratus lamborum (**Figure 7**) [10].

3.3 Spread of local anesthetic after injection

The mechanism by which the quadratus lumborum block produces analgesia is much more complicated than other fascial plane blocks. After a local anesthetic is injected anteriorly to the quadratus, it can spread cranially along the endothoracic fascia to reach the paravertebral space in the upper lumbar and thoracic regions through the lateral and medial arcuate ligaments of the diaphragm to reach the somatic and sympathetic trunk in the thoracic region [11].

3.4 Indications for QLB block

QLB block can be used for pain management in a wide range of surgical procedures, for example:

Abdominal: Laparotomy-Abdominoplasty – Open and laparoscopic appendectomy – Cholecystectomy.

Obstetric and gynecological: Cesarean section-Total abdominal hysterectomy.

Urologic Open prostatectomy-Renal transplant surgery.

Orthopedics: Iliac crest-bone graft Hip surgery.

Contraindications: patient refusal, allergy to local anesthetic, infection at injection site, and abnormal coagulation profile.

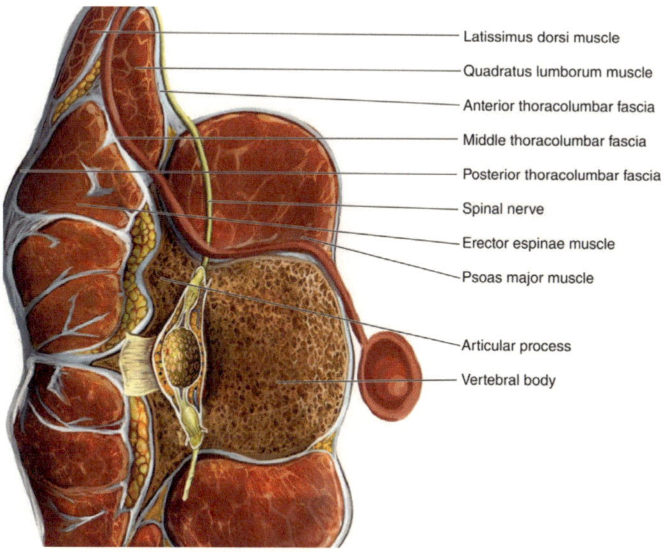

Figure 7.
Important relations of QL muscle. Note. Image from: https://www.nysora.com/topics/abdomen/ultrasoundguided-transversus-abdominis-plane-quadratus-lumborum-blocks/

3.5 Technique

3.5.1 Patient preparation: As before

Performing the Block: An in-plane needle approach is used for all QLB techniques. The patient is preferentially placed in a lateral position for better sonographic identification and more steadiness in handling the needle and ultrasound probe. In thin patients, the block can be done in a supine position and elevation of flanks using a wedge under the hip (**Figure 8**).

A low-frequency (2 to 6 Hz) curved probe is used to perform the block. The probe is placed horizontally over the iliac crest and then directed laterally to observe the tapered abdominal muscle layers and the appearance of the QL muscle, the fascia transversalis, which is identified as a hyperechoic line separating the muscle layers from the perinephric fat and abdominal contents. Sometimes movement of the bowel, kidney, and perinephric fat can be observed with respiration, making it easier to identify landmarks (**Figure 9**) [8].

Variants of QLBs: there are four subtypes of the block depending on the site of local anesthetic injection (**Figure 10**).

Lateral Quadratus Lumborum Block (previously known as type 1): Local anesthetic is applied anterolateral to the QLM and lateral to the transversus abdominis muscle. The needle entry point is anterior to the probe, then introduced in a plane to penetrate the transversus abdominis aponeurosis lateral to the QLB muscle.

Posterior Quadratus Lumborum Block (previously known as type 2): The needle entry point is anterior to the probe, then introduced in a plane to reach the dorsal aspect of the QLM, local anesthetic is injected posterior to the QLB muscle between it and the erector spinae muscle.

Anterior Quadratus Lumborum Block (previously known as type 3): The needle is inserted posteriorly to the probe, and the needle is passed anterolaterally through the

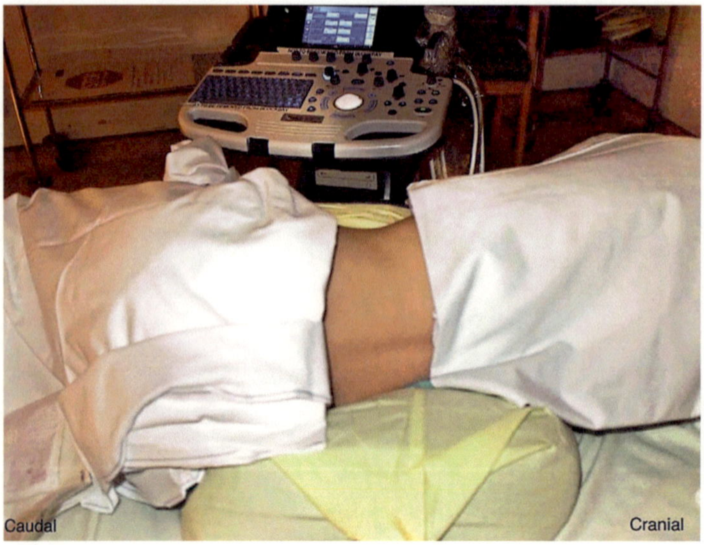

Figure 8.
Patient positioning before QLB block. Note. Image from: "Quadratus Lumborum Blocks" Anesthesia tutorial of the week 433, September 2020, p. 5.

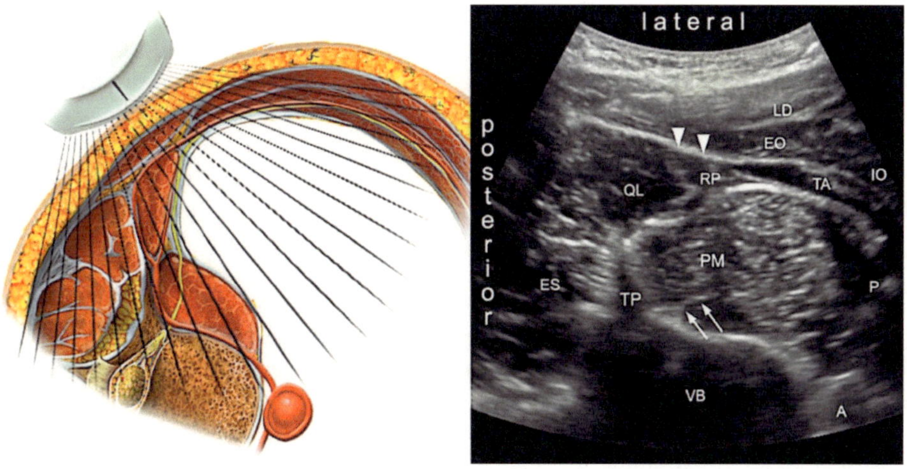

Figure 9.
Cross-section with orientation of ultrasound probe and ultrasound image obtained. EO: external oblique – IO: internal oblique – TA: transversus abdominus – LD latissimus dorsi – QL quadratus lamborum TP = transverse process; VB = vertebral body (L4); IO = internal oblique; EO = external oblique; RP = retroperitoneal space; P = peritoneal space; A = aorta; arrows = lumbar plexus; arrow heads = transversus abdominis aponeurosis. Note. Image from: https://www.nysora.com/topics/abdomen/ultrasoundguided-transversus-abdominis-plane-quadratus-lumborum-blocks/

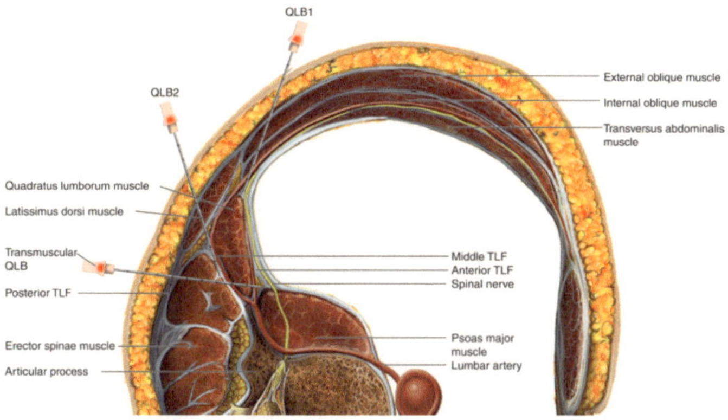

Figure 10.
Site of injection of types of QLBs. Note. Image from: https://www.nysora.com/topics/abdomen/ultrasoundguided-transversus-abdominis-plane-quadratus-lumborum-blocks/

posterior layer of the thoracolumbar fascia, the QLB muscle, and the anterior layer of the thoracolumbar fascia until it reaches this endpoint between the psoas muscle and the QLB. (Called the transmuscular approach by Børglum et al) [12].

Intramuscular block: In this case, the local anesthetic is injected into the QL muscle. As with the lateral block, the needle is inserted from anterior to posterior, penetrating the thoracolumbar fascia, and then the muscle itself, where the local anesthetic is deposited.

The volume of local anesthetic required to perform the block is 20–30 ml. It is important to ensure that the total dose of local anesthetic applied does not exceed the maximum toxic dose, especially when performing the block on both sides.

Complication of QL block: Incomplete understanding of sonographic anatomy and incompetent block performance give rise to complications, which may include kidney injury, especially right kidney (lower position), bowel injury, vascular injury, block failure, and local anesthetic toxicity, especially after injecting both sides. Undesired femoral nerve block, especially with anterior QL block, has been documented and manifests as quadriceps weakness. Paravertebral spread of local anesthetic may lead to hypotension. [13]

3.6 Erector spinae block

The erector spinae plane block is a relatively new, versatile technique that has rapidly gained popularity due to its simplicity, fewer complications, and effective pain control in various surgical techniques. Credit goes to Forero and his colleagues, who first performed the block in 2016 on patients with thoracic neuropathic pain and patients undergoing video-assisted thoracic surgery, documenting a strong analgesic effect.

Anatomy: Erector spinae muscle is actually a group of muscles arranged in three columns (iliocostalis, longissimus, and spinalis) [14] that run the length of the spine from sacrum to skull base and lie on either side of spinous processes of the vertebrae superficial to lamina and transverse processes, extending throughout cervical, thoracic, and lumbar regions (**Figure 11**). The idea of the block is that the needle is inserted just lateral to the midline and advanced to contact the transverse process, where the local anesthetic is administered and spread along this fascial plane in a craniocaudal fashion.

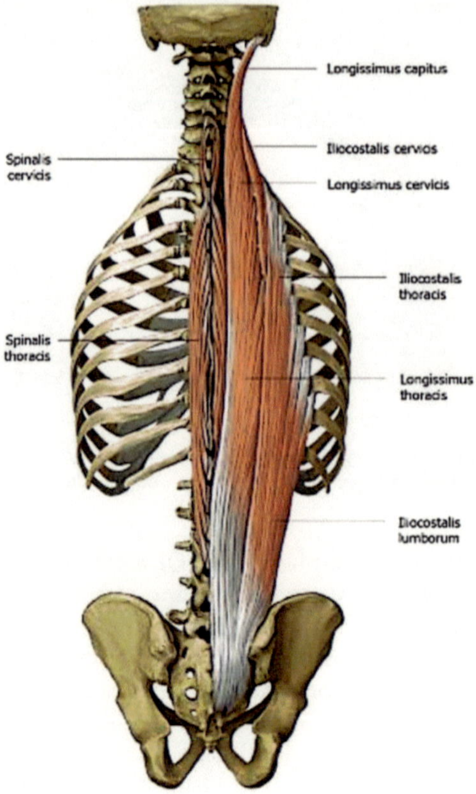

Figure 11.
Anatomy of erector spinae muscle. Note. Image from "Erector spinae muscles" by A. Rad, 2023, (https://www.kenhub.com/en/library/anatomy/erector-spinaemuscles).

3.7 Technique

3.7.1 Patient preparation: As before

Performing the Block: The block can be performed in sitting or lateral position, the block can be performed at any level of spine and the usual starting points are T5 for thoracic indications, T10 for abdominal indications, and L3 for lumbar spine surgery. Linear transducers are usually appropriate for the majority of patients; however, curved probes can be used in obese patients. The probe is placed in a parasagittal orientation in the thoracic region; ribs will appear with rounded acoustic shadow, and pleura is clearly sliding on either side. If the probe is moved medially transition to transverse process will appear, unlike rib transverse process, which is more superficial and square in appearance, and the pleura is less apparent or not seen at all (**Figure 12**).

After identifying the TP needle is inserted in plane to contact the transverse process at the corner. A test injection of 1–2 ml of saline is used to confirm the needle position, seeing the muscle lift by the fluid is a sign of success. A total volume of 30 ml of local anesthetic is used (**Figure 13**).

3.8 Mechanism of action of ESP block

The mechanism of action of erector spinae block is an area of debate. Data derived from cadaveric studies and imaging modalities confirm diffusion of local anesthetic to dorsal ramus [15], anesthetizing skin and paraspinal structures skin, muscle, and periosteum, and this explains effective pain control in spine surgeries. Another interesting mechanism was described by Daniele and his colleagues, who performed a dissection and histotopographic pilot study and concluded that there is a considerable anterior diffusion of dye along the course of blood vessels and dorsal ramus through the costotransverse foramen to reach the anterior paravertebral space and the intercostal nerves (**Figure 14**) [17]. This mechanism is supported by the results of other cadaveric studies, which demonstrated dye diffusion to paravertebral space and acknowledged ESP as an alternative to paravertebral block [14]. On the other hand,

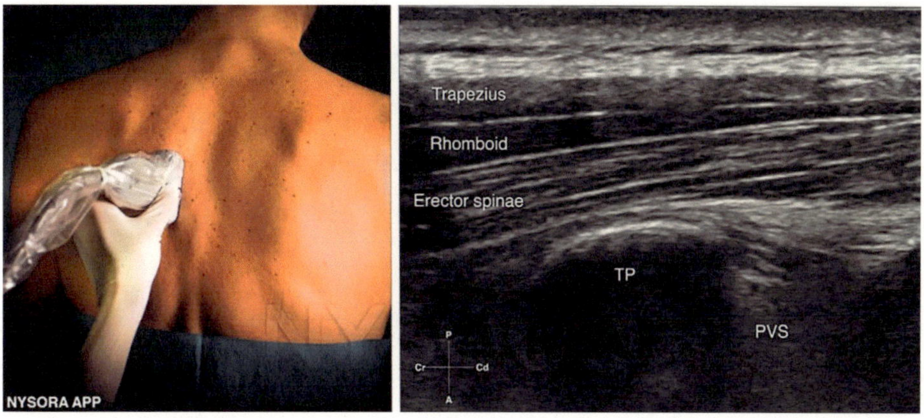

Figure 12.
Patient positioning and sonoanatomy of erector spinae muscle (TP: transverse process – PVS: paravertebral space). Note. Image from "Erector Spinae Plane Nerve Block" (Erector Spinae Plane Nerve Block - Nysora).

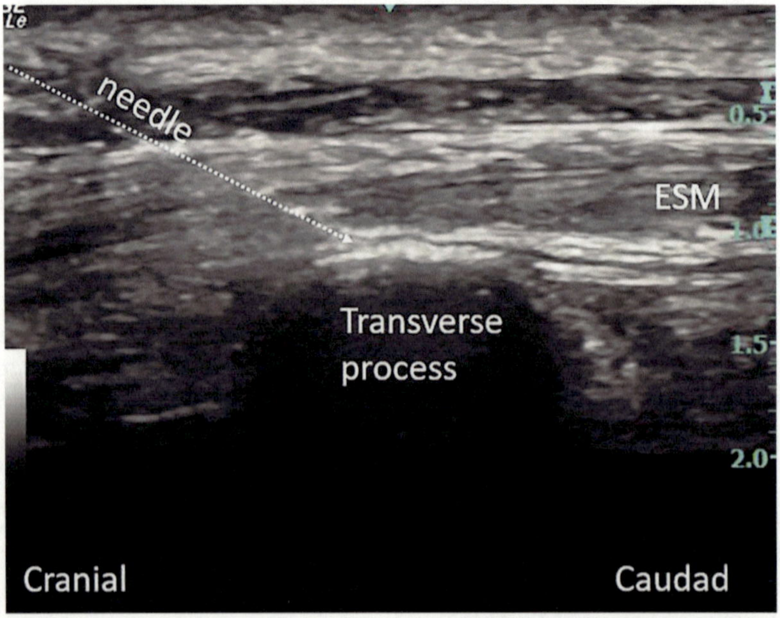

Figure 13.
Correct needle position and test dose showing slight elevation of the muscle from underlying transverse process. Note. Image from ASRA pain medicine update, how I do it erector Spinae block for rib fractures: the Penn state health experience, by H.C. Eng, and K. J. Chin. 2020 (https://www.asra.com/news-publications/asra-newsletter/newsletter-item/asranews/2020/05/01/how-i-do-it-erector-spinae-block-for-rib-fractures-the-penn-state-health-experience).

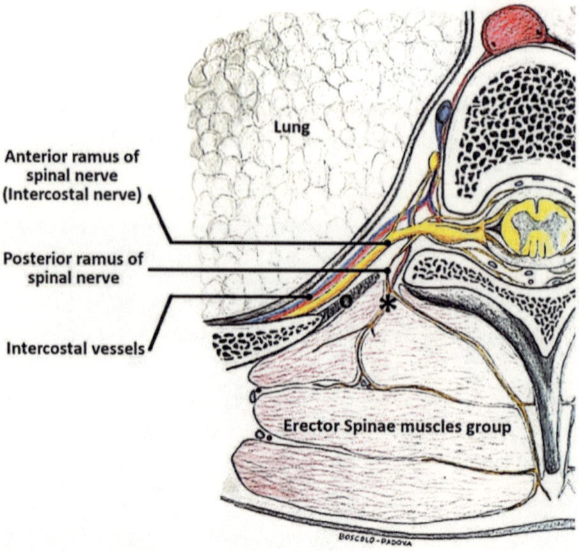

Figure 14.
Cross-section of thoracic vertebra showing intercostal space with corresponding nerve and vessels. The dorsal ramus of the spinal nerve and its accompanying blood vessels pass through the costotransverse foramen (asterisk), to supply erector spinae muscles. Note. Adapted from: Ref. [16].

it is also obvious that the three muscles that form the erector spine plane block do not form a single plane and that it is even questionable whether they form a fascia that could define this block.

3.9 Indications for ESP block

- *Rib Fracture:* a very painful condition that may cause significant complications, especially in patients with respiratory disorders.
- *Thoracic Surgery* including video-assisted thoracoscope and surgeries requiring lateral thoracotomies.
- *Cardiac surgery,* where the use of high doses of anticoagulant agents makes traditional regional anesthesia problematic.
- *Abdominal surgery*: ESP block is superior to TAP block and rectus sheath block in controlling visceral pain due to the paravertebral spread of local anesthetic.
- *Lower Limb Surgery* in hip fracture produces significant analgesia and reduce opioid consumption.

Contraindications: patient refusal, allergy to local anesthetic, infection at injection site.

Clinical pearls

- To avoid intramuscular injection the tip off the needle should be at the tip of transverse process.
- If the muscle returns to its original position after the injection, this is a good sign that the block has been successful.
- In the thoracic region, use saline hydrolocation to keep track of the needle tip in the thoracic region to avoid the risk of pneumothorax.

3.10 Pectorlais (PECS) blocks

PECS blocks are relatively new thoracic fascial blocks, first performed by Blanco in 2011 [14], that target the pectoral and intercostal nerves to provide analgesia for surgical procedures involving the anterior chest wall. In the PECS I block, local anesthetic is injected between the pectoralis major and minor muscles, whereas PEC II requires two injections, the first identical to PECS I and the second between the pectoralis major and serratus anterior muscles.

Anatomy: innervation of the chest wall is derived from: (**Figure 15**)

- Anterior divisions of the fourth, fifth, and sixth intercostal nerve.
- Intercostobrachial nerve, a cutaneous branch from second intercostal nerve that innervates the apex of axilla.
- Medial pectoral nerve (C8-T1) and Lateral pectoral nerve (C5-7) supplying pectoralis major and minor.

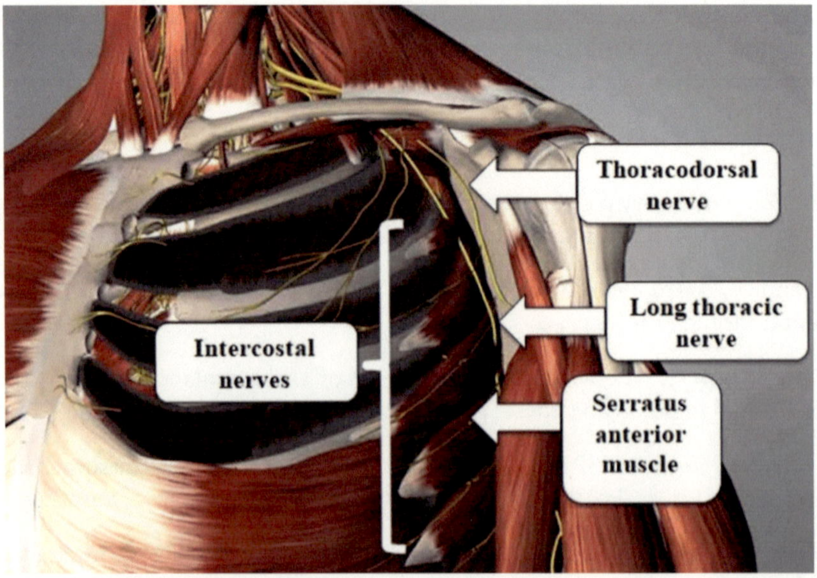

Figure 15.
Innervation of chest wall. Note. Image from: Ref. [18].

- The long thoracic nerve (C5-7) supplies the serratus anterior muscle.
- The thoracodorsal nerve (C6-8) supplies latissimus dorsi and involve in more extensive procedures.
- Anterior divisions of intercostal nerves supply the skin over the sternum and cutaneous branches of cervical plexus supply the skin just below the clavicle. (not involved in our topic).

3.11 Technique

3.11.1 PECS I block

3.11.1.1 Patient preparation: As before

Performing the Block: The block can be performed in supine position, linear probe is used with arm abducted 90 degree to stretch pectoralis muscles. The probe is placed just below the clavicle to visualize pectoralis major and minor muscles and axillary vessels. Usually an artery is seen which is pectoral branch of thoracoacromial artery and considered a good landmark as it close to medial and lateral pectoral nerves (**Figures 16** and **17**). Using in plane approach, needle introduced in cranio-caudal direction to fascial plane between the two pectoralis muscles and 10-15 ml of bupivacaine is injected.

3.11.2 Indications of PECS I block

The PECS I block affects the medial and lateral pectoral nerves and is therefore valuable in breast reconstruction surgery using submuscular implants and tissue expanders, modified radical mastectomy [20], insertion of prostheses such as porta-caths and implantable pacemakers.

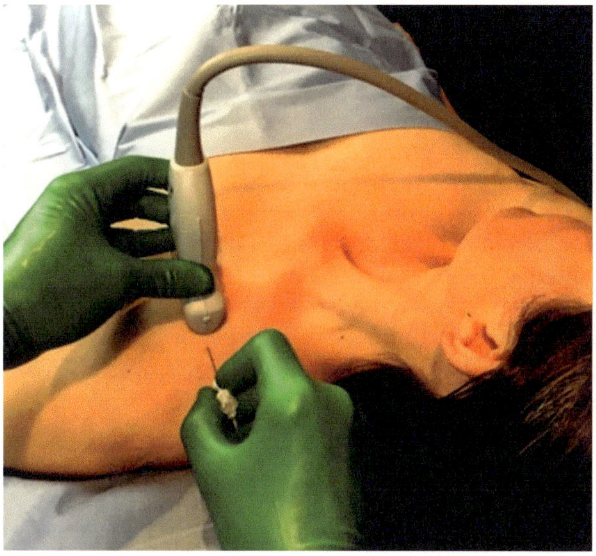

Figure 16.
Patient positioning and probe orientation in PECS I.

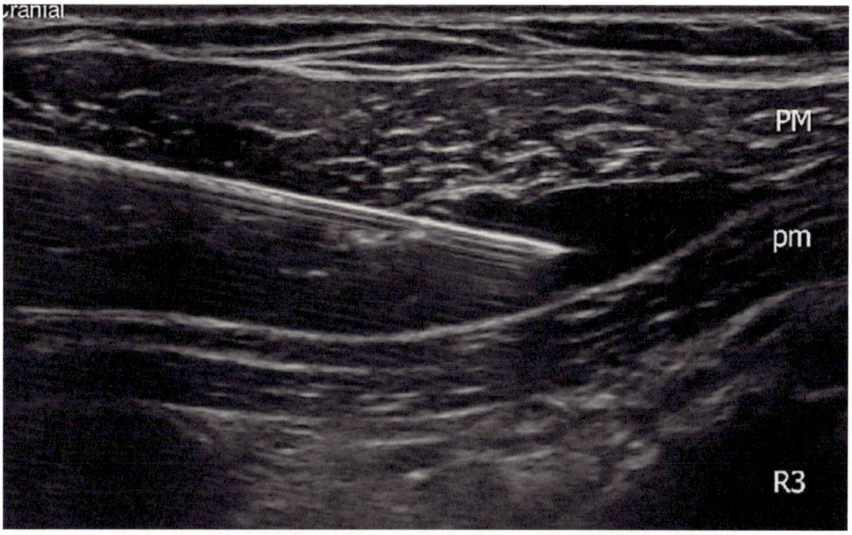

Figure 17.
Sonoanatomy of PECS I (PM: Pectoralis major – pm Pectoralis minor – R3: Third rib). Note. Image from: Ref. [19].

3.11.3 PECS II block

Performing the Block: The first step in this block is the usual PECS I injection, then the probe tilted medially to be parallel to the deltopectoral groove to bring the axillary vessels in view. The rib located over the axillary vein is the second rib. At this point, the probe is moved downward and laterally counting the ribs till the fourth rib is visualized where the serratus anterior appears overlying the rib and underneath the pectoralis minor muscle. The plane between the last two muscles is the target for PECS II block, where 15–20 ml of local anesthetic is injected (**Figures 18** and **19**).

3.11.4 Indications of PECS II block

The indications for PECS II are similar to those for PECS I. However, in PECS II, the local anesthetic injectate diffuses in a wider plane, blocking the long thoracic nerve, the thoracodorsal nerve, and the intercostal nerves from T2 to T6. This makes it an appropriate choice in breast surgeries with axillary dissection or sentinel lymph node biopsy. The block can be combined with the supraclavicular block in upper arm fistula surgery [21] as the intercostobrachial block, which is a branch from T2, is consistently effective.

3.11.5 Clinical pearls

- In the event that the two blocks are to be performed, it is preferable to commence with PECS II, given that it is more profound and, upon withdrawal of the needle, it readily falls into the plane of PECS I.

- It is recommended that repeated aspiration be performed before injection in order to prevent complications, given that the fascial planes in the thorax are relatively more vascular.

- It is imperative that the trajectory of the needle be aligned with the superior aspect of the fourth rib in order to circumvent the potential for injection into the intercostal space and consequently reduce the risk of pneumothorax.

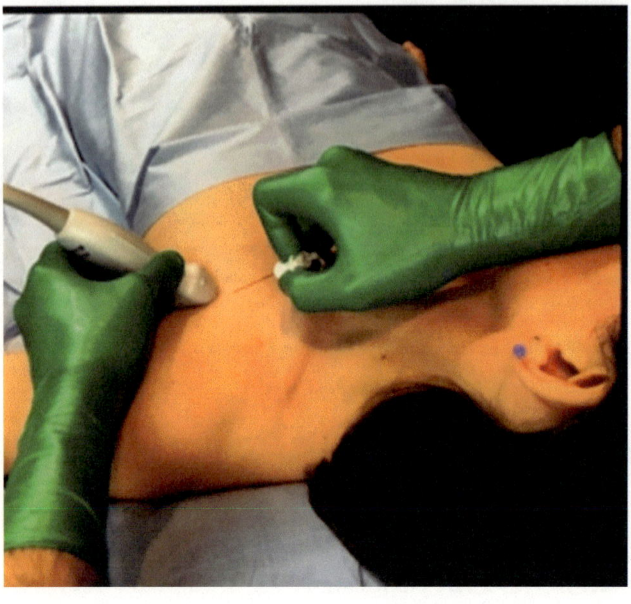

Figure 18.
Patient positioning and probe orientation in PECS II.

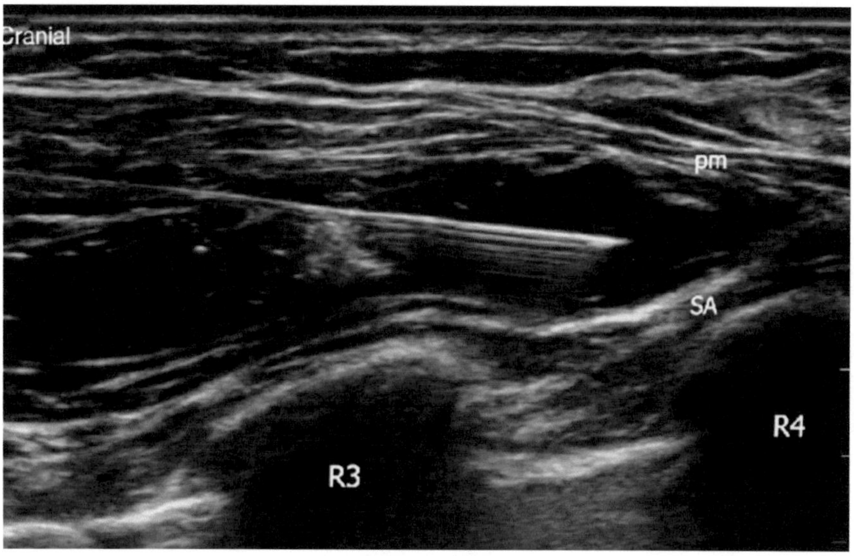

Figure 19.
Sonoanatomy of PECS II (pm Pectoralis minor – SA: Serratus Anterior-R3: Third rib – R4: Fourth rib). Note. Image from: Ref. [19].

3.12 Serratus plane block (SPB)

In 2016, Blanco and his colleagues introduced a unique regional anesthetic technique (serratus plane block) [22] aiming at anesthetizing nearly the whole hemithorax by injecting local anesthetic superficial and deep to serratus muscle and providing a safer and more feasible surrogate for thoracic paravertebral block which is more sophisticated and requires well-trained anesthesiologist to evade its hazardous complications.

Anatomy: Upon exiting the intervertebral foramen, each thoracic nerve subsequently divides into a ventral ramus and a dorsal ramus, which then runs posteriorly to supply the paraspinal muscles and the overlying skin. The ventral ramus continues laterally in the intercostal space as the intercostal nerve, which runs in the neurovascular plane within the costal groove between the innermost and internal intercostal muscles. In the vicinity of the midaxillary line, the lateral cutaneous branch arises and permeates the overlying intercostal and serratus muscles, subsequently dividing into anterior, and posterior branches. Thereafter, the nerve runs anteriorly, and in close proximity to the sternum, subsequently penetrating the intercostal muscles and the pectoralis major muscle to ultimately terminate as the anterior cutaneous nerve (**Figure 20**).

Serratus anterior is a broad muscle that takes its origin as digitations from outer surface of first to ninth rib and is inserted along superior angle, medial border, and superior angle of the scapula. Its main action is protraction of the scapula.

3.12.1 Injecting superficial or deep to serratus?

The initial study conducted by Blanco involved four volunteers, each of whom received two injections. One injection was administered in a superficial location relative to the muscle, while the other was delivered in a deep location on the opposite

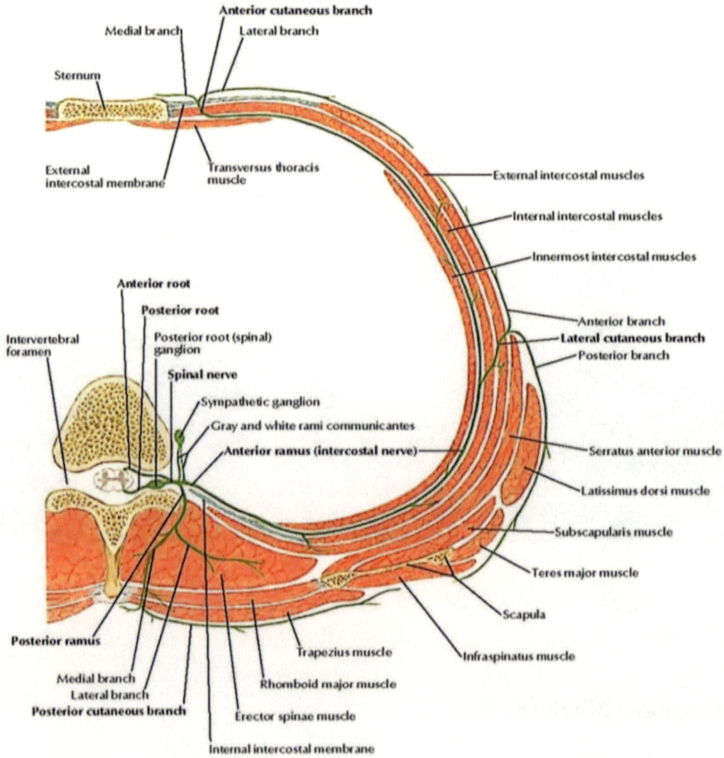

Figure 20.
Cross-section showing origin, course, relations, and branches of intercostal nerve. Note. Image from typical thoracic spinal nerve: cross section anatomy, by Netter, 2018 (https://www.pediagenosis.com/2018/12/typical-thoracic-spinalnerve-cross.html).

side of the muscle. The study's findings indicated that the duration of paresthesia of the motor and intercostal nerves was longer in the superficial block, and the territory of sensory loss was identical (from T2 to T9) in both the superficial and deep injection sites. Subsequent studies yielded conflicting results. For instance, some studies demonstrated no difference in analgesic efficacy between the two injections in ambulatory breast cancer surgery [23, 24]. Some studies have indicated that the superficial block may be more effective than the deep block in terms of analgesic potency, as evidenced by lower pain scores and opioid requirements in patients undergoing mastectomy with axillary clearance [25]. However, other authors have proposed that the deep block may offer superior pain relief compared to the superficial block [26]. It is evident that there is still a need for further research to conclusively determine the optimal approach for regional anesthesia in this context.

3.12.2 Technique

3.12.2.1 Patient preparation: As before

Performing the Block: The block was performed in the supine position with the arm abducted at a right angle to facilitate the positioning of the probe. The high-frequency linear probe is positioned at the midaxillary line, at the fifth intercostal space (see **Figure 21**). The scanning process can be conducted in a manner consistent with that employed for PECS blocks. The probe is positioned in a parasagittal orientation just beneath the clavicle, where the pectoralis major and pectoralis minor muscles can be observed. The probe is then directed inferiorly and laterally, resulting in the gradual fading of the pectoralis major and the emergence of the serratus anterior, which is seen over the latissimus dorsi muscle. The ribs are counted until the fifth rib in the midaxillary line is identified (**Figure 22**). The thoracodorsal artery is visible between the serratus and latissimus muscles and can be used as an additional landmark to identify the plane correctly.

The in-plane technique involves inserting the needle from the superior to the inferior direction, then backward, to inject local anesthetic between the serratus and latissimus muscles (superficial serratus block) or deep to the serratus muscle over the fifth rib (deep serratus block).

3.12.3 Indications of SPB block

A comparison of the two techniques reveals that the serratus plane block produces a greater extent of blockade from T2 to T9. The analgesic effect is a result of the lateral cutaneous branches of the intercostal nerves being anesthetized, as determined by a cadaveric study [28]. The remaining three nerves that consistently undergo blockade are the intercostobrachial nerve, the long thoracic nerve (which is motor to the serratus muscle), and the thoracodorsal nerve (which is motor to the latissimus dorsi muscle) [29]. This information is pertinent when discussing the block with the surgeon and the patient in order to ensure that both parties are aware that transient winging may occur as a result of long thoracic nerve blockade.

SPB is indicated in the context of breast surgery with axillary dissection, thoracic surgeries (including the insertion of pacemakers), and pain management in rib fractures [30].

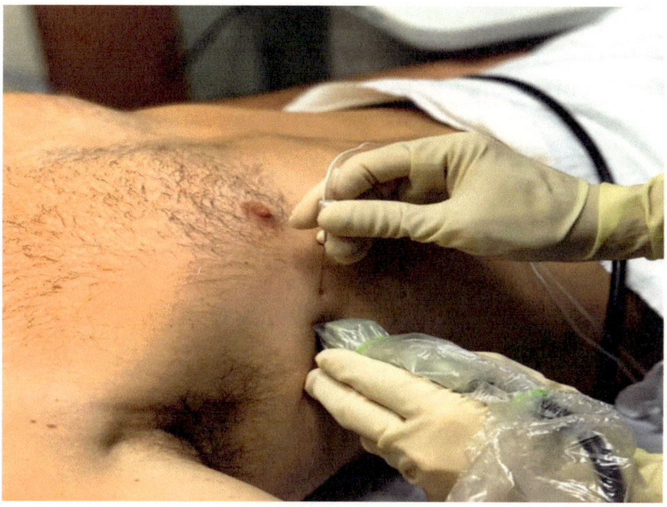

Figure 21.
Patient positioning and probe orientation in Serratus plane block.

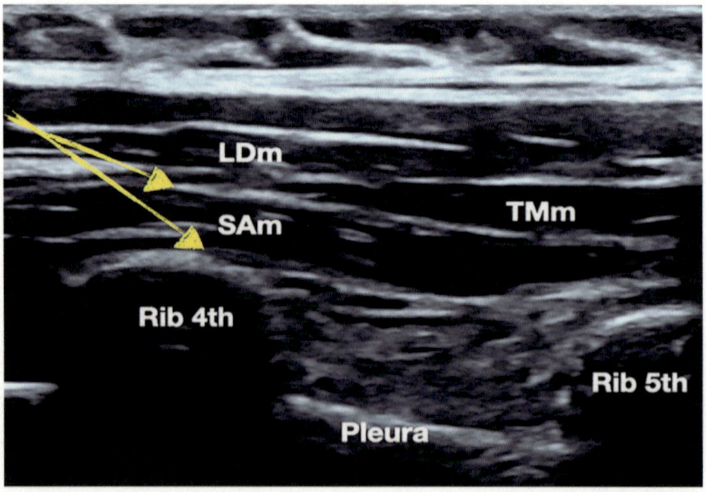

Figure 22.
Sonoanatomy of serratus plane block (Sam: Serratus Anterior-LDm Latissimus dorsi muscle – TMm: Teres major muscle). Note. Image from: Ref. [27].

3.12.4 Complications of SPB block

Pneumothorax may occur especially in the deep approach, and other general complications such as hematoma, infection, failed block, and local anesthetic toxicity.

3.13 Fascia Iliaca compartment block

The fascia iliaca block has emerged as a highly efficacious method for providing analgesia to the extensive lower limb region. It is regarded as an anterior approach for lumbar plexus block, with the objective of achieving blockade of three of its terminal branches: the femoral nerve (FN), the lateral femoral cutaneous nerve (LFCN) and the obturator nerve (ON). This is achieved through the deposition of local anesthetic deep into the fascia iliaca. Although the psoas compartment block or posterior lumbar plexus is more efficient, as it blocks the lumbar plexus at the roots of these nerves, it is technically more advanced and carries a greater potential for complications, such as epidural spread and intravascular injection [31]. Consequently, the fascia iliaca block has been adopted as a safer substitute.

The performance of the block has been enhanced over time, with the earliest iteration dating back to 1973. This was when Winnie presented the "three-in-one" block [32] as an anterior inguinal paravascular injection of 20 ml of local anesthetic, which blocks the three nerves. Subsequently, in 1989, Dalens described a novel injection technique at the junction of the lateral one-third and medial twothirds of the inguinal ligament (the landmark technique), recommending it for use in children [33]. This technique was subjected to further modification and adjustment through ultrasound guidance until 2011, when Hebbard and his colleague described the recent anatomical adjustment of the block (ultrasound-guided suprainguinal fascia iliaca block) [34].

Anatomy: The lower limb receives nerve supply from lumbosacral plexus. The major nerves are FN (L2-3-4), ON (L2-3-4), LFCN (L2-3), and sciatic nerve (L4-5 S1-2-3) (**Figure 23**).

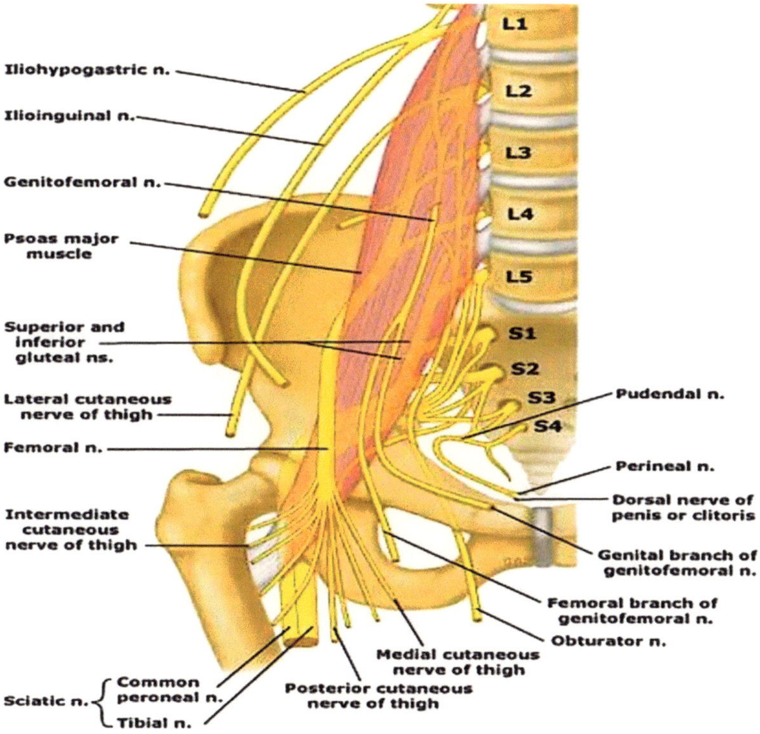

Figure 23.
Origin, course, and relations of major nerves supplying lower limb. Note. Image from: Ref. [35].

The femoral nerve has its origin in the posterior divisions of the anterior rami of the L2, L3, and L4 vertebrae. It descends from the lateral border of the psoas muscle and runs downward between it and the iliacus muscle. It passes beneath the inguinal ligament, which is covered by the fascia iliaca, in order to enter the thigh in a position lateral to the femoral artery. It provides motor innervation to the knee extensors and sensory innervation to the front and medial side of the thigh and the medial side of the leg.

The obturator nerve has its origin in the anterior divisions of the anterior rami of L2, L3, and L4 and descends from the medial border of the psoas muscle, lateral to the internal iliac vessels. It passes through the obturator foramen to enter the thigh. Its main functions are to supply the hip adductors and to provide sensory input to a small area on the inner side of the thigh, which can extend to just proximal to the knee.

The lateral femoral cutaneous nerve has its origin in the L2-3 vertebrae and passes over the lateral aspect of the psoas muscle, subsequently traversing the iliacus muscle, which is covered by the iliacus fascia and oriented in a direction that leads toward the anterior superior iliac spine. It then passes beneath the inguinal ligament and pierces the fascia iliaca, ultimately reaching the thigh, where it divides into its terminal branches.

Fascia iliaca: a broad fibrous band that lines the posterior abdomen and pelvis, covering psoas major, and iliacus muscle, attached laterally to iliac crest, anterior superior iliac spine, medially to vertebral column, and pectineal fascia. Above the inguinal ligament, the femoral vessels lie superficial to the fascia iliaca while the FN, ON, and LFCN are situated deep to it [36].

Fascia iliaca compartment: it is a potential space which is located between fascia iliaca anteriorly and iliacus and psoas muscle posteriorly, inner side of iliac crest medially and fascia covering quadratus lamborum laterally [36] (**Figure 24**).

3.13.1 Technique

The landmark technique involves the patient lying in the supine position with a line drawn connecting the anterior superior iliac spine (ASIS) and pubic tubercle, which is then divided into thirds. The point of injection is located 1 cm below the junction of the medial 2/3 and lateral 1/3 of the line. The needle is inserted at a right angle, and once it passes the skin, the angle is adjusted to approximately 60 degrees while directing the tip cranially. The needle is advanced until two pops are felt, indicating the piercing of the fascia lata and fascia iliaca. Local anesthetic injection is performed after negative aspiration (**Figure 25**).

3.13.1.1 Ultrasound-guided infrainguinal FICB

The utilization of ultrasound enables the accurate identification of tissue planes and the related structures. The utilization of ultrasound increases the success rate by ensuring the accurate deposition of local anesthetic in the targeted plane, thereby reducing the risk of complications such as block failure due to faulty pops and/or intramuscular injections.

In the supine position, a high-frequency ultrasound probe is placed at the inguinal crease in a transverse plane to localize the femoral artery, iliopsoas muscle with fascia iliaca covering, and femoral nerve between them, with the sartorius seen more laterally (**Figure 26**). The needle is then inserted in the plane from the lateral to the medial aspect, targeting the fascia iliaca at the junction of the medial aspect of the sartorius and the psoas muscle. It is expected that no resistance will be encountered during the injection and that the injectate will spread both laterally and medially to reach the femoral nerve.

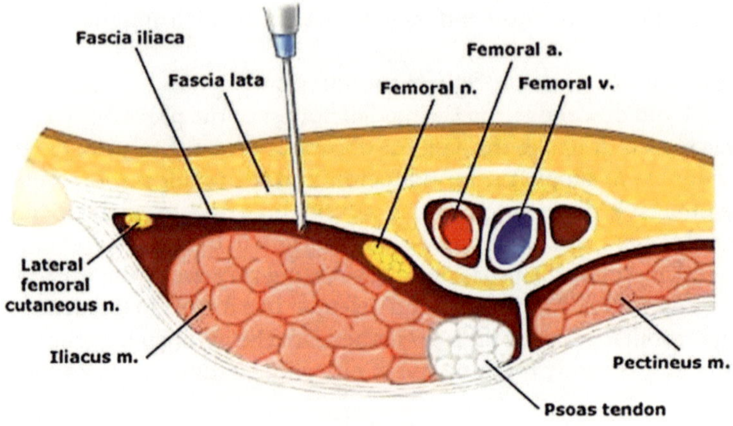

Figure 24.
Fascia iliaca compartment. Note. Image from: Ref. [37].

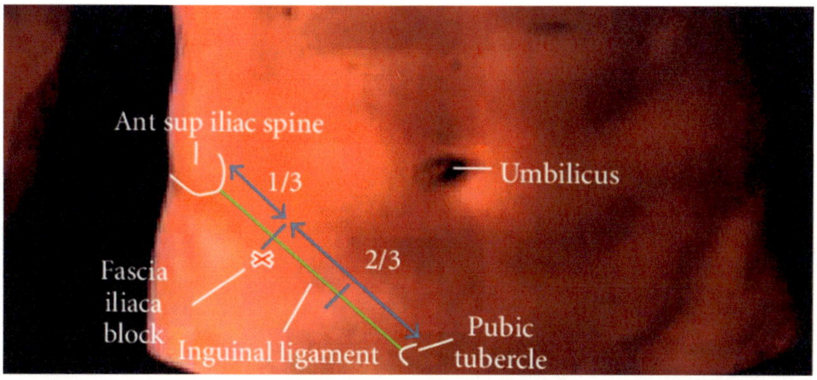

Figure 25.
Landmark technique for fascia iliaca block. Note. Image from: Ref. [38].

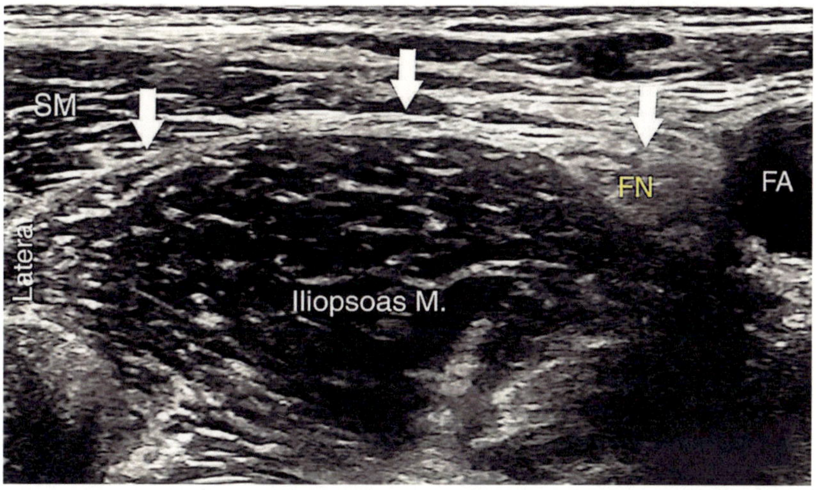

Figure 26.
Sonoanatomy of Infrainguinal fascia iliaca block FN: femoral nerve FA: femoral artery – SM: sartorius muscles. Arrows point to fascia iliaca covering iliopsoas muscle, the plane between them is the target of local anesthetic. Note. Image from ultrasound-guided fascia iliaca nerve block, by A. Atchabahian, 2024 (https://www.nysora.com/techniques/lowerextremity/ultrasound-guided-fascia-iliaca-block).

3.13.1.2 Ultrasound-guided suprainguinal FICB

The scanning process commences with the identification of the anterior superior iliac spine, after which the probe is positioned in a parasagittal orientation in a medial position relative to it. The probe is frequently rotated in a clockwise direction from its parasagittal orientation, so that it is perpendicular to the inguinal ligament. The bow-tie sign of the internal oblique and sartorius muscles is identified. The iliopsoas muscle is observed to be hypoechoic in consistency with the overlying hyperechoic fascia iliaca directly beneath the bow tie. An additional vascular landmark is the deep circumflex iliac artery, which can be seen in a superficial position relative to the fascia iliaca.

The needle is introduced with an in-plane targeting of the fascia iliaca, and a popping sound is audible when the fascia is penetrated. A large volume of fluid (30-40 ml) is required to spread in this potential space and reach the desired nerves. The peeling of the fascia iliaca from the underlying iliopsoas muscle is an indicator of success (**Figures** 27 and **28**).

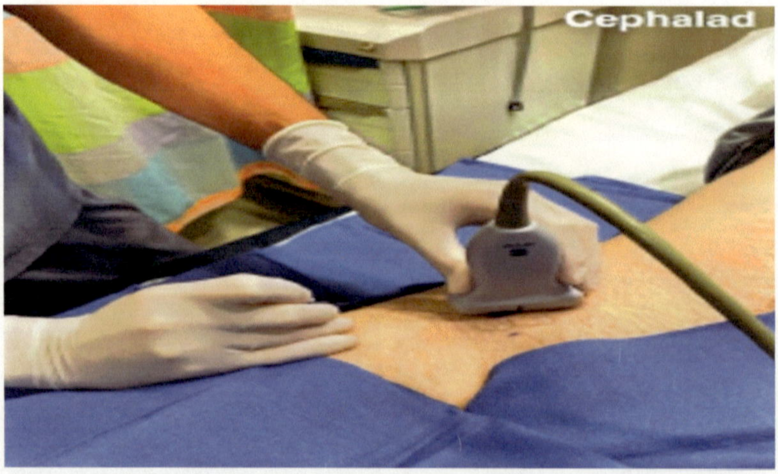

Figure 27.
Transducer position in suprainguinal FICB, perpendicular to the inguinal ligament. Note. Image from "Fascia Iliaca Compartment Block: An Update," by J. Major and M. Narayanan, 2023, Anesthesia Tutorial of the week 489.

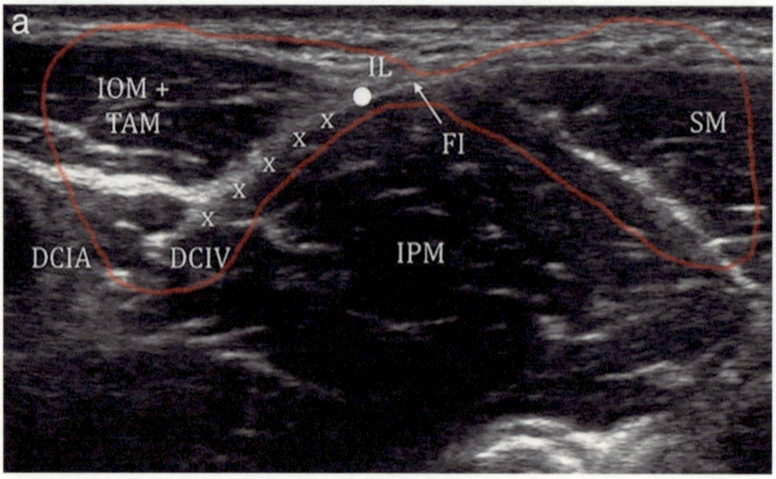

Figure 28.
Sonoanatomy of suprainguinal FICB. The X marks indicate the correct plane, and the white circle indicates the needle entry point. The bow-tie sign is outlined with the red line (IPM: iliopsoas muscle – DCIA-V: deep circumflex iliac artery and vein – FI: Fascia iliaca – IL: Inguinal ligament-SM: Sartorius muscle – IOM: internal oblique muscle). Note. Image from "fascia iliaca compartment block: an update," by J. Major and M. Narayanan, 2023, Anesthesia tutorial of the week 489.

3.13.2 Indications of FICB block

- Surgical procedures involving hip either fractures or arthroplasty and analgesia femur or knee surgeries

3.13.2.1 Which is more superior supra or infra inguinal approach?

In the Infrainguinal approach, the local anesthetic may incompletely cover the targeted nerves, resulting in partial block of obturator and lateral cutaneous nerve. On the contrary, suprainguinal involves injecting local anesthetic in a higher and more proximal location, resulting in more extensive spread and more reliable blockade of the three nerves and the articular branches of femoral and obturator nerves before they leave. This hypnosis is supported by a volunteer study which showed reliable anesthesia of medial, lateral, and anterior aspects of the thigh in 80% of suprainguinal compared to 30% in the infrainguinal group [39] and more consistent cranial spread of local anesthetic toward the lumbar plexus in suprainguinal approach than the Infrainguinal one as evaluated by MRI. So, it is recommended that the suprainguinal approach be adopted, provided that the anesthesiologist has the appropriate experience.

Conflict of interest

The authors declare no conflict of interest.

Author details

Mohammed Khamis
Faculty of Medicine Ain Shams University, Cairo, Egypt

*Address all correspondence to: mohammedkhamis891@gamil.com

References

[1] Chin KJ, Versyck B, Elsharkawy H, Gomez MF, Sala-Blanch X, Reina MA. Anatomical basis of fascial plane blocks. Regional Anesthesia & Pain Medicine. 2021;**46**(7):581-599

[2] Black ND, Stecco C, Chan VW. Fascial plane blocks: More questions than answers? Anesthesia & Analgesia. 2021;**132**(3):899-905

[3] Rafi AN. Abdominal field block: A new approach via the lumbar triangle. Anesthesia. 2001;**56**(10):1024-1026

[4] McDonnell JG, O'Donnell BD, Tuite D, Farrell T, Power C. The regional abdominal field infiltration (RAFI) technique: Computerised tomographic and anatomical identification of a novel approach to the transversus abdominis neuro-vascular fascial plane. Anesthesiology. 2004;**101**:A899

[5] Tran TM, Ivanusic JJ, Hebbard P, Barrington MJ. Determination of spread of injectate after ultrasound-guided transversus abdominis plane block: A cadaveric study. British Journal of Anaesthesia. 2009;**102**(1):123-127

[6] Sethi D, Garg G. Analgesic efficacy of ultrasound-guided transversus abdominis plane block for laparoscopic gynecological surgery. Anesthesia and Pain Medicine. 2022;**17**:67-74

[7] Blanco R. 271. Tap block under ultrasound guidance: The description of a "no pops" technique. Regional Anesthesia & Pain Medicine. 2007;**32**:130

[8] Elsharkawy H, El-Boghdadly K, Barrington M. Quadratus lumborum block: Anatomical concepts, mechanisms, and techniques. Anesthesiology. 2019;**130**(2):322-335

[9] Willard FH, Vleeming A, Schuenke MD, Danneels L, Schleip R. The thoracolumbar fascia: Anatomy, function and clinical considerations. Journal of Anatomy. 2012;**221**(6):507-536

[10] Beveridge TS, Power A, Johnson M, Power NE, Allman BL. The lumbar arteries and veins: Quantification of variable anatomical positioning with application to retroperitoneal surgery. Clinical Anatomy. 2015;**28**(5):649-660

[11] Dam M, Moriggl B, Hansen CK, Hoermann R, Bendtsen TF, Børglum J. The pathway of injectate spread with the transmuscular quadratus lumborum block: A cadaver study. Anesthesia and Analgesia. 2017;**125**(1):303-312

[12] Børglum J, Moriggl B, Jensen K, Lønnqvist PA, Christensen AF, Sauter A, et al. Ultrasound-guided transmuscular quadratus lumborum blockade. British Journal of Anesthesia. 2013;**111**(eLetters)

[13] Gupta A, Sondekoppam R, Kalagara H. Quadratus lumborum block: A technical review. Current Anesthesiology Reports. 2019;**9**:257-262

[14] Pourkashanian A, Narayanan M, Venkataraju A. The erector spinae plane block: A review of current evidence. Update in Anesthesia. 2020;**35**:27-33

[15] Pawa A, King C, Thang C, White L. Erector spinae plane block: The ultimate 'plan A'block? British Journal of Anesthesia. 2023;**130**(5):497-502

[16] Berto FB et al. Anatomical basis of erector spinae plane block: A dissection and histotopographic pilot study. Journal of Anesthesia. 2020;**35**:111

[17] Bonvicini D, Boscolo-Berto R, De Cassai A, Negrello M, Macchi V, Tiberio I, et al. Anatomical basis of erector spinae plane block: A dissection and histotopographic pilot study. Journal of Anesthesia. 2021;**35**:102-111

[18] Ueshima H et al. How to use pectoral nerve blocks effectively-an evidence-based update. Asian Journal of Anesthesiology. 2019;**57**:30

[19] Kim H et al. Surgical excision of the breast giant fibroadenoma under regional anesthesia by Pecs II and internal intercostal plane block: A case report and brief technical description. Korean Journal of Anesthesiology. 2016;**70**:78

[20] Blanco R, Fajardo M, Maldonado TP. Ultrasound description of Pecs II (modified Pecs I): A novel approach to breast surgery. Revista espanola de anestesiologia y reanimacion. 2012;**59**(9):470-475

[21] Purcell N, Wu D. Novel use of the PECS II block for upper limb fistula surgery. Anesthesia. 2014;**69**(11):1294

[22] Blanco R, Parras T, McDonnell JG, Prats-Galino A. Serratus plane block: A novel ultrasound-guided thoracic wall nerve block. Anesthesia. 2013;**68**(11):1107-1113

[23] Bhoi D, Jain D, Chhabra A, Mohan VK, Talawar P, Kataria K. Analgesic efficacy of superficial versus deep serratus plane block for modified radical mastectomy under general anaesthesia: A randomised comparative study. Indian Journal of Anaesthesia. 2022;**66**(Suppl 6):S307-S313

[24] Abdallah FW, Cil T, MacLean D, Madjdpour C, Escallon J, Semple J, et al. Too deep or not too deep?: A propensity-matched comparison of the analgesic effects of a superficial versus deep serratus fascial plane block for ambulatory breast cancer surgery. Regional Anesthesia & Pain Medicine. 2018;**43**(5):480-487

[25] Tan KW, Masri SN, Musthafa QA, Azidin AM, Kamil AN, Izaham A, et al. Analgesic efficacy of the superficial versus deep serratus plane blocks for mastectomy with axillary clearance: A randomized controlled trial. Medicine. 2022;**101**(35):e30515

[26] Edwards JT, Langridge XT, Cheng GS, McBroom MM, Minhajuddin A, Machi AT. Superficial vs. deep serratus anterior plane block for analgesia in patients undergoing mastectomy: A randomized prospective trial. Journal of Clinical Anesthesia. 2021;**75**:110470

[27] Sharma R. Chest wall nerve blocks for cardiothoracic, breast surgery, and rib-related pain. Current Pain and Headache Reports. 2022;**26**:47

[28] Mayes J, Davison E, Panahi P, Patten D, Eljelani F, Womack J, et al. An anatomical evaluation of the serratus anterior plane block. Anesthesia. 2016;**71**(9):1064-1069

[29] Elwen F, Desai N, Parras T, Blanco R, Duran J. Serratus Plane Block. Anaesthesia Tutorial of the week. 2020:427

[30] Durant E, Dixon B, Luftig J, Mantuani D, Herring A. Ultrasound-guided serratus plane block for ED rib fracture pain control. The American Journal of Emergency Medicine. 2017;**35**(1):197.e3-197.e6

[31] Auroy Y, Benhamou D, Bargues L, Ecoffey C, Falissard B, Mercier F, et al. Major complications of regional anesthesia in France: The SOS regional anesthesia hotline service. The

Journal of the American Society of Anesthesiologists. 2002;**97**(5):1274-1280

[32] Winnie AP, Ramamurthy S, Durrani Z. The inguinal paravascular technic of lumbar plexus anesthesia: The “3-in-1 block”. Anesthesia & Analgesia. 1973;**52**(6):989-996

[33] Dalens B, Vanneuville G, Tanguy A. Comparison of the fascia iliaca compartment block with the 3-in-1 block in children. Anesthesia & Analgesia. 1989;**69**(6):705-713

[34] Hebbard P, Ivanusic J, Sha S. Ultrasound-guided supra-inguinal fascia iliaca block: A cadaveric evaluation of a novel approach. Anaesthesia. 2011;**66**(4):300-305

[35] Foreman M et al. Differentiating lumbar spinal etiology from peripheral plexopathies. Biomedicines. 2023;**11**:4

[36] Range C, Egeler C. Fascia iliaca compartment block. Anaesthesia Tutorial of the week. 2010:193

[37] Attaia JZ. Effects of adjuvant in potentiating the analgesic effect of fascia iliaca compartment block. Journal of Anesthesia and Surgery. 2017;**4**:87

[38] Singh SK. The loss of resistance nerve blocks. ISRN Anesthesiology. 2011;**2011**:7

[39] Vermeylen K, Desmet M, Leunen I, Soetens F, Neyrinck A, Carens D, et al. Supra-inguinal injection for fascia iliaca compartment block results in more consistent spread towards the lumbar plexus than an infra-inguinal injection: A volunteer study. Regional Anesthesia & Pain Medicine. 2019;**44**(4):483-491

Section 8

Anesthesiologic Management of Hemorrhagic Shock

Chapter 10

General Anaesthesia in the Context of Haemorrhagic Shock and Trauma

Fabrizio G. Bonanno

Abstract

In a patient with haemorrhagic shock, the interference of general anaesthesia (GA) with physiology homeostasis is more significative and relevant than the one in a not deranged patient about to undergo elective surgery, haemorrhagic shock (HS) being by definition a scenario with deranged cardiovascular and cellular respiratory physiology, manifesting with hypotension and hypoperfusion. Considering the absence of studies assessing the effects of standard GAs in HS or trauma, as a corollary, it can be recommended to achieve a general anaesthesia tailored to the patient's actual physiology, specifically a titrated-to-response anaesthesia (TRA), in any situation of HS with or without trauma. Schemes of induction and maintenance for GA, optimalized for advanced hypotensive or critical HS, have been drafted, based on experience with TIVA in critical airway, and emergency not shocked patients have been adapted to the deteriorating physiology of a progressing HS. Recommendations for damage-control-anaesthesia (DCA) in trauma, particularly to face/neck trauma and burns, have also been given.

Keywords: haemorrhagic shock, face/neck trauma and burns, titrated-to-response anaesthesia, damage control anaesthesia, total intravenous anaesthesia

1. Introduction

General anaesthesia entails a transient disruption to the physiology of a patient, with the objective of achieving a state of sedation and loss of consciousness. This is achieved from the outset, through the cessation of protective airway reflexes triggered by the sympatho-adrenal response to oropharyngeal manipulations and endotracheal intubation. Additionally, the response to sensory and pain stimuli associated with surgery, namely anaesthesia and analgesia, is prevented throughout the procedure. Facilitating endotracheal intubation (ETI), the most common method of protecting the airways from stomach regurgitation and improving ventilation, is an additional benefit for ensuring the safety and efficacy of general anaesthesia (GA).

This can be achieved through the use of short-acting muscle relaxant via a neuromuscular blocking drug. However, this sequence of objectives has the disadvantage of causing local anaesthesia and paralysis of the laryngeal reflexes and a general depression of respiratory and cardiovascular homeostasis.

In order to tailor GA, identification of the actual shock level dynamics and progression in a patient before GA is the first essential appraisal step.

A 'physiological classification' of haemorrhagic shock has been proposed since 2010, based conceptually upon the right definition of shock, the body's natural haemostatic mechanisms, the new developments in the microcirculation/arteriolar system, the concept of 'cardiac/circulatory reserve' and the basic physiological considerations such as the significance of fluid-resistant hypotension.

That classification has been revised twice to include the indications for the management of pre- or established CA by exsanguination (**Table 1**) [1]. The revised 'physiological classification of HS' frames the current haemodynamic situation, dictates the timely management and fits with 'titrated hypotensive resuscitation' +/– iatrogenic vasoconstriction's tactics and titrated-to-response anaesthesia and damage control surgery strategies (**Table 2**).

The term 'damage control resuscitation' (DCR) encompasses the combined implementation of three distinct techniques: (i) titrated hypotensive resuscitation (THR) +/– iatrogenic vaso-constriction, (ii) titrated-to-response anaesthesia (TRA) and damage control anaesthesia (DCA), and (iii) damage control surgery (DCS).

The assessment of an HS hinges on an evaluation of its physiological compensation capacity and its level. Stage III is characterized by hypotension and failure to compensate due to arteriolar system failure in intra-parenchymal bleeding or in the case of extra-parenchymal bleeding that is not self-contained. Stage IV defines a critical pre-cardiac arrest situation in equilibrium, maintained at the maximum limit that the body can sustain. In this state, a minimal solution of continuity in that equilibrium can lead to pump arrest by exsanguination or by a cardiac or cerebrovascular event before it. In contrast to the focus on rapid anaesthesia induction in stage III HS GA, where the primary concern is the stabilization of the patient in the context of ongoing haemorrhage and associated physiological deterioration, in stage IV, the objective should be to minimize any interference with the critical physiological balance.

Stable HS	• Stage I: Mild/Stable: only skin signs and tachycardia
Stabilized compensated HS	• Stage II: Moderate/Stabilized: shock responsive to fluid test load of 7 mL Kg/bw (−10/20% in obese) or 10% TBV × 1–2 within max 5–10 min with BP normalization and reverse tachycardia trend
Progressive, Unstable	• Stage III: Hypotensive shock not responsive to fluid test load of 20% TBV or transient response ≤20 min
Critical HS: (a) Impending CA; (b) Imminent CA	• Stage IV: (a) TBV loss of >30% with heart or brain ischemic signs or TBV > 40% in elderly; (b) TBV loss >50% or absent central pulses but present life signs in young
Cardiac Arrest by Exsanguination	• Stage V. Cardiac Arrest by Exsanguination: No vital signs and life signs

HS, hemorrhagic shock; TBV, total blood volume; SAP, systolic arterial pressure.

Table 1.
Revised diagnostic classification of hemorrhagic shock [1].

Stage I: Mild, stable, not-hypotensive HS: Oral or iv fluids suffice; blood can be spared except in susceptible patients such as the ones with pre-existing anaemia or cardiopathy where PRC are added to reach Hb ≥ 9 g/dL. Investigate with VBG and basic X-ray; interventional radiology, laparoscopy, thoracoscopy. Plan NOM or surgery within max 6–8 hours.
Stage II: Moderate, stabilized, compensated HS: IV crystalloids and PRC to test compensation. Investigate with Xr, EchoFast and/or IV contrast CT; interventional radiology, laparoscopy, thoracoscopy; surgery within maximum 4–6 hours from injury; consider NOM.
Stage III: Severe, hypotensive, unstable, decompensated, progressive, advanced HS: Indoors: no investigation should be entertained in the presence of severe shock and the patient should be taken as fast as possible to theatre except basic X-ray prn, VBG and E-Echofast Outdoors: THR tactics if known arterial bleeding; scoop and run or continuous transfusion and iatrogenic vasoconstriction if venous, mixed or unknown bleeding source.
Stage IV: Critical/in extremis shock, impending/imminent cardiac arrest by exsanguination: There is not yet a recommendable preoperative management of critical/in extremis HS with impending or imminent cardiac arrest by exsanguination. Do only 'clinical appraisal and sonar'! Outdoors: Scoop & Run tactics until source control, or continuous blood transfusion if pt. with IHD or CVE. Indoors: Stand-by surgery.
Stage V: Cardiac arrest by exsanguination: ERT/St.y: Primarily or added to an initial ERT/ALT/TACC or as continuation of an ERL/AACC within 5–10 min from CA, up to 20–30 min if penetrating thoracic injury, and in a patient oxygenated within 5 min from CA. A second team is required for DCS outside the chest.

NOM, nonoperative management; PRC, packed red cells; CA, cardiac arrest; St-y, sternotomy; TACC, thoracic aorta cross-clamping; ERT, emergency resuscitative thoracotomy; ALT, anterolateral thoracotomy; THR, titrated hypotensive resuscitation; IHD, ischemic heart damage; CVE, cerebrovascular event; DCS, damage control surgery; AACC, abdominal aorta cross-clamping.

Table 2.
Overall management of HS stages [1].

2. Titrated-to-response anaesthesia

2.1 Logistics

GA for HS with or without trauma can be administered in a war/warfare field, in a bush hospital, in a mass casualty, in the ER or, more frequently, in the OT. If the patient ventilates and oxygenates satisfactorily, GA is deferred in the OT.

The comprehensive checklist of requisite equipment and tools includes the following: oxygen, high-flow nasal cannula, Venturi face mask, CPAP mask, non-rebreather masks with reservoir and positive-end-expiratory-pressure (PEEP) valve, nasal masks, oropharyngeal (Guedel and Choi) and nasopharyngeal cannulae, and tubes. A bag-valve mask with a PEEP valve, a supraglottic airway (SGA) in a variety of sizes, nasotracheal tubes, endotracheal tubes (ETT) and direct laryngoscopes (Miller and McIntosh) in a range of sizes, a video laryngoscopy (VL) set, and surgical instruments. Additionally, the following devices and pharmaceuticals are available: Surgical airway devices (SAD), percutaneous trans-tracheal jet ventilation and high-frequency jet ventilation, cricothyroidotomy, percutaneous tracheotomy, open-standard tracheostomy and a series of drugs (alfentanil, sufentanil, remifentanil, ketamine racemic and left isomer). Additionally, the anaesthetic machine, non-invasive ventilation (NIV) portable machine, portable ventilators, intravenous fluids and blood, and phenylephrine are required. A set of peripheral venous cannulae of different sizes is also necessary for anaesthesia and transfusions.

While central venous lines for transfusion and pressure measurements, and arterial lines, are beneficial, they are not obligatory. Their purpose is to facilitate rapid massive transfusions or venous return evaluation and arterial real-time pressure monitoring. However, regardless of the expertise of the practitioner, Echo snap imaging can be crucially time-saving and lifesaving.

2.2 Position of the patient before GA

The standard sniff position, with the head extended at the atlanto-occipital joint and the patient lying on a cushion between 3 and 7 cm thick, is the optimal position for facilitating endotracheal intubation (ETI) and is the position that is typically used, except in cases of cervical spine injury (CSI), when the patient's head position is not manipulated. In the case of pregnant patients, the trunk should be tilted to the left.

In the context of obesity, a ramped position is required, with the head positioned 25° up and additional PEEP of 7.5–10 cm H_2O for manual ventilation/oxygenation. This approach offers a superior laryngeal view and results in a 20–25% higher PaO_2 and SaO_2 with a longer desaturation time and functional residual capacity (FRC) maintenance [2–4].

Chin lift and jaw thrust are standard maneuvers in the usual patient. Stabilization of the head and neck and traction of any kind without manipulations are enough for HS GA induction on patients with evident or likely CSI.

'*All airway interventions are associated with some degree of movement of the cervical spine; in general, these are very small and whether these are clinically significant in terms of impingement of the spinal cord is unclear. Manual in-line stabilization does not effectively immobilize the cervical spine and increases the likelihood of difficult and failed tracheal intubation. Video-laryngoscopy appears to cause a similar degree of cervical spine displacement and is an appropriate alternative approach. Direct laryngoscopy does cause a slightly greater degree of cervical spinal movement during tracheal intubation than video-laryngoscopy, but this does not appear to increase the risk of spinal cord compression. The risk of spinal cord injury during tracheal intubation appears to be minimal even in the presence of gross cervical spine instability. Depending on the clinical situation, practitioners should choose the tracheal intubation technique with which they are most proficient and that is most likely to minimize cervical spine movement*' [5].

SGA and VL obviate the need of any head/neck manipulation.

2.3 Pre-anaesthetic glance appraisal and management of the patient

2.3.1 Arterial pressure

In elderly patients with hypertension, particularly in the presence of traumatic brain injury (TBI), any reduction in pressure within the typical normal range should be regarded as mere hypotension. Furthermore, a systolic arterial pressure (SAP) of 110–120 should be considered indicative of shock [6, 7].

It is frequently possible to counteract pre-existing hypotension prior to intubation by administering blood or blood products for the treatment of haemorrhagic shock, intravenous fluids and timely use of vasopressors. In the presence of spinal or neurogenic shock, a fluid bolus or infusion of vasoconstrictors, such as ephedrine or vasopressin/anti-diuretic hormone, is frequently employed to buffer or slow the neurogenic-mediated vasodilation. It is imperative that ongoing fluid therapy be maintained prior to induction and that vasopressors be continued as an infusion throughout the THA procedure. In the event that the patient is brought to the operating room with a vasoconstrictor infusion under titrated hypotensive resuscitation, the infusion is to be left running.

2.3.2 Pre-oxygenation

The treatment of hypercapnia prior to anaesthesia is conducted either before or during the pre-oxygenation phase. An elevation in PCO_2 is frequently associated with the presence of hypertension.

Pre-oxygenation is a standard step before GA. The tidal volume breath for 3 min at 100% O_2 on a non-rebreather bag-valve-mask and the 8 deep breaths at 10 L/min in 1 min are techniques suitable for most patients. Similarly, O_2 at 15 L/min nasal cannula is an appropriate method for most patients [8, 9]. Pre-oxygenation with 100% oxygen extends the safe period of inevitable apnoea to 8 minutes after induction and muscle relaxation with a neuro-muscular blocker (NMBD) when used before endotracheal intubation (ETI). It ensures sufficient functional residual capacity (FRC) before or during the procedure.

In HS, excess of oxygen is deleterious too [10].

In normo-oxygenating patients with HS grade III, it is recommended that patients with stage IV HS be maintained on air oxygen at a level not exceeding PaO_2. It is advised that oxygen levels should not exceed 40–60% unless acute respiratory failure from chest contusion is in progress, in which case it should be titrated to 90–94% SaO_2 and the PF ratio maintained at a level not below 200 [10].

In cases where a patient presents with a non-invasive ventilation (NIV) device (i.e., a high-flow nasal cannula delivering >60 L/min of oxygen, a bilevel positive airway pressure (BiPAP) or continuous positive airway pressure (CPAP)) for hypoxemia resulting from pre-existing respiratory failure, thoracic trauma, obesity, or a difficult airway, it is recommended to allow for a minimum of three minutes of supported pre-oxygenation, which will extend the apnoea time [11–15].

2.3.3 Stomach status

In the absence of acute hypoxia, it is advisable to empty the stomach to the greatest extent possible. The author recommends pre-emptying the stomach with a nasogastric tube and positioning the patient laterally. It is advised that the 45–90° semi-sitting-sitting position is avoided in a hypotensive patient.

The use of a pre-induction sonar to the epigastrium and a reliable anamnesis-taking technique permit the recognition of a safe or potentially dangerous induction with stomach insufflation.

2.3.4 Imaging

The use of an echo facility for indirect imaging of neck anatomy [16], cardiac output measurement and early identification of pericardial tamponade or pneumothorax allows for the rapid acquisition of images and provides invaluable information to the anaesthetist about to anaesthetize a hypotensive patient with progressive haemorrhage.

The primary application of this technique remains the evaluation of gastric status, specifically whether the stomach is full or empty. An empty stomach is optimal for any general anaesthetic. Pre-induction echocardiography can provide crucial information on endotracheal tube (ETT) positioning, neck post-traumatic conformation and gastric status [17–19].

2.3.5 Things not to do in an emergency GA

In a GA for emergency surgery and trauma surgery or haemorrhagic shock, no premedication is administered, in contrast to the routine practice in elective anaesthesia/surgery. In particular, drugs used electively, such as midazolam, are contraindicated in emergency DCA/DCS as they may produce hypoventilation and hypotension, have a slow onset and discrete half-life, and interfere with subsequent monitoring and management. The use of fibre-optic bronchoscopy (FOB) for the induction of anaesthesia is considered to be an inefficient and laborious process in emergency situations.

Waking up the patient following difficult ventilation or intubation during a drill is 'no option in GA on a patient needing emergency surgery'.

It is inadvisable to perform volatile GA induction in the context of emergency surgery, given the imperative for speed and the necessity of promptly identifying any potential unexpected complications. It is this author's opinion that the procedure can nevertheless be attempted in the IV stage of critical HS, where the lack of interference with circulation and direct brain targeting results in fewer complications than other techniques that may affect the delicate equilibrium. To the best of my knowledge, this procedure has never been attempted previously. Pre-oxygenation with 100% oxygen plus IV induction is currently regarded as the safest option.

2.4 Induction

Patients may receive general anaesthesia with an endotracheal tube (ETT) or a supraglottic airway device (SGA) *in situ*, or breathing spontaneously through a simple oropharyngeal cannula. Additionally, general anaesthesia induction and total intravenous anaesthesia (TIVA) can be achieved with the use of special nasal cannulae, nasal masks and nasotracheal tubes [20–22].

The term 'induction' is used to describe the process of initiating a state of amnesia, sedation and anaesthesia. Concurrently, the aim is to prevent the sympathoadrenal response to upper airway manipulation (contact pressure), to safeguard the airway during a state of diminished consciousness and to ensure that oxygen levels are maintained at an optimal level during apnoea periods. An ETT offers the optimal protection and advantages; however, the patient may also be left breathing spontaneously with or without an SGA, depending on the filling of the stomach. An ETT serves three purposes: energy sparing, airway protection from face/neck trauma/bleeding and gastric aspiration, and an easier and safer control of the airway and breathing under GA.

In standard logistics, these questions must be answered rapidly before induction: firstly, whether the stomach is empty or not; secondly, whether the patient can be manually ventilated; thirdly, whether the patient can be easily intubated with anticipated difficulties; and fourthly, how to prepare for an unanticipated difficult or impossible intubation.

2.4.1 Induction methods

2.4.1.1 Rapid sequence induction intubation (RSII)

Rapid sequence induction intubation (RSII) represents the most common practice for initiating general anaesthesia in emergency surgical procedures. It entails a rapid succession of steps involving the administration of an induction drug, a neuromuscular blocking drug (NMBD), and endotracheal intubation.

Other two optional tactics are the *stepped sequence induction intubation (SSII)* and the *delayed sequence induction intubation (DSII)* (**Table 3**).

RSII is the standard and most frequent tactic in hypotensive shock. It is employed to protect the airway in cases where the stomach is not empty, despite the absence of evidence indicating that it reduces the risk of aspiration or other complications associated with airway management [23, 24].

In the event of an unsuccessful initial attempt at endotracheal intubation (ETI), the patient should be manually ventilated with pressures of less than 15 to 20 cm H_2O. This is a harmless ventilation technique that avoids inflation of the stomach in the event that it is not empty [25, 26]. The provision of positive pressure ventilation for high-risk patients during the pre-oxygenation period and between the induction of anaesthesia and the commencement of laryngoscopy has been demonstrated to reduce the incidence of hypoxemia [27–29]. For patients at high risk of hypoxemia and low risk of aspiration (e.g., those without vomiting, hematemesis, or hemoptysis), there is an indication for pre-oxygenation with non-invasive BiPAP ventilation with 100% FiO_2 for 5 minutes whenever feasible [30]. In patients at high risk of hypoxemia and high risk of aspiration, there is an indication for pre-oxygenation with 60 L/min of 100% FiO_2 via a high-flow nasal cannula or with supplemental oxygen via a standard face mask and nasal cannula [31].

In *SSII*, manual ventilation interposes after induction before NM blockade.

It is recommended that a stepped sequence induction intubation be performed in some emergency general anaesthesia (GA) situation for valid reasons. The capacity to manually ventilate the lungs via a face mask serves to assess the viability of rescuing a paralyzed patient in the event of anticipated or unanticipated challenging intubation scenarios, while simultaneously oxygenating a hypoxemic patient prior to induction. This may be particularly relevant in cases involving patients with poor respiratory reserves, sepsis or high metabolic requirements, who have decompensated during the intubating attempts of a difficult intubation.

Induction-intubation sequences		
Rapid Sequence Induction/Intubation	Stepped Sequence Induction/Intubation	Delayed Induction/Intubation Induction/Intubation
Induction drug NMB ETI	Induction drug Manual Ventilation NMB ETI	Ket. im induction NMB ETI/SGA
• Emerg Surg with stomach possibly not empty • Intestinal Obstruction - drain with SNG before RSII • Face and Neck injury or burns - patient sitting and no O_2 direct fm ventilation • Compensated HS	• TBI • Anticipated DA • Hypoxaemic patient • Septic patient • Advanced Hypotensive HS	• Patients uncooperative, vomiting or in psychosis • Uncooperative children

ETI, endo-tracheal intubation; FM, face mask; HS, hemorrhagic shock; CVE, cerebrovascular event; TBI, traumatic brain injury; SGA, supra-glottic ventilation device; DA, difficult airway.

Table 3.
Induction-intubation sequences in GA for HS and trauma.

In DSII, ketamine allows for induction within a 5–10-minute timeframe in patients who are uncooperative and require urgent surgical intervention.

2.4.2 Intubation drill

2.4.2.1 Peri-oxygenation/manual ventilation

It is recommended that oxygen be administered between attempts of endotracheal intubation (ETI) in continuity with pre-induction oxygenation.

The presence of difficult or ineffective mask ventilation represents a threatening situation that can be anticipated [32, 33]. A body mass index (BMI) greater than 26 kg/m^2, an age greater than 55 years, a history of macroglossia/snoring/apnoea, the presence of a beard, edentulousness/limited jaw protrusion, a Mallampati grade III or IV, and a thyromental distance of less than 6 cm are considered independent risk factors for inadequate, unstable, difficult-to-impossible mask ventilation (MV) [24].

The use of a gauze between the mask and the face may facilitate face mask ventilation, thereby assisting the anaesthesiologist in maintaining an open airway in cases where the anaesthesiologist has small hands, which may impede their ability to hold the chin and the mask with one hand.

Manual face mask ventilation can be contraindicated in cases of face and neck trauma [34–37].

In the event that a patient is unable to be adequately ventilated with a face mask, an SGA may be employed as an alternative means of ventilation.

SGA prevents the tongue from obstructing the oropharynx and, when correctly positioned, can effectively ventilate the lungs in a manner that is more efficient than that achieved by a face mask. An SGA can be inserted blindly, but not in an awake patient, where it would trigger local reflexes (gagging, coughing and vomiting) and a systemic sympatho-adrenal autonomic response (an increase in blood pressure, heart rate and respiratory rate). Among the SGA, the intubating laryngeal mask airway [38] and the intubating gel [39, 40] allow passage of a nasogastric tube and FOB, and the AIR-Q is suited as the only ventilation conduit during general anaesthesia [41].

In cases where ETI is not feasible and the patient can be ventilated between steps or has been adequately pre-oxygenated, FOB-assisted and VL have now superseded ILMA on the ETI function [42].

In certain cases, patients with a mouth opening of less than 2.5 cm (the average for an adult), a glottis that is off midline, a history of neck radiotherapy and post-fibrotic distorted anatomy, as well as lesions to the oropharynx or epiglottis, supraglottic stenosis and other factors, may not be suitable for ventilation with an SGA [43].

In the event of the ineffectiveness or impossibility of MV with an SGA following induction, the rapid neuro-muscular blockade and ETI serve to prevent death by asphyxial hypoxia. A rare but life-threatening event, difficult or failed mask ventilation after the administration of induction drugs and a neuro-muscular blocking agent (NMBA) is not typically caused by mechanical factors. Rather, it can manifest in one of two ways: either as an excess of sympatho-adrenal reflexes, which can be dampened by an excess of induction drug over relaxing the upper airway smooth muscle tone, or as a reflex spasm, which can occur when there is not enough relaxation due to an inadequate dosage of the induction drug. In the event of an unknown silent lesion in the airways, both scenarios have the potential to transform a potential partial stenosis into a complete or significant occlusion. This can result in inadequate or impossible ventilation resp. intubation [24, 44].

When both ventilatory tactics and ETI rescue tactics fail, a stab CTY followed by a 5–6 Fr ETT is lifesaving. If post-traumatic swelling by oedema or haematoma obscures landmarks, then an open Trach-y is what saves life [34].

A bougie-aided LMA insertion has higher rate of successful placement than digital insertion aid [45]. The blind technique of ETI through an ILMA has however been superseded by VL with a not-hyperangulated laryngoscope [46]. VL compared to DL is associated with higher odds of first-pass intubation success among ED trauma patients and has the same frequency of hypoxic events and time to successful intubation than DL. VDL requires a slightly longer execution time than DL [46–49] but is invaluable in the presence of an obvious CSI.

2.4.2.2 Induction agents

It is essential that the induction drug is effective and targeted (hypnosis and dampening of laryngeal reflexes), with no under- or overdosage; it should have a rapid and predictable onset to achieve the primary goals of rapid loss of consciousness (LOC) and avoidance of consciousness. This is the rationale behind the decision of numerous anaesthetists to await the feasibility of both LOC and ventilation before the administration of an NMBD, such as the stepped RSII, in order to ascertain that the dosage is neither excessive nor inadequate. Moreover, it is essential that the procedure achieves other significant secondary objectives, including the enhancement of intubation conditions in the context of inadequate paralysis, the minimization of haemodynamic disturbances and the attenuation of the sympathetic responses to laryngoscopy and tracheal intubation [24]. The administration of a fixed, predetermined dose of an induction agent carries the inherent risk of either underdosing, which may result in the potential for awareness, or overdosing, which may precipitate severe haemodynamic changes.

A stepped RSII should be performed as a matter of routine whenever there are indications of difficult ventilation or intubation. Severe hypotension during intubation in a patient with hypovolaemic HS can result in cardiac arrest and death. The mechanisms that contribute to peri-intubation hypotension include vasodilation from induction medications, decreased sympathetic tone from sedation and decreased venous return from increased intra-thoracic pressure with positive pressure ventilation. In addition, other major causes of intra-operative hypotension that should be addressed before induction include hemopneumothorax and pericardial tamponade [50–53].

At present, in order to reverse pre-existing hypotension prior to intubation, fluids, blood products and vasopressors (phenylephrine 100 mcg by IV push) are administered for GA in cases of haemorrhagic shock.

In patients at risk of hypotension, induction agents that contribute to hypotension must be avoided. An opioid may be employed as an induction agent and for the maintenance of anaesthesia throughout the surgical procedure. The titration of the induction drug to the point of loss of consciousness circumvents the potential issues associated with under- or overdosing. Furthermore, if the drug is administered in excess or in insufficient quantities, an NMBA in an RSII may be administered following the establishment of unconsciousness, thereby mitigating the risks associated with unexpected difficulties or impossibilities in ventilation [24, 44, 54, 55].

Alfentanil, the fastest-acting synthetic opioid, is the optimal choice for induction in patients with cardiac disease, given its efficacy and minimal interference with cardiovascular functions. It exhibits the most rapid onset of analgesia and time to peak effect, as well as the shortest distribution and elimination half-life [51, 56–59]. In bolus, it works safely at dosages of 10–50 mcg/kg (1–3 mcg/Kg/min in infusion).

Sufentanil (0.3 mcg/Kg) bolus [60, 61] is an effective induction agent in coronary artery disease.

Remifentanil (0.3–0.5 mcg/Kg/min) is the most suitable opioid in infusion for maintenance due to the shortest half-life [62], and the benefits on ischemic myocardium [63] and in neuro-surgical anaesthesia [64].

Etomidate (0.15–0.3 mg/Kg) is best suited for induction in cardiopathic patients as it hardly interferes with cardiovascular dynamics and its rapid onset action [51, 65, 66]. Etomidate was associated with worse intubating conditions than propofol when laryngoscopy was performed 1 minute after rocuronium [67]. Adrenal suppression even after a single bolus makes it c.i. in septic shock [68]. Etomidate is as safe also in TBI and HS + TBI [69].

The use of *ketamine* at a dose of 2 mg/kg administered intravenously is an effective induction agent, as it does not depress the myocardium and maintains or increases vasomotor tone and airways tone, with a tendency to normalize or increase blood pressure. The disadvantages are significant, including an increase in oxygen consumption (VO_2) and heart rate in an organ that is dependent on flow to increase oxygen delivery. At a basic regimen, ketamine extracts 75% of the oxygen delivered (DO_2). Therefore, ketamine is a suitable induction drug only for healthy patients and those with mild haemorrhagic shock. Indeed, in HS, it should only be employed for interventions on compensated (mild to moderate) shock in healthy, non-coronaropathic patients with a heart rate not exceeding 120 bpm. Ketamine has been effectively utilized in warfare, in both rural and urban settings, as an induction agent with and without supplementary oxygen, as well as in TIVA in elective and emergency patients, both with and without oxygen [70–74]. Ketamine iv is safe and effective, as it picks up in 1 minute.

Succinylcholine can be used to deal with the rare laryngospasm caused by ketamine [70, 71]. The new (L) isomer of ketamine, S (+)-ketamine, is expected to become an invaluable anaesthetic for critical illness due to its lesser chronotropic and neurotropic effects in comparison to the classical racemic mixture. Furthermore, it may extend the use of ketamine in patients with cardiac disease and traumatic brain injuries (TBIs) with or without haematoma (HS) [69, 75–78]. S(+)Ketamine is beneficial also in septic shock for its vasoconstricting effect [65]. The claimed effect of ketamine raising ICP has been challenged; as a matter of fact, it does not raise it and even may have beneficial effects [79, 80].

Propofol at a dose of ≤0.75 mg/kg has been demonstrated to be more effective than other induction agents in blunting the sympathetic reflex on endotracheal intubation (ETI). Furthermore, it has been shown to have a beneficial effect on intracranial pressure (ICP) following traumatic brain injury (TBI). However, the main disadvantage of propofol is the potential for hypotension and pain on injection. Consequently, it is recommended for use only in GA for TBI or TBI with compensated mild or moderate haemorrhagic shock [51, 64].

A similar drug, ciprofol, has a lower incidence of pain on injection and hypertension [81]. Propofol reduces mean arterial pressure but, when mitigated with adequate fluid resuscitation and vasopressors or drugs such as ketamine, is associated with improved neuro-protection.

A *ketamine/propofol admixture* (ketamine 0.75 mg/kg; propofol 1.5 mg/kg) in non-trauma patients has the same post-induction mean arterial pressure response than propofol (2 mg/kg) on its own [82]. Ketamine/propofol admixture (0.5 mg/kg of ketamine and 0.5 mg/Kg propofol), compensating each other's potential drawbacks, in emergency intubations in ICU on medical patients, has the same post-induction MAP response to intubation of etomidate [66].

A further advantage of ketamine and propofol is that they can be appropriately used as induction agents and continued in a TIVA.

Thiopentone, propofol, ketamine and etomidate all have been used for the induction in patients with raised ICP. Barbiturates are contraindicated in HS and are used only in the induction of patients with TBI without shock.

2.4.2.3 Neuro-muscular blockade

The objective is to facilitate intubation against laryngeal reflex and prevent a rise in systolic pressure, heart rate and laryngospasm. This is achieved by seeking myorelaxation through hypnosis and unconsciousness. There are two options for achieving this: neuro-muscular blocking drugs (NMBDs), such as suxamethonium or rocuronium, or a synthetic opioid at high doses without NM blockade.

Opioids have two potential drawbacks in emergency or critical scenarios, due to their repressive effect of repressing ventilation and blood pressure, which is faster than the effect of facilitating the ETI, and the interference with maintenance regimes. For these reasons, opioids, if used, must have the shortest action time and duration. Fentanyl 2 mcg/Kg is the most powerful drug to curb the haemodynamic and facilitate intubation conditions. Its respiratory and haemodynamic effect would need to be controlled.

Suxamethonium is a depolarizing neuro-muscular blocking agent with a dosage range of 1–1.5 mg/kg. It is the fast- and short-acting myorelaxing agent for endotracheal intubation (ETI), inducing myorelaxation within the first minute and a spontaneous reversal in approximately five to ten minutes. Furthermore, it is the optimal pharmacological agent to address potential complications associated with the synthetic opioid during induction, including the occurrence of thoracic rigidity [23, 24].

Suxamethonium-induced fasciculation increases oxygen consumption during apnoea, which may become relevant in the event of pre-existent partial airway obstruction.

A prolonged block renders a non-depolarizing NMBD such as rocuronium (1–1.5 mg/kg and an onset of action in the order of 2 min) a less optimal option in critical trauma GA. However, rocuronium-induced neuro-muscular blockade has a unique advantage compared to suxamethonium. It can be reversed with sugammadex at 16 mg/kg in a faster fashion than the spontaneous recovery from suxamethonium [83, 84]. *Rocuronium* finds the main indication and advantage in an unanticipated difficult airway scenario during an SSII or in TBI or pre-existent unknown silent stenosis when the rare event of a situation of pre-existent unknown stenosis after myo-relaxation of an RSII would make ventilation and intubation difficult to impossible [44]. With a rapid reversal of the NMBD, the muscle would regain tone and allow ventilation.

2.4.2.4 Endotracheal intubation

It is recommended that a maximum of two or three attempts by one or two experienced airway operators should be permitted before defining a difficult intubation. The ability to perform the procedure successfully is contingent upon the skill, experience and expertise of the airway operators, as well as their mental promptness. These factors are essential for the prevention, early identification and successful, timely ETI.

A 'minimum number' of 50 GA for emergency surgery, of 100 combined emergency/elective GA and of 10 cardiac arrest airways management should give reassurance, confidence, reliability, safety and predictable success rate.

On the issue about which adjunct facilitates quick intubation, whether it is an armoured ETT with stylet or a bougie that increases chances of quick intubation [85], the author prefers an ETT armoured with a stylet in all emergency or critical anaesthesia (*pers obs*).

The following factors have been identified as potential risk indicators for difficult endotracheal intubation (ETI): prior history of difficult intubation, inability to extend the head and pronate the mandible, mouth opening <4 cm in an adult, thyro-mental distance < 6 cm in an adult, sterno-hyoid length short neck < 8 cm in an adult, stridor, thick neck for oedema, haemathoma or obesity, Mallampati III & IV, Cormack-Lehane IIb, II, IV. The presence of an altered mental status precludes many critically ill patients from undergoing the classic airway assessments, such as Mallampati scoring, due to the limitations imposed by these conditions [86, 87].

In a predicted difficult airway, one skillful airway operator with the assistance of two nurses is a prudent set-up [88].

The practice of applying *cricoid pressure* with the peak inspiratory pressure (PIP) up to 40 cm H_2O for the prevention of gastric inflation with gas is currently regarded as a controversial measure. However, when applied in a moderate, prudent and safe manner, it is not possible to ascertain its efficacy in advance. Consequently, its recommendation remains a topic of contention, as the protection it affords against regurgitation, optimal cord visualization and ventilation cannot be guaranteed.

The application of backward, upward and rightward pressure to the cricoid cartilage against the cervical vertebrae of 1 kg in an awake patient and 3 kg in an anaesthetised patient, with the head and neck in extreme extension, is hypothesized to prevent gastric insufflation and regurgitation while simultaneously facilitating ETI. The current standard sniffing position, which is typically employed for standard ETI, may not yield the same degree of success in occluding the oesophagus as intended, but rather the hypopharynx. If gastric insufflation is prevented, gastric regurgitation is not. Furthermore, ventilation and oxygenation are made less effective, and in an awake patient, reflex gagging and vomiting can be triggered. However, external laryngeal manipulation may provide a superior and more comprehensive visualization of the laryngeal inlet on ETI when performed with caution and moderation.

While the tube entry can be successfully completed with clear vision of the epiglottis and a free margin of tissues around it, particularly in the super space, complications may arise when only the epiglottis is visible and the tube covers it during the introduction. In such instances, it is advisable to employ a BURP manoeuvre or to utilize an ETT with stylets from the outset in order to minimize the risk of missing the epiglottis.

Oesophageal intubation represents the most significant risk associated with failed intubation. In addition to the failure of direct oxygenation, the potential for ventilating into the stomach with regurgitation of its contents into the airways would only serve to compound or contribute to hypoxemia. A continuous capnography waveform with end-tidal values of CO_2 ($EtCO_2$) is the gold standard for confirming ventilation of the lungs. In a series of emergency intubations, clinical examination identified a maximum of 90% of malpositioning compared to capnography. However, clinical methods demonstrated a superior, faster predicted value in cardiac arrest ETI [89].

Over the past decade, the use of wave capnography (WC) has become a standard adjunct to any ETT circuit and is now mandatory in emergency, intensive care unit (ICU) and cardiac arrest ETI. In this context, it is of the utmost importance to monitor the quality of the resuscitation and the prognosis. Wave capnography has a sensitivity and specificity of 100% in confirming the position of ETT compared to clinical appraisal in the field or to sonar. However, it remains a tool that is slower to signal when compared to clinical appraisal and sonar. Consequently, it has limitations in several shock and cardiac arrest scenarios and is unable to identify unintentional bronchial intubation. Nevertheless, it remains invaluable during resuscitation to signal ROSC, as routine in settings like the ICU, in patients in a coma to gauge CO_2, or during GA to troubleshoot ETT displacement [90, 91].

When both tracheal intubation and manual ventilation are impossible, ventilate with any ESA (PTJV, CTY, PCTy or OSTy).

2.5 Managing the difficult airway and recognizing the critical airway

In 2013, the American Society of Anesthesiologists (ASA) defined a difficult airway (DA) as 'a clinical situation in which a conventionally trained anaesthesiologist experiences difficulty with face mask ventilation or difficulty with tracheal intubation or both.' This definition is, in the author's view, the most convenient and conceptually useful [92]. A maximum of 2–3 attempts should be done by two anaesthetists before considering ETI impossible.

In a study on non-obstetric patients, 2.5% of patients required two laryngoscopies to achieve tracheal intubation and that 1.8% required more than three [93].

Factors associated to difficult manual face mark ventilation or difficult SGA ventilation or to ETI are known [32, 33, 43, 86, 87]. The presence of any of the associated factors defines consensually the 'anticipated difficult airway'.

As a challenging mask ventilation can be addressed through the use of SGA or ETI, a challenging SGA ventilation can be managed through ETI, and a difficult ETI can be resolved with SGA, the aforementioned comprehensive generic definition provides a clear delineation. The distinction between a difficult airway that remains manageable without percutaneous or surgical access and a critical advanced stage of deterioration of the airways that requires an emergency surgical airway (ESA) due to the inability to ventilate and the subsequent life-threatening hypoxia remains clear. In the event that both manual ventilation and ETI are not viable options, the situation is defined as a 'critical airway', which is a condition necessitating the use of a surgical or percutaneous airway device for oxygenation and ventilation. A 'can intubate, can't ventilate' scenario is defined as a situation in which the patient can be intubated but not ventilated with ETT due to a number of potential causes, including lung collapse (pneumothorax resulting from tracheal, bronchial or lung rupture), bronchospasm or oesophageal intubation. The management of this scenario is dependent on the underlying cause. The use of clinical acumen, $EtCO_2$ monitoring and sonar allows for the identification of the etiology. The recommended approach is TTJV, bronchodilators, immediate redo-ETI and rapid chest drainage. This can be performed in 30–60 seconds using the quick measured stab and intercostal drainage insertion technique. In cases where an ETT is unable to ventilate and oxygenate the patient, the scenario may be considered a physiological difficult airway [34].

2.5.1 Are definitions such as anticipated and unanticipated difficult airway and anatomical or physiological difficult airway of any practical usefulness?

Some authors have questioned the practical value of definitions such as 'anticipated or unanticipated difficult airway' in the context of the mandatory awareness and vigilance for risks that operators must maintain regardless of whether a difficult airway is expected or not. Indeed, the predictive criteria for difficult airways may demonstrate high sensitivity, but low specificity and positive predictive value [94].

In a comprehensive review, out of 3391 difficult intubations, 3154 (93%) were unanticipated with only 2% of positively predicted DAs; difficult mask ventilation was unanticipated in 94% of cases with only 1.5% of positively predicted difficult mask ventilation [95].

The incidence of a difficult airway with sole impossibility of intubation is 1:2000 in elective cases and up to 1:100 in emergencies, rising to 1:300 in obstetric GA. The incidence of DA with inability to ventilate and intubate is 1:5000 in routine anaesthesia, necessitating an emergency surgical airway in 1:50000 elective GA. In the emergency department, an emergency surgical airway (ESA) may be required in 1 in 200 cases of emergency anaesthesia with a difficult airway. An inadequately or mismanaged DA has been identified as a significant factor in up to 25% of anaesthesia-related deaths [96].

In a study on parturients undergoing GA for caesarean section, the risk of difficult airway by failed intubation is around 1:300 and was found around 10 times higher than the same risk in a general mix surgical population [97].

In a study on non-obstetric patients, 2.5% of patients required two laryngoscopies to achieve tracheal intubation and that 1.8% required more than three [93].

Difficulty with intubation occurs more frequently during obstetric anaesthesia, but that the frequency of very difficult intubation is similar in obstetric and non-obstetric surgical populations. These numbers haven't changed over the years [96, 98].

The rate of failed intubations is dependent on a number of factors, including the circumstances of the procedure (e.g., indoor or outdoor setting), the context of the procedure (e.g., elective or emergency) and the experience and expertise of the attending healthcare professional. For instance, data indicates that anaesthetists performing procedures in outdoor settings have a low failure rate (less than 2–3%), while emergency physicians and paramedics have reported failure rates above 10% and as high as 20% or more. In cases of cardiac arrest, the failure rate for physicians performing procedures outdoors has been reported to be less than 10%, while in trauma cases, the rate is less than 1% [99, 100].

A difficult airway is an anatomical and mechanical problem. The term 'physiological difficult airway' is discouraged as it is not an accurate description of the situation when there is pre-existent hypoxemia and hypotension. These two physiological concomitant or pre-existent abnormalities simply abut into the terminal tunnel of the pyramidal/funnelled mental process of a DA, which is 'safe ventilation and oxygenation'.

To extrapolate conceptually those variables as autonomous packaged information during the mental processing of an airway crisis implies using a binary approach [101]. The binary mental approach distracts and makes one lose mental speed and focus that in some circumstances can be lethal to the patient when the target aim is oxygenation/ventilation anyhow [35, 102, 103].

In essence, the mind should concentrate on the primary objective and consider only the background variables that are not conducive to achieving this goal. Any conceptualization hinders the ability to make rapid decisions based on priorities, such as ensuring adequate oxygenation through ventilation and sufficient Hb presence.

The outcome of managing an unanticipated difficult airway scenario is significantly influenced by human factors such as leadership with an appropriate level of assertiveness, situation awareness and decision-making. It is not possible to distil the complexities of difficult airway management into a single algorithm or theoretical teaching. Even the best anaesthetic teams supported by the best guidelines will still experience difficulties in performing optimally if the systems in which they operate are flawed [42, 104, 105].

2.5.2 Critical airway

The critical airway, described a decade ago, represents a more expansive conceptualization of the difficult airway, encompassing only GA. It delineates a scenario of imminent clinical hypoxaemia, necessitating prompt ESA, including PTJV as a temporizing technique, as a lifesaving surgical airway. This may occur during GA inductions or ex novo [34, 35].

2.5.3 Special cases of difficult airway inductions

Other circumstances [34] may necessitate the induction of an ESA, including injuries to the face and neck, burns, agitation, vomiting, paediatrics, intestinal obstruction and unconsciousness.

In the event of a patient vomiting at the time of induction, they should be placed in the lateral position and returned to the supine position following the administration of either ketamine or etomidate via intravenous induction.

In the case of patients who have sustained injuries to the face and burns, it is recommended that they be pre-oxygenated in a sitting position with a face mask placed in proximity to the mouth. The induction of anaesthesia should be conducted in a sitting position with ketamine administered intravenously. Once unconsciousness has been achieved, the patient should be placed in a supine position to complete the rapid sequence induction with endotracheal intubation or a laryngeal mask airway. It is not uncommon for patients who have sustained injuries to the neck or head to present with these conditions.

In the event that a patient has an intestinal obstruction or ileus, it is advisable to drain the stomach in a sitting position prior to induction. This can be achieved by placing a nasogastric tube in situ. In general, SGA is indicated for the ventilation of facial trauma in the absence of laryngeal trauma, where the use of a face mask is contraindicated. The use of an SGA in facial injuries prevents the entry of blood into the lower airways; however, it should not be employed in cases of neck trauma. The application of positive pressure ventilation in these circumstances would result in the displacement of foreign bodies, blood or secretions into the smaller airways [34–37].

Failure or contraindication to SGA in neck injuries seeing ventilation preludes to PCT, OTY or ETT to be kept standby [34].

In patients with severe traumatic brain injury (TBI) who are already unconscious, it is recommended that the Glasgow Coma Scale (GCS) and laryngeal reflexes be tested before induction. In such cases, ETI is indicated if the GCS is >8 or if hypotensive HS is present in elderly patients. The most appropriate approach for these patients is selective serial intubation and inflation (SSII). Difficult patients who are highly agitated should be pre-medicated with ketamine.

Actively vomiting patients require NGT drainage of the stomach in lateral position and ketamine with no neuro-muscular blockade for induction (*pers obs*).

Nursing support is indispensable.

The concurrent administration of both an antiemetic and a ketamine has the potential to elicit adverse effects. In patients with intestinal obstruction, a sitting position is preferable; however, it is contraindicated in hypotensive shock with paralytic ileus.

In patients who are in a state of distress and require immediate medical intervention, as well as in individuals with head and neck trauma and burns, and in those with an anticipated difficult airway, ketamine is a highly beneficial and advantageous medication that can be safely administered.

In patients with significant neck injuries or burns, ketamine should be used for its ability to maintain airway and vascular tone in situations of high risk, including critical airway and respiratory arrest resulting from the conversion or completion of a pathological partial stenosis or narrowing of the airways, or the introduction of a foreign body into the lower airways [34–37].

Patients who have received a dissociative dose of ketamine, following pre-oxygenation with a high-flow non-rebreather mask or non-invasive positive pressure ventilation (NIPPV), are paralyzed and intubated. In patients who require emergency airway management and who will not tolerate pre-oxygenation and peri-intubation procedures due to uncooperative psychotic vomiting or in children, delayed sequence induction intubation (DSII) represents an invaluable alternative [106].

2.6 Maintenance

2.6.1 Drugs

At present, satisfactory and safe general anaesthesia with or without airway protection can be maintained under total intravenous anaesthesia (TIVA) with oxygen plus ketamine or a synthetic opioid (e.g., remifentanil or propofol, all of which have the shortest half-life and emergence time) [57, 62, 71].

The use of TIVA with remifentanil presents certain advantages over ketamine in terms of sedation and ischemic preconditioning, as well as a reduced impact on heart rate. Conversely, propofol is only considered a safe option for general anaesthesia in cases of traumatic brain injury.

Oxygen should be kept within a maximal limit of 40 perhaps up to 60% $PaO2$, unless respiratory insufficiency is present [10–15].

Ketamine is an effective anaesthetic for both induction and maintenance of anaesthesia. However, it has been observed that ketamine increases oxygen consumption ($VO2$) and heart rate in an organ, the heart, which is dependent on flow to increase oxygen delivery. Furthermore, at a basic regimen, it has been demonstrated that ketamine extracts 75% of the oxygen delivered ($DO2$). In HS, ketamine can be used as an induction agent for interventions on compensated (mild to moderate) shock in normal or healthy patients, provided that their heart rate does not exceed 120 beats per minute.

Ketamine is the sole anaesthetic agent that does not depress the myocardium, the vasomotor tone and the airway tone. Consequently, it has been successfully employed in war-outdoor scenarios as TIVA on elective surgery and on emergency patients not in HS, without the addition of oxygen, on patients breathing air-oxygen only [71].

The doses that have been used in not shocked patients, breathing spontaneously air-oxygen or intubated, hint to 50–100 mcg/Kg/min as suitable dosage for maintenance of ketamine TIVA [72–74].

The conduct of TIVA during maintenance is strictly dependent on stimuli during surgery: the above dosages appear to suffice in emergency and HS and all scenarios where speed is determinant.

The new (L) isomer of ketamine, S (+)-ketamine, promises, in virtue of lesser chronotropic and neurotropic effects as compared to the classical racemic mixture, to become an invaluable drug in anaesthesia for critical illness, extending ketamine usage in cardiopathic patients [75–78].

2.6.2 Maintenance of neuro-anaesthesia

There is no significant difference in gross lines between TBI GA and HS GA. The brain is more susceptible to hypoxaemia and hypercapnia than other organs, and the heart is similarly vulnerable to hypoxaemia. Both organs can benefit from hypothermia conditions, with the brain after ROSC post-CA and the heart in ECLS. This is particularly relevant in cases of extreme resuscitation following hypovolaemic and normovolaemic CA.

All TBI GA is, by definition, a DCA that is designed to prevent the production or exacerbation of any secondary injury. The distinction lies in the self-regulated cerebral microcirculation, which becomes dysregulated in the presence of trauma. The local and systemic deleterious effects of hypotension, hypertension, hypoxemia and hypercapnia are identical in HS and TBI.

The objective of TBI management is to prevent or mitigate secondary brain damage from hypoxia, which can result from either systemic hypotension or a loco-regional mass effect. While hypotension can be managed by intervening on the systemic macrocirculation, mass effect necessitates surgical or percutaneous decompression, preceded and followed by postural and medical methods (hyperosmolar therapies, sedation, therapeutic coma, hyperventilation and therapeutic hypothermia).

Sedation with BZD and hypocapnia up to and not lower than 28 mmHg constitutes a significant aspect of specific ICP management.

In cases where intracranial hypertension requires urgent relief, surgical intervention for traumatic brain injury (TBI) can be safely performed concurrently with orthopaedic and limb and trunk surgery. Otherwise, the surgical procedure is monitored during the general surgery or orthopaedic operation and addressed at the conclusion of the procedure under the same GA protocol.

BZD is beneficial in TBI GA as one of the options for decreasing ICP and as a co-adjuvant in GA maintenance for surgery of combined HS and TBI, provided that systemic pressures have been restored.

The management of traumatic brain injury (TBI) and concomitant neck injury or trunk lesions requires a high level of expertise and careful consideration of the patient's positioning. In the majority of cases, controlling the source of haemorrhage is of greater importance than managing TBI, unless there is evidence of mass effect on the brain before or during surgery. In such instances, the two procedures are carried out simultaneously.

Propofol has a rapid onset and a relatively short-acting effect. It is hypotensive, blunts the sympathetic reflex on endotracheal intubation (ETI) and is suitable for GA for traumatic brain injury (TBI) due to its known efficacy in decreasing endocranial pressures at doses that do not reduce mean arterial pressure (MAP) and cerebral perfusion pressure (CPP). In head injury with TBI, it is to be used judiciously at dosages sufficient to decrease intracranial pressure (ICP) but not CPP. This makes propofol usable only in compensated head injury with TBI [64]. In contrast to inhalation agents, propofol has been demonstrated to reduce both cerebral blood flow (CBF) and the cerebral metabolic rate of oxygen (CMRO2). Furthermore, it has been shown to lower ICP, improve CPP and provide an adequate neuro-protective effect during cerebral ischemia. In comparison to etomidate and barbiturates, propofol has been observed to decrease mean arterial pressure (MAP) to a greater extent than etomidate and to a lesser extent than thiopental. Additionally, propofol can be utilized for both induction and maintenance due to its efficacy in dampening the laryngeal reflex and its rapid onset and short half-life. It remains the primary agent for amnesia in neuro-anaesthesia.

However, propofol lacks sufficient analgesic and sedative properties, which is why it is most effective when used in TIVA in conjunction with other drugs that have a higher analgesic and sedative impact. Due to its lack of analgesic properties, opioids are frequently combined with it. Midazolam is co-administered to alleviate anxiety [64].

Cerebral blood flow (CBF) and cerebral metabolic rate of oxygen ($CMRO_2$) are interdependent. Given that the skull is a closed space, any increase in CBF will result in an increase in ICP, which may subsequently affect CPP and, in turn, $CMRO_2$. It is essential to reduce $CMRO_2$ and ICP while maintaining MAP/CPP.

It is imperative to reduce ICP prior to, during and following the intervention, employing a range of techniques and strategies, to prevent secondary brain damage.

A reverse Trendelenburg position at 30° following haemorrhagic source control and the restoration of pressures is beneficial during GA for combined trauma where craniotomy or craniectomy follows in succession to surgery for source control. The anaesthetist and neurosurgeon are responsible for overseeing the procedure.

Mannitol and HTS are both employed to reduce ECP during surgery. In cases of TBI where neither craniotomy nor craniectomy is necessary, HTS is the preferred option, with consideration given to the limits of its administration in terms of dosage and time [64]. Conversely, in the event that concomitant surgical intervention is indicated in the context of DCS, it is imperative to implement ICP and intra-arterial monitoring, with the subsequent administration of mannitol contingent upon the initial HTS bolus.

The use of TIVA with propofol in conjunction with other pharmaceutical agents has been demonstrated to result in a significantly greater reduction in intracranial pressure (ICP) compared to the administration of inhalation agents in patients presenting with a GCS score of less than 8, evidence of brain oedema, and a midline shift exceeding 5 mm, in preparation for an emergency craniotomy.

However, the risk of awareness is higher with TIVA than with gaseous anaesthesia maintenance. Monitoring of TIVA with somatosensory-evoked potentials (SSEP), motor-evoked potentials (MEP) and electromyography (EMG) is essential for the detection of awareness. The interference of inhalation agents on the evoked potential monitoring, which is not affected by IV agents, makes TIVA the preferred choice for TBI surgery when awareness is a risk factor and monitoring is required [64].

The use of TIVA with 'propofol and remifentanil' or 'propofol and rocuronium', with 'propofol and ketamine infusions with or without an opioid such as remifentanil', or with 'propofol/remifentanil/rocuronium', has been demonstrated to be an appropriate method of anaesthesia in neuro-anaesthesia, with no decrease in SAP or increase in ICP [51, 64].

Rocuronium is the preferred alternative to succinylcholine as it does not result in an increase in endocranial pressure and can be reversed with sugammadex.

In the current era, the utilization of propofol and remifentanil infusion has rendered the administration of muscle relaxants unnecessary for intubation in the presence of traumatic brain injury (TBI) with mass effect.

Furthermore, the administration of diazepam, in lieu of the hypotensive midazolam, can be employed after the establishment of airway and source control with a normalized blood pressure, in order to buffer the neurotropic, extrapyramidal and chronotropic effects of ketamine. The administration of benzodiazepines for the purpose of sedation during the maintenance phase of treatment has been observed to exert a more pronounced direct influence on the functioning of an injured brain than in the absence of injury. The primary disadvantage, apart from the counteractable hypotensive and hypoventilating effects, is the interference with frequent neurological examinations. Midazolam is frequently administered in conjunction with propofol and opioids to mitigate the anxiety associated with sedation. Midazolam should only be used in GA maintenance following the stabilization of pressures and source control. Barbiturates may be used as an induction agent in TBI without HS.

Glycopyrrholate bolus is effective in controlling increased salivation without crossing the blood–brain barrier or increasing the heart rate, in contrast to atropine. The fascia, membrane and skin are sensitive to pain and increase autonomic reflexes and tachycardia [71].

Dexmedetomidine has recently become a popular choice as a sole anaesthetic agent, offering sedation without the adverse effects of hypoventilation.

Dexmedetomidine has been demonstrated to provide sedation that is comparable with propofol and remifentanil in a range of surgical and interventional contexts, yet with a reduced incidence of respiratory adverse events, and to possess analgesic properties that obviate the necessity for opioids, while concomitantly engendering improvements in stability of haemodynamics and ventilation/respiration.

Dexmedetomidine has been employed as a sole agent for conscious sedation during awake craniotomies and in intensive care unit (ICU) sedation.

In the case of shorter procedures, such as computed tomography (CT), the preferred option is conscious or deep sedation with short-acting drugs, such as intravenous (IV) midazolam. However, if hypotension is a potential issue, dexmedetomidine can be a valuable alternative.

Furthermore it has been extensively employed for sedation during awake intubation, demonstrating comparable safety and efficacy to propofol and remifentanil combinations. The benefits of utilizing intravenous anaesthetic agents in awake intubation include reduced local anaesthetic requirements, cough reflex suppression, anxiety alleviation and the provision of sedation.

Dexmedetomidine, likewise propofol and remifentanil target controlled infusion (TCI), has gained popularity as TIVA in awake surgery conscious sedation [107].

It has been demonstrated that an awake craniotomy/craniectomy with or without scalp block is a feasible procedure and has been successfully completed in the absence of HS.

Two techniques are available: the 'asleep-awake-asleep' technique and the 'awake-awake-awake' technique. The objective of TIVA in awake craniotomy is to guarantee optimal patient comfort without disrupting neurophysiological monitoring and to ensure adequate ventilation and patency of the airways throughout the procedure.

2.6.3 Volatile anaesthetics

There is no study yet on safety efficacy and outcomes of volatile agents on maintenance of GA in HS, despite the appealing safety and efficacy with the least haemodynamic interference. Because of the interference with monitoring of TBI TIVA [64], gas should be used only in critical HS with no TBI.

Volatile anaesthetics such as desflurane, isoflurane and sevoflurane are potentially suitable for use in Stage IV HS [1], with minimal systemic effects compared to IV drugs. This reduces the risk of disrupting the critical equilibrium of the patient's actual compensatory physiology.

In patients with multiple injuries or multiple episodes of severe haemodynamic instability, agents with a low blood-gas partition coefficient (e.g., desflurane and sevoflurane) are preferred to permit rapid titration.

The minimum effective dose for induction in a Stage IV HS is yet to be determined. However, it can be reasonably assumed that it should be maintained at <0.5 MAC. As blood pressure improves to a level exceeding 90 mmHg systolic, inhalation agents are increased to a concentration of half the minimum alveolar concentration (MAC) or greater.

The gaseous agents exert a modulatory effect on inflammatory processes, thereby protecting the heart and brain from ischemia–reperfusion injury. This is achieved by opening and activating the mitochondrial K-ATP channels [51, 108, 109].

Pre-exposure of brain to isoflurane induces ischemic tolerance. Isoflurane preconditioning protects myocardium against infarction via activation of K(ATP) channels [110]. More ominously, it is possible that it provides post-ischemic neuroprotection as well [111].

2.6.4 Monitoring of TIVA

MEP, SSEP and EMG during neuro-anaesthesia with TIVA are commonly monitored [64].

In the context of trauma, the shock index is not a reliable indicator due to the potential influence of pain, the inflammatory response, hypoxemia or hypercapnia on the pulse. However, it remains a valuable parameter in the assessment of non-traumatic haemorrhage [1, 112].

Subsequently, GA maintenance can be conducted with 'TIVA on demand' in a 'titrated-to-response anaesthesia' (TRA), with due consideration of the pain-sensitive structures encountered during the various body ingress sites. It is only the skin incision and fascia incision and stretching, such as serosa and capsules, that elicit pain and thus warrant a sufficient level of circulating anaesthetic [71].

The era of flat anaesthetics and surgery is over, and it is time we go toward a tailored-to-individual physiology restoration in real time.

3. General anaesthesia schemes

Schemes for GA (**Tables 4** and **5**), optimalized for advanced hypotensive or critical HS, have been drafted.

The scheme has been developed based on the experience gained from the use of TIVA in non-HS/trauma scenarios [62, 71]. It is designed to ensure the safe and least interfering GA, taking into account the physiological imperatives and the characteristics and properties of the pertinent drugs or gases. However, there is a need for a rapid and safe induction, a safe and least interfering yet efficacious maintenance, and special considerations for scenarios of combined HS and TBI (**Table 6**).

A question was posed on Research Gate several years ago: 'Should we administer analgesic drugs to intubate a patient during cardiac arrest?' [113]. The participants in

Drugs for GA in stable compensated HS	
Induction	**Maintenance**
• Oxygen • Etomidate • Suxamethonium	Remifentanil TIVA (Mild/Moderate HS, in cardiopathic or HR >120/min)
• Oxygen • Ketamine • Suxamethonium	S(+)-Ketamine/Remifentanil TIVA (Mild/Moderate HS not in cardiopathic or HR > 120/min)
• Oxygen • Propofol • Rocuronium	Propofol/Remifentanyl +/-Rocuronum TIVA (Mild&/Moderate HS in CVA or TBI patients)

GA, general anesthesia; HS, hemorrhagic shock; HR, heart rate; CVA, cerebrovascular accident; TBI, traumatic brain injury.

Table 4.
Drugs for GA for stable compensated HS stage I & II.

Drugs for Ga in advanced HS			
GA	HS Stage III	HS Stage IV	HS Stage 5 - CA ECLS + DCS during or post ROSC
Induction	40–60% FiO_2 ⇧ ⇨ 90–94 SaO_2 VASOCONSTRICTION INFUSION + ALFENTANYL/ ETOMIDATE	Air OXYGEN + ALFENTANYL/ ETOMIDATE or? SEVOFLURANE/ DESFLURANE	100% O_2 + SUFENTANIL
Maintenance	REMIFENTANIL TIVA +/– VASOCOSTRICTION INFUSION followed by REMIFENTANIL TIVA after source control and restoration of MAP/SAP	REMIFENTANIL TIVA or? ISOFLURANE +40–60% FiO_2 ⇧ ⇨ 90–94 SaO_2 after source control and restoration of pressures	REMIFENTANIL TIVA

CA, cardiac arrest; ECLS, extracorporeal life-support; DCS, damage control surgery; TIVA, total intra-venous anaesthesia; FiO_2 = fraction of inspired Oxygen; ROSC = return of spontaneous circulation.

Table 5.
Drugs for GA for advanced HS stages III, IV, V.

Induction	**Maintenance**
• Oxygen Etomidate	Remifentanil CIVA (Mild/Moderate HS, in cardiopathic or HR >120/min)
• Oxygen Ketamine	S(+)-Ketamine CIVA or Remifentanil CIVA (Mild/Moderate HS, not in cardiopathic patients or HR > 120/min)
• Oxygen Propofol	S(+) Propofol/Remifentanil+/– Rocuronium (Mild&/Moderate HS in CVA or TBI patients)

Table 6.
GA in stable compensated HS.

the discussion expressed a preference for a positive answer. If the indication for extracorporeal cardiopulmonary resuscitation (E-CPR) via extracorporeal life support (ECLS) is correctly applied and timed, until a patient is deemed to be in irreversible coma and suitable for organ donation, any autonomic stimulation, such as endotracheal intubation (ETI) and deep chest compressions (DCS), should be avoided, and the patient should receive an intravenous or intra-tracheal opioid drug before ETI and a top-up before sternotomy and laparotomy for DCS and/or resuscitation by ECLS.

Sufentanil is an appropriate choice for providing profound and long-lasting analgesia. The author has previously employed it in a successful medical CA resuscitation before ETI, after ROSC, with no adverse effects on the surviving patient.

Author details

Fabrizio G. Bonanno
Department of Surgery, Polokwane Provincial Hospital, Polokwane, South Africa

*Address all correspondence to: f.g.bonanno@gmail.com

References

[1] Bonanno FG. Management of hemorrhagic shock according to the revised "physiological classification"—Update 2024. In: New Visions in Medicine and Medical Science. Vol. 4. Bengal, India: B P International; 5 Apr 2024. pp. 136-181. DOI: 10.9734/bpi/nvmms/v4/12052F. P-ISBN: 978-81-971983-5-9. E-ISBN:978-81-971983-7-3

[2] Collins JS, Lemmens HJ, Brodsky JB, Brock-Utne JG, Levitan RM. Laryngoscopy and morbid obesity: A comparison of the "sniff" and "ramped" positions. Obesity Surgery. 2004;**14**:1171-1175

[3] Dixon BJ, Dixon JB, Carden JR. Preoxygenation is more effective in the 25 degrees head-up position than in the supine position in severely obese patients: A randomized controlled study. Anesthesiology. 2005;**102**:1110-1115

[4] Gander S, Frascarolo P, Suter M. Positive end-expiratory pressure during induction of general anesthesia increases duration of non-hypoxic apnea in morbidly obese patients. Anesthesia and Analgesia. 2005;**100**:580-584

[5] Wiles MD. Airway management in patients with suspected or confirmed traumatic spinal cord injury: A narrative review of current evidence. Anaesthesia. 2022;**77**:1120-1128. DOI: 10.1111/anae.15807

[6] Berry C, Ley EJ, Bukur M, Malinoski D, Margulies DR, Mirocha J, et al. Redefining hypotension in traumatic brain injury. Injury. 2012;**43**:1833-1837. DOI: 10.1016/j.injury.2011.08.014

[7] Brenner M, Stein DM, Hu PF, Aarabi B, Sheth K, Scalea TM. Traditional systolic blood pressure targets underestimate hypotension-induced secondary brain injury. Journal of Trauma and Acute Care Surgery. 2012;**72**:1135-1139

[8] Taya SK, Siddik-Sayyid SM, El-Khatib MF, Dagher CM, Hakki MA, Baraka AS. Nasopharyngeal oxygen insufflation following pre-oxygenation using the four deep breath technique. Anaesthesia. 2006;**61**:427-430

[9] Tanoubi I, Drolet P, Donati F. Optimizing preoxygenation in adults. Canadian Journal of Anaesthesia. 2009;**56**(6):449-466. DOI: 10.1007/s12630-009-9084-z. Epub 2009 Apr 28

[10] Bonanno FG. Pathways to reduce late mortality in hemorrhagic shock. In: Contemporary Approach to Trauma and Emergency Surgery. Rijeka, Croatia/London, UK: IntechOpen; 2024. DOI: 10.5772/intechopen.1004934. Available from: https://www.intechopen.com/online-first/1172459

[11] Baillard C, Fosse JP, Sebbane M. Noninvasive ventilation improves preoxygenation before intubation of hypoxic patients. American Journal of Respiratory and Critical Care Medicine. 2006;**174**:171-711

[12] Vourc'h M, Asfar P, Volteau C, Bachoumas K, Clavieras N, Egreteau P-Y, et al. High-flow nasal cannula oxygen during endotracheal intubation in hypoxemic patients: A randomized controlled clinical trial. Intensive Care Medicine. 2015;**41**:1538-1548. DOI: 10.1007/s00134-015-3796-z

[13] Jaber S, Monnin M, Girard M. Apnoeic oxygenation by high-flow nasal cannula oxygen combined with

non-invasive ventilation preoxygenation for intubation of hypoxaemic patients in the intensive care unit: the single-centre, blinded, randomised controlled OPTINIV trial. Intensive Care Medicine. 2016;**42**:1877-1887

[14] Baillard C, Prat G, Jung B. Effect of preoxygenation using non-invasive ventilation before intubation on subsequent organ failures in hypoxaemic patients: A randomised clinical trial. British Journal of Anaesthesia. 2018;**120**(2):361-367

[15] Frat J-P, Ricard J-D, Quenot J-P, Pichon N, Demoule A, Forel J-M, et al. Non-invasive ventilation versus high-flow nasal cannula oxygen therapy with apnoeic oxygenation for preoxygenation before intubation of patients with acute hypoxaemic respiratory failure: A randomised, multicentre, open-label trial. The Lancet Respiratory Medicine. 2019;**7**(4):303-312. DOI: 10.1016/S2213-2600(19)30048-7

[16] Ezri T, Gewürtz G, Sessler DI, Medalion B, Szmuk P, Hagberg C, et al. Prediction of difficult laryngoscopy in obese patients by ultrasound quantification of anterior neck soft tissue. Anaesthesia. 2003;**58**(11):1111-1114. DOI: 10.1046/j.1365-2044.2003.03412.x

[17] Bouvet L, Albert ML, Augris C. Real-time detection of gastric insufflation related to facemask pressure-controlled ventilation using ultrasonography of the antrum and epigastric auscultation in non-paralyzed patients: A prospective, randomized, double-blind study. Anesthesiology. 2014;**120**:326-334

[18] Mishra PR, Bhoi S, Sinha TP. Integration of point-of-care ultrasound during rapid sequence induction in trauma resuscitation. Journal of Emergencies, Trauma, and Shock. 2018;**11**:92-97

[19] van de Putte P, van Hoonacker J, Perlas A. Gastric ultrasound to guide anesthetic management in elective surgical patients non-compliant with fasting instructions: A retrospective cohort study. Minerva Anestesiologica. 2018;**84**(7):787-795. DOI: 10.23736/S0375-9393.17.12305-9

[20] Craig RG, Howie AJ, Acheson S, Wilde R. Nasal high-flow oxygen and total intravenous anaesthesia for tubeless airway assessment and surgery in spontaneously breathing children. Journal of Anesthesia & Intensive Care Medicine. 2019;**9**(3):555764. DOI: 10.19080/JAICM.2019.09.555764

[21] Vijitpavan A, Kooncharoensuk Y. High flow versus conventional nasal cannula for oxygenation and ventilation maintenance during surgery with intravenous deep sedation by propofol: A randomized controlled study. BMC Anesthesiology. 2021;**21**:214. DOI: 10.1186/s12871-021-01432-4

[22] Zadkar S, Ranjitha YS, Mishra P, Saraf R. High-flow nasal cannula (HFNC) oxygenation for sclerotherapy of facial and upper airway vascular malformations in pediatric patients: Case series. Journal of Anaesthesiology Clinical Pharmacology. 2023;**39**(2):309-312. DOI: 10.4103/joacp.joacp_238_21. Epub 2022 May 13

[23] Neilipovitz DT, Crosby ET. No evidence for decreased incidence of aspiration after rapid sequence induction. Canadian Journal of Anaesthesia. 2007;**54**(9):748-764. DOI: 10.1007/BF03026872

[24] El-Orbany M, Connolly LA. Rapid sequence induction and intubation: Current controversy. Anesthesia and Analgesia. 2010;**110**:1318-1325

[25] Ruben H, Knudsen EJ, Carugati G. Gastric inflation

in relation to airway pressure. Acta Anaesthesiologica Scandinavica. 1961;**5**:107-114

[26] Davies JM, Weeks S, Crone LA, Pavlin E. Difficult intubation in the parturient. Canadian Journal of Anaesthesia. 1989;**36**:668-674

[27] Clements P, SJ WA, McCluskey A. Should patients be manually ventilated during rapid sequence induction of anaesthesia? British Journal of Hospital Medicine (London, England). 2009;**70**:424

[28] Brown JPR, Werrett G. Bag-mask ventilation in rapid sequence induction. Anaesthesia. 2009;**64**:784-785

[29] Casey JD, Janz DR, Russell DW, Vonderhaar DJ, Joffe AM, Dischert KM, et al. PreVent investigators and the pragmatic critical care research group. bag-mask ventilation during tracheal intubation of critically ill adults. The New England Journal of Medicine. 2019;**380**(9):811-821. DOI: 10.1056/NEJMoa1812405. Epub 2019 Feb 18

[30] Frat J-P, Ricard J-D, Quenot J-P, Pichon N, Demoule A, Forel J-M, et al. Non-invasive ventilation versus high-flow nasal cannula oxygen therapy with apnoeic oxygenation for preoxygenation before intubation of patients with acute hypoxaemic respiratory failure: A randomised, multicentre, open-label trial. The Lancet Respiratory Medicine. 2019;**7**(4):303-312. DOI: 10.1016/S2213-2600(19)30048-7

[31] Vourc'h M, Asfar P, Volteau C, Bachoumas K, Clavieras N, Egreteau P-Y, et al. High-flow nasal cannula oxygen during endotracheal intubation in hypoxemic patients: A randomized controlled clinical trial. Intensive Care Medicine. 2015;**41**:1538-1548. DOI: 10.1007/s00134-015-3796-z

[32] Langeron O, Masso E, Huraux C. Prediction of difficult mask ventilation. Anesthesiology. 2000;**92**:1229-1236

[33] Kheterpal S, Martin L, Shanks AM. Prediction and outcomes of impossible mask ventilation. Anesthesiology 2009; 110:891-897.al. The Lancet Respiratory Medicine. 2019;**7**(4):303-312. DOI: 10.1016/S2213-2600(19)30048-7

[34] Bonanno FG. The critical airway in adults: The facts. Journal of Emergencies, Trauma, and Shock. 2012;**5**(2):153-159. DOI: 10.4103/0974-2700.96485

[35] Bonanno FG. An appraisal on emergency tracheostomy. Injury Extra. 2007;**38**:346-349

[36] Glapa M, Kourie JF, Doll D, Degiannis E. Early management of gunshot injuries to the face in civilian practice. World Journal of Surgery. 2007;**31**:2104-2110

[37] Jose A, Nagori SA, Agarwal B. Management of maxilla-facial trauma in emergency. An update of challenges and controversies. Journal of Emergencies, Trauma, and Shock. 2016;**9**:73-80

[38] Gerstein NS, Braude DA, Hung O, Sanders JC, Murphy MF. The fast-trach intubating laryngeal mask airway: An overview and update. Canadian Journal of Anaesthesia. 2010;**57**:588-601

[39] Singh A, Bhalotra AR, Anand R. A comparative evaluation of ProSeal laryngeal mask airway, I-gel and supreme laryngeal mask airway in adult patients undergoing elective surgery: A randomised trial. Indian Journal of Anaesthesia. 2018;**62**:858-864

[40] Kim MH, Lee JH, Choi YS, Park S, Shin S. Comparison of the laryngeal mask airway supreme and the i-gel in paralysed elderly patients: A randomised

controlled trial. European Journal of Anaesthesiology. 2018;**35**(8):598-604. DOI: 10.1097/EJA.0000000000000700

[41] Attarde VB, Kotekar N, Shetty SM. Air-Q intubating laryngeal airway: A study of the second generation supraglottic airway device. Indian Journal of Anaesthesia. 2016;**60**:343-348

[42] Frerk C, Mitchell VS, McNarry AF. Difficult airway society 2015 guidelines for management of unanticipated difficult intubation in adults. British Journal of Anaesthesia. 2015;**115**:827-848

[43] Atlas GM. A comparison of fiberoptic compatible oral airways. Journal of Clinical Anesthesia. 2004;**16**:66-73

[44] Mendonca C. Sugammadex to rescue a 'can't ventilate' scenario in an anticipated difficult intubation: Is it the answer? Anaesthesia. 2013;**68**:795-799

[45] Taneja S, Agarwalt M, Dali JS, Agrawal G. Ease of proseal laryngeal mask airway insertion and its fibreoptic view after placement using gum elastic Bougie: A comparison with conventional techniques. Anaesthesia and Intensive Care. 2009;**37**:435-440

[46] Aziz MF, Dillman D, Fu R, Brambrink AM. Comparative effectiveness of the C-MAC video laryngoscope versus direct laryngoscopy in the setting of the predicted difficult airway. Anesthesiology. 2012;**116**:629-636. DOI: 10.1097/ALN.0b013e318246ea34

[47] Kovacs G, Sowers N. Airway management in trauma. Emergency Medicine Clinics of North America. Feb 2018;**36**(1):61-84. DOI: 10.1016/j.emc.2017.08.006

[48] Li T, Jafari D, Meyer C, et al. Video laryngoscopy is associated with improved first-pass intubation success compared with direct laryngoscopy in emergency department trauma patients. JACEP Open. 2021;**2**:e12373. DOI: 10.1002/emp2.12373

[49] Trent SA, Kaji AH, Carlson JN, McCormick T, Haukoos JS, Brown CA, et al. Video laryngoscopy is associated with first-pass success in emergency department intubations for trauma patients: A propensity score matched analysis of the national emergency airway registry. Annals of Emergency Medicine. 2021 Dec;**78**(6):708-719. DOI: 10.1016/j.annemergmed.2021.07.115

[50] Nicholls BJ, Cullen BF. Anesthesia for trauma. Journal of Clinical Anesthesia. 1988;**1**(2):115-129. DOI: 10.1016/0952-8180(88)90031-1

[51] Sikorski RA, Koerner AK, Fouche-Weber GSM Jr. Choice of general anesthetics for trauma patients. Current Anesthesiology Reports. 2014;**4**:225-232

[52] Perbet S, De Jong A, Delmas J, Futier E, Pereira B, Jaber S, et al. Incidence of and risk factors for severe cardiovascular collapse after endotracheal intubation in the ICU: A multicenter observational study. Critical Care. 2015;**19**:257. DOI: 10.1186/s13054-015-0975-9

[53] Russell DW, Casey JD, Gibbs KW, Ghamande S, Dargin JM, Vonderhaar DJ, et al. Effect of fluid bolus administration on cardiovascular collapse among critically ill patients undergoing tracheal intubation: A randomized clinical trial. Journal of the American Medical Association. 2022;**328**(3):270-279. DOI: 10.1001/jama.2022.9792

[54] Scholz J, Steinfath M, Schulz M. Clinical pharmacokinetics of alfentanil,

fentanyl and sufentanil. An update. Clin Pharmacokinet. 1996;**31**(4):275-292. DOI: 10.2165/00003088-199631040-00004

[55] Mireskandari SM, Abulahrar N, Darabi ME, Rahimi I, Haji-Mohamadi F, Movafegh A. Comparison of the effect of fentanyl, sufentanil, alfentanil and remifentanil on cardiovascular response to tracheal intubation in children. Iranian Journal of Pediatrics. 2011;**21**(2):173-180

[56] Miller DR, Martineau RJ, O'Brien H, Hull KA, Oliveras L, Hindmarsh T, et al. Effects of alfentanil on the hemodynamic and catecholamine response to tracheal intubation. Anesthesia and Analgesia. 1993;**76**(5):1040-1046. DOI: 10.1213/00000539-199305000-00023

[57] Ahonen J, Olkkola KT, Hynynen M, Seppälä T, Ikävalko H, Remmerie B, et al. Comparison of alfentanil, fentanyl and sufentanil for total intravenous anaesthesia with propofol in patients undergoing coronary artery bypass surgery. British Journal of Anaesthesia. 2000;**85**(4):533-540. DOI: 10.1093/bja/85.4.533

[58] Hancı V. Tracheal intubation without use of muscle relaxants: Comparison of remifentanil and alfentanil. Anesthesia and Pain Medicine. 1 Jan 2012;**1**(3):210-211. DOI: 10.5812/kowsar.22287523.3599

[59] Kaya PK, Sivrikaya GU, Hanci A. Alfentanil use in rapid sequence induction. Comprehensive Medicine. 2023;**15**(3):205-210. DOI: 10.14744/cm.2023.66376

[60] Choi BH, Lee YC. Effective bolus dose of sufentanil to attenuate cardiovascular responses in laryngoscopic double-lumen endobronchial intubation. Anesthesia and Pain Medicine. 2016;**6**(2):e33640. DOI: 10.5812/aapm.33640

[61] Yang Y, Teng X, Zhu J. Sufentanil blunts the myocardial stress induced by tracheal intubation in older adult patients with coronary heart disease better than equipotent fentanyl. Annals of Palliative Medicine. 2020;**9**(6):3909-3914. DOI: 10.21037/apm-20-1813

[62] Bonanno FG. Issues of critical airway management (Which anesthesia; which surgical airway?). Journal of Emergencies, Trauma, and Shock. 2012;**5**(4):279-284. DOI: 10.4103/0974-2700.102353

[63] Qiao S, Mao X, Wang Y, Lei S, Liu Y, Wang T, et al. Remifentanil preconditioning reduces postischemic myocardial infarction and improves left ventricular performance via activation of the janus activated kinase-2/signal transducers and activators of transcription-3 signal pathway and subsequent inhibition of glycogen synthase kinase-3beta in rats. Critical Care Medicine. Mar 2016;**44**(3):e131-45. DOI: 10.1097/CCM.0000000000001350

[64] Kannabiran N, Bidkar PU. Total intravenous anesthesia in neurosurgery. Journal of Neuroanaesthesiology and Critical Care. 2018;**5**(3):141-149. DOI: 10.1055/g-0038-1673544

[65] Jabre P, Combes X, Lapostolle F, Dhaouadi M, Ricard-Hibon A, Vivien B, et al. Etomidate versus ketamine for rapid sequence intubation in acutely ill patients: A multicentre randomised controlled trial. Lancet. 2009;**374**:293-300. DOI: 10.1016/s0140-6736(09)60949-1

[66] Smischney NJ, Nicholson WT, Brown DR, Gallo De Moraes A, Hoskote SS, Pickering B, et al. Ketamine/propofol admixture vs etomidate for

intubation in the critically ill: KEEP PACE Randomized clinical trial. Journal of Trauma and Acute Care Surgery. 2019;**87**(4):883-891

[67] Skinner HJ, Biswas A, Mahajan RP. Evaluation of intubating conditions with rocuronium and either propofol or etomidate for rapid sequence induction. Anaesthesia. 1998;**53**(7):702-706. DOI: 10.1046/j.1365-2044.1998.396-az0506.x

[68] Dean P. Should etomidate be used for rapid-sequence intubation induction in critically ill septic patients? Probably not. The American Journal of Emergency Medicine. 2008;**26**(6):728-729; author reply 729-30. DOI: 10.1016/j.ajem.2008.04.010

[69] Mansvelder FJ, Bossers SM, Loer SA, Bloemers FW, Van Lieshout EMM, Den Hartog D, et al. BRAIN-PROTECT collaborators. Etomidate versus Ketamine as Prehospital Induction Agent in Patients with Suspected Severe Traumatic Brain Injury. Anesthesiology. 2024;**140**(4):742-751. DOI: 10.1097/ALN.0000000000004894

[70] Gofrit O, Leibovici D, Shemer J, Henig A, Shapira S. Ketamine in the field: The use of ketamine for induction of anaesthesia before intubation in injured patients in the field. Injury. 1997;**28**:41-43. DOI: 10.1016/s0020-1383(96)00140-4

[71] Bonanno GF. Ketamine in war/tropical surgery (a final tribute to the racemic mixture). Injury. 2002;**33**:323-327

[72] Morris C, Perris A, Klein J, Mahoney P. Anaesthesia in haemodynamically compromised emergency patients: Does ketamine represent the best choice of induction agent? Anaesthesia. 2009;**64**:532-539

[73] Meo G, Andreone D, De Bonis U, Cometto G, Enrico S, Giustetto G, et al. Rural surgery in southern Sudan. World Journal of Surgery. 2006 Apr;**30**(4):495-504. DOI: 10.1007/s00268-005-0093-y

[74] Kurdi MS, Theerth KA, Deva RS. Ketamine: Current applications in anesthesia, pain, and critical care. Anesthesia, Essays and Researches. 2014;**8**(3):283-290. DOI: 10.4103/0259-1162.143110

[75] Adams HA, Werner C. Vom Razemat zum Eutomer: (S)-Ketamin—Renaissance einer Substanz? Anaesthesist. 1997;**46**:1026-1042

[76] Adams HA. Endokrine Reaktionen nach S-(+)-Ketamin. Der Anaesthesist. 1997;**46**:S30-S37. DOI: 10.1007/pl00002462

[77] Kienbaum P, Heuter T, Pavlakovic G, Michel MC, Peters JS. (+)-Ketamine increases muscle sympathetic activity and maintains the neural response to hypotensive challenges in humans. Anesthesiology. 2001;**94**:252-258

[78] Trimmel H, Helbok R, Staudinger T, Jaksch W, Messerer B, Schöchl H, et al. S (+)-ketamine: Current trends in emergency and intensive care medicine. Wien Klin Wochensch. 2018;**130**:356-366

[79] Zeiler FA, Teitelbaum J, West M, Gillman LM. The ketamine effect on ICP in traumatic brain injury. Neurocritical Care. 2014;**21**(1):163-173 14

[80] Wang X, Ding X, Tong Y, et al. Ketamine does not increase intracranial pressure compared with opioids: meta-analysis of randomized controlled trials. Journal of Anesthesia. 2014;**28**(6):821-827

[81] Akhtar SMM, Fareed A, Ali M, Khan MS, Ali A, Mumtaz M, et al.

Efficacy and safety of Ciprofol compared with Propofol during general anesthesia induction: A systematic review and meta-analysis of randomized controlled trials (RCT). Journal of Clinical Anesthesia. 2024;**94**:111425. DOI: 10.1016/j.jclinane.2024.111425

[82] Smischney NJ, Beach ML, Loftus RW, Dodds TM, Koff MD. Ketamine/propofol admixture (ketofol) is associated with improved hemodynamics as an induction agent: a randomized, controlled trial. Journal of Trauma and Acute Care Surgery. 2012;**73**:94-101

[83] Lee C, Jahr JS, Candiotti KA, Warriner B, Zornow MH, Naguib M. Reversal of profound neuromuscular block by sugammadex administered three minutes after rocuronium: a comparison with spontaneous recovery from succinylcholine. Anesthesiology. 2009;**110**(5):1020-1025. DOI: 10.1097/ALN.0b013e31819dabb0

[84] Sørensen MK, Bretlau C, Gätke MR, Sørensen AM, Rasmussen LS. Rapid sequence induction and intubation with rocuronium-sugammadex compared with succinylcholine: a randomized trial. British Journal of Anaesthesia. 2012;**108**(4):682-689. DOI: 10.1093/bja/aer503. Epub 2012 Feb 6

[85] Driver BE, Prekker ME, Klein LR, Reardon RF, Miner JR, Fagerstrom ET, et al. Effect of use of a bougie vs endotracheal tube and stylet on first-attempt intubation success among patients with difficult airways undergoing emergency intubation: a randomized clinical trial. JAMA. 2018;**319**:2179-2189. DOI: 10.1001/jama.2018.6496

[86] El-Ganzhouri AR, McCarthy RJ, Tuman KJ. Preoperative airway assessment: Predictive value of a multivariate risk index. Anesthesia and Analgesia. 1996;**82**:1197-1204

[87] Levitan RM, Everett WW, Ochroch EA. Limitations of difficult airway prediction in patients intubated in the emergency department. Annals of Emergency Medicine. 2004;**44**:307-313

[88] Casey JD, Semler MW, High K. How I manage a difficult intubation. Critical Care. 2019;**23**:177

[89] Takeda T, Tanigawa K, Tanaka H, Hayashi Y, Goto E, Tanaka K. The assessment of three methods to identify tracheal tube placement in the emergency setting. Resuscitation. 2003;**56**:153-157

[90] Whitaker DK, Benson JP. Capnography standards for outside the operating room. Current Opinion in Anaesthesiology. 2016;**29**:485-492

[91] Cook TM. The winds of change–Progress in the implementation of universal capnography. Anaesthesia. 2016;**71**:363-368

[92] Apfelbaum JL, Hagberg CA, Caplan RA, Blitt CD, Connis RT, Nickinovich DG, et al. American society of anesthesiologists task force on management of the difficult airway. Practice guidelines for management of the difficult airway: An updated report by the American society of anesthesiologists task force on management of the difficult airway. Anesthesiology. 2013;**118**(2):251-270. DOI: 10.1097/ALN.0b013e31827773b2

[93] Rose DK, Cohen MM. The airway: Problems and predictions in 18,500 patients. Canadian Journal of Anesthesia. 1994;**41**:372-83.11

[94] Yentis SM. Predicting difficult intubation—Worthwhile

exercise or pointless ritual? Anaesthesia. 2002;**57**(2):105-109. DOI: 10.1046/j.0003-2409.2001.02515.x

[95] Nørskov AK, Rosenstock CV, Wetterslev J, Astrup G, Afshari A, Lundstrøm LH. Diagnostic accuracy of anaesthesiologists' prediction of difficult airway management in daily clinical practice: A cohort study of 188 064 patients registered in the Danish anaesthesia database. Anaesthesia. 2015;**70**:272-281

[96] Cook TM, MacDougall-Davis SR. Complications and failure of airway management. British Journal of Anaesthesia. 2012;**109**:i68-i85

[97] Rocke DA, Murray WB, Rout CC, Gouws EB. Relative risk analysis of factors associated with difficult intubation in obstetric anesthesia. Anesthesiology. 1992;**77**:67-73

[98] Huitink JM, Bouwman RA. The myth of the difficult airway: Airway management revisited. Anaesthesia. 2015;**70**(3):244-249. DOI: 10.1111/anae.12989

[99] Lyon RM, Ferris JD, Young DM. Field intubation of cardiac arrest patients: A dying art? Emergency Medicine Journal. 2010;**27**:321-323

[100] Lockey D, Crewdson K, Weaver A. Observational study of the success rates of intubation and failed intubation airway rescue techniques in 7256 attempted intubations of trauma patients by pre-hospital physicians. British Journal of Anaesthesia. 2014;**113**:220-225

[101] Trunkey DD. Initial treatment of patients with extensive trauma. The New England Journal of Medicine. 1991;**324**:1259-1263

[102] Bonanno FG. Techniques for emergency tracheostomy. Injury. 2008;**39**(3):375-378. DOI: 10.1016/j.injury.2007.09.025

[103] Chrimes N. The vortex: A universal 'high-acuity implementation tool' for emergency airway management. British Journal of Anaesthesia. 2016;**117**(Suppl. 1):i20-i27. DOI: 10.1093/bja/aew175. Epub 2016 Jul 20

[104] Reason J. Human error: Models and management. British Medical Journal. 2000;**320**:768-770

[105] Shaw J, Frerk C, Russell J. A commentary on human factors aspects of cases reported to NAP4. In: Cook T, Woodall N, Frerk C, editors. 4th National Audit Project of the Royal College of Anaesthetists and the Difficult Airway Society. Major Complications of Airway Management in the United Kingdom. London: RCA; 2011. pp. 193-201

[106] Weingart SD, Trueger NS, Wong N. Delayed sequence intubation: A prospective observational study. Annals of Emergency Medicine. Apr 2015;**65**(4):349-355. DOI: 10.1016/j.annemergmed.2014.09.025. [Epub 2014 Oct 23]

[107] Garavaglia MM, Das S, Cusimano MD, et al. Anesthetic approach to high-risk patients and prolonged awake craniotomy using dexmedetomidine and scalp block. Journal of Neurosurgical Anesthesiology. 2014;**26**(3):226-233

[108] DeHert SG, Turani F, Mathur S, Stowe DF. Cardioprotection with volatile anesthetics: Mechanisms and clinical implications. Anesthesia and Analgesia. 2005;**100**:1584-1593

[109] Head BP, Patel P. Anesthetics and brain protection. Current Opinion in Anesthesiology. 2007;**20**:395-399

[110] Kersten JR, Schmeling TJ, Pagel PS, Gross GJ, Warltier DC. Isoflurane mimics

ischemic preconditioning via activation of K(ATP) channels: Reduction of myocardial infarct size with an acute memory phase. Anesthesiology. 1997;**87**(2):361-370

[111] Lee JJ, Li L, Jung HH, Zuo Z. Postconditioning with isoflurane reduced ischemia-induced brain injury in rats. Anesthesiology. 2008;**108**:1055-1062

[112] Ushida T, Kotani T, Imai K, Nakano-Kobayashi T, Nakamura N, Moriyama Y, et al. Shock index and postpartum hemorrhage in vaginal deliveries: A multicenter retrospective study. Shock. 2021;**55**:332-337

[113] ResearchGate. Should we administer analgesic drugs to intubate a patient during cardiac arrest? Q. by Andrea Caglià, May 6th, 2014.h

Section 9

Tracheostomata in Anesthesiology

Chapter 11

The Tracheotomized Patient for Anesthesia

Torsten Richter

Abstract

The increasing number of tracheostomized patients means that it is becoming more and more necessary to be aware of the special aspects associated with this type of airway access. For an anesthetic treatment, it is essential to know the different surgical procedures for creating a tracheostoma, the possible complications associated with them, and the types of cannulas that can be used. To minimize risk, knowledge of how to proceed in the event of life-threatening complications is required. Breathing through a tracheostoma leads to altered physiological parameters. Selecting a suitable tracheostomy tube helps to meet the various requirements and also to avoid complications.

Keywords: tracheostomy, percutaneous dilatational tracheostomy, tracheal tube, tracheostomy complication, t-tube, Montgomery-tube, speaking valve, tracheostomy complications

1. Introduction

Thanks to the ever-improving possibilities of intensive care medicine, even long-lasting critical illnesses can be bridged. Temporary or permanent tracheostomata is created as a result of prolonged or long-term ventilation, pharyngo-laryngeal tumor, or other space requirements, such as trauma and dysphagia. In this way, more efficient airway care (airway suctioning), better oral care, and a reduction in the work of breathing can be achieved in ventilated patients. A tracheostomy increases the potential to improve patient liberation from mechanical ventilation [1] and also creates the possibility of initiating contact. Due to the removal of the laryngeal tube, phonation is possible after a tracheostomy, and therefore, speech is possible under certain conditions.

It has been estimated that 250,000 tracheostomy procedures are performed annually [2]. In Germany, 42,364 patients were tracheotomized in 2023 [3]. About 85,000 tracheostomies were performed per year between 2002 and 2017 in the United States [4]. This means that the probability of caring for tracheotomized patients as an anesthetist is high.

The aim of this chapter is to prepare the reader for the safe handling of a tracheostomized patient, to point out possible pitfalls and complications, and to give an overview of the different types of tracheostoma care in order to be able to care for these patients knowledgeably.

2. The tracheostomized patient

Before taking over a tracheostomized patient, the following questions should be answered:

1. Why does this patient have a tracheostomy?
2. When was the tracheostomy performed?
3. Which tracheostomy technique was used?
4. What is in the tracheostoma?
5. What does the tracheostoma look like?

2.1 Why was a tracheostomy performed?

The above-mentioned indications for a tracheostomy often result in important secondary findings. If a tracheostomy was placed due to a difficult airway, has the patient possibly undergone a tracheostomy due to swelling or another mass (e.g., edema, hypopharyngeal tumor, laryngeal carcinoma)? In connection with this, there may be a relevant drug or radiation therapy treatment. An operation may have been performed in connection with this, such as a tumor removal with flap surgery or a laryngectomy. The relevance of this information arises, for example, from the fact that oropharyngeal oxygenation or intubation would no longer be possible after a laryngectomy.

The answer to the question of "why" therefore has a decisive influence on the approach to anesthesia planning. Indications such as COPD-related or long-term ventilation-induced tracheostomata in neurodegenerative diseases, for example, provide indications of the severity of the concomitant disease and increase awareness of associated potential complications. Patients with more sickness are at higher risk of complications [4].

2.2 When was the tracheostomy performed?

The time at which the stability of the tracheostoma shaft can be assessed is important. This question is closely linked to the question of whether the tracheostoma is a standard surgical tracheostoma or a tracheostoma created by a dilated puncture tracheostomy, as this can make it extremely difficult to change the tracheostomy tube (see next section [2.3]). The timing of the tracheostomy has an impact on anesthesia planning and the classification of potential complications to be expected.

2.3 How was the tracheostomy performed?

In principle, there are two approaches, a conventional surgical standard tracheostomy (usually between the 2nd and 3rd tracheal ring) and a percutaneous dilatative tracheostomy.

During a surgical tracheostomy, the pretracheal tissue is dissected under vision. The cartilage segments are specifically removed to create a round tracheal opening. A tracheostoma shaft is often formed so that the outer skin is fixed to the trachea. This creates a funnel-shaped tracheostoma, which means that the constrictions are smaller compared to a dilatational tracheostomy, and a tracheostomy tube can usually be changed on the 2nd postoperative day after insertion (see **Figure 1**). Epithelialization therefore makes it easier to change the tracheostomy tube and protects the surrounding tissue from secretions from the trachea. The spontaneous closure of a tracheostoma created in this way may take longer than with a non-epithelialized tracheostoma.

A conventional surgical tracheostoma can also be created without epithelialization. The individual layers of the cervical fascia and the musculature are directly adjacent to the tracheostoma shaft and therefore allow tissue to be separated using inserted materials, such as a tracheostomy tube, before the tracheostoma shaft is finally healed.

Every percutaneous dilatational tracheostomy (PDT) creates a non-epithelialized tracheostoma (**Figure 1**). Deviating arteries can be injured during the puncture, which can lead to massive bleeding complications [5–8]. However, the tracheal ring structures are not surgically removed but displaced anterograde (according to Fantoni) or retrograde, depending on the direction of dilatation. In the retrograde approach of PDT, dilatation can be performed differentially by using a guide wire dilating forceps, balloon, screw, or bougie [9]. This perforation of the anterior tracheal wall and the associated dislocation of the fractured parts of the tracheal ring can potentially cause problems, such as mechanically induced bleeding (e.g.,

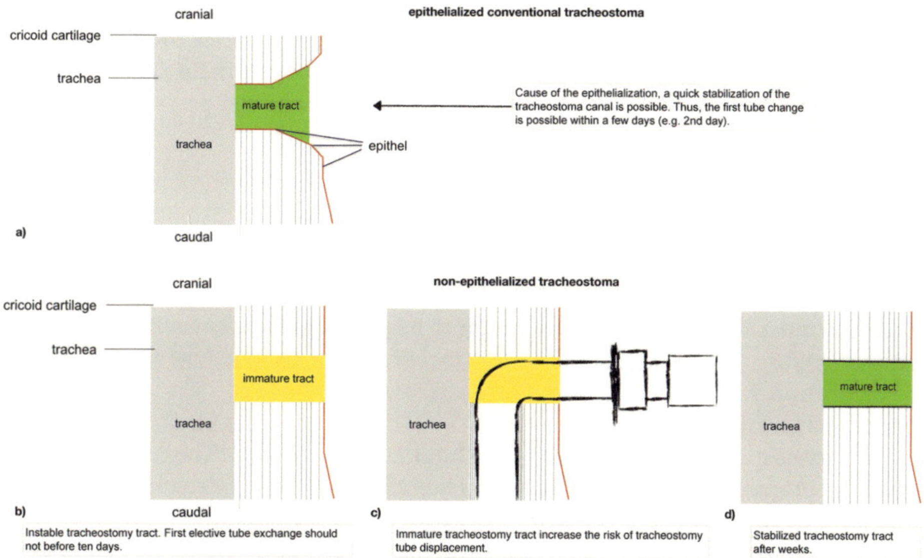

Figure 1.
Schematic sagittal view of (a) an epithelized and (b)–(d) non-epithelized tracheostoma. A non-epithelialized tracheostoma shaft takes longer to heal until a resilient stability of the shaft is achieved. An initial tracheostomy tube change after percutaneous dilatational tracheotomy is therefore recommended after 10–14 days. Initially, the pretracheal layers are easy to displace. Therefore, changing the tracheostomy tube before stability is reached (d) can result in the potential risk of the tracheostomy tube becoming displaced (c). It is clear that if the tracheostomy tube is positioned pretracheally, (c) airway loss occurs and, when ventilated, pronounced soft tissue emphysema develops.

after anterograde bougie bleeding from the brachiocephalic trunk [10] or intubation problems even a long time after puncture tracheotomy due to depressed cartilage fragments [11]). Furthermore, changing the tracheostomy tube can be difficult and painful.

Another important aspect is that the usually narrow tracheostoma shaft is not stable in the first week after insertion. If the tube is removed during this time, reinserting the tube can be extremely difficult and not successful. It is particularly feared that the cannula will come to rest in front of the trachea, as the preformed tracheal cannula can very easily penetrate a pretracheal layer (compare **Figure 1**). If ventilation is performed via the supposedly correctly placed tracheostomy tube in this incorrect position, this can result in the impossibility of ventilation, subacute emphysema, hemorrhage, pneumothorax, and pneumomediastinum [12–17]. Intubation should therefore be unproblematic in PDT patients so that the airway can be secured with this approach if necessary. For this reason, a PDT should not be performed in patients with a difficult airway or inflexible cervical spine.

Another problem is the occasional occurrence of primary off-center puncture stomas that are not positioned in the desired target zone [18]. As a consequence, changing the cannula can be difficult or painful for the awake patient. This may require a tracheostoma revision operation. If the puncture is too cranial, there is also a risk of inflammation of the cricoid cartilage with stenosis formation. If the puncture is too caudal, this can jeopardize adequate cannula supply, as the distal end of the cannula comes to rest below the carina, and changing the cannula can be considerably more difficult. There is also an increased risk of mechanical damage to mediastinal vessels [19–21].

Furthermore, the length of the tracheostoma tube, its course, and the localization height of the tracheostoma have a significant influence on the subsequent tracheostomy tube management (see **Figure 2**). These factors can determine the subsequent care in terms of who normally changes the cannula. The spectrum for this ranges from the patient themselves, to trained family members, to specialized personnel (ENT physicians).

2.4 What is inside?

This question is essential for anesthesia planning. If regional anesthesia or sedation is used, a possible escalation of the anesthesia procedure to positive pressure ventilation must also be considered in order to be prepared for all eventualities. This section therefore discusses the options for tracheostoma care and how positive pressure ventilation can be established.

What is inside? - *Nothing*.

The tracheostoma has no contents and should become closed. The tracheostoma may be the original size or only a few millimeters in diameter. The tracheostoma is either open or covered with a dressing (e.g., plaster). If the remaining size is appropriate and indicated, a blocked cannula can be placed again. Otherwise, depending on the size of the residual lumen, a gauze pad, a foil plaster, and appropriate external counterpressure are advisable for preoxygenation and mask ventilation in order to seal the leak until the tracheal tube has been placed.

What is inside? - *Tracheostomy tube*.

In *addition to knowing* the *type of cannula*, the following information is also essential:

When was the *last cannula change*?

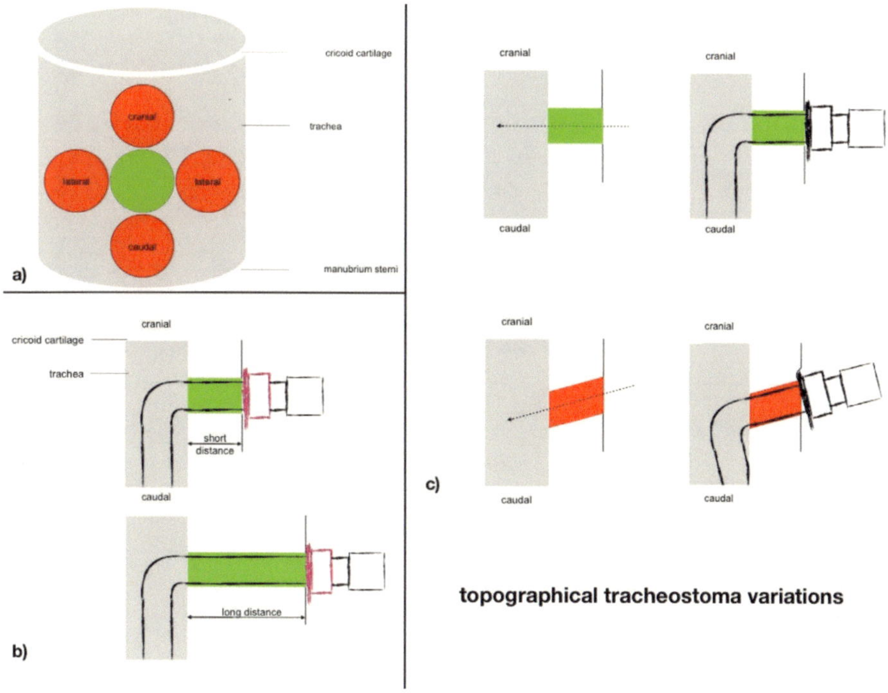

Figure 2.
Schematic representation of possible puncture sites and tracheostoma shaft courses. (a) Frontal view: In percutaneous dilatational tracheostomy (PDT), the entry points (red) may deviate from the desired puncture site (median, 2nd-3rd tracheal ring) into the trachea. (b) Sagittal view: The probability of a problematic puncture with PDT increases with the length of the pretracheal tissue to be penetrated. Therefore, the indication for PDT in very obese patients should be carefully weighed. The length of the tracheostoma shaft has a direct impact on the subsequent tracheal cannula management. (c) Sagittal view: above: normal tracheostoma shaft with correctly placed tracheal cannula; below: example of an oblique (from cranial to caudal) puncture and tracheostoma placement. In this case, the internal orifice may already be located intrathoracally. This results in a dangerous proximity to the mediastinal vessels. The inserted tracheal cannula leads to pressure on the ventral tracheal wall with the risk of mucosal injury, ulceration, and tracheoarterial fistula formation.

Was it *easy or difficult to change* the cannula?
Which *cannula type?*
Which *cannula size?*

In principle, *flexible or rigid* tracheostomy tubes can be used. They may or may not have an *adapter suitable* for connection to a ventilator. Furthermore, they may or may not be *blockable* or may or may not have an internal insert (inner cannula). The blockage can be an inflatable cuff filled with air or water or can consist of foam. Tracheostomy tubes can have channels for secretion suction above the blockage.

The inner cannula can either open or close an endotracheal opening in the cannula cranially. Furthermore, a valve mechanism can be attached to the outer end of the tracheostomy tube, which, in the event of expiration, discharges the air endotracheally rather than via the tracheostoma in order to enable phonation. The inner cannula has or has no adapters to other devices (e.g., ventilator tube). The principles of the individual cannulas are summarized in **Figure 3**.

Phonation can even be achieved in ventilated patients with a PassyMuir® valve (**Figure 4**). Under certain conditions, phonation can also be achieved in ventilated patients with a barely blocked or unblocked cannula if the cannula is well adjusted. The principle is summarized in **Figure 4**.

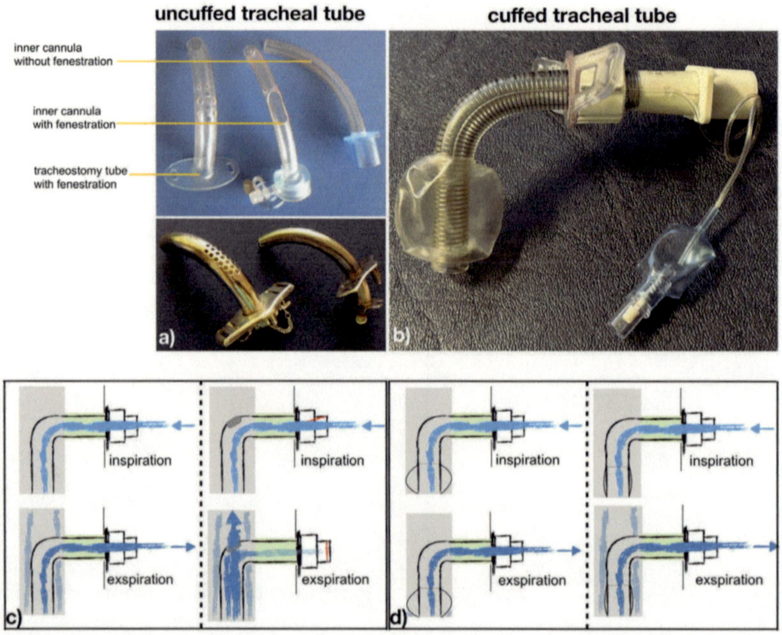

Figure 3.
Illustration of a tracheal cannula without cuff (left, a)) and with inflatable cuff (right, b)). (a): The fenestration of the tracheal cannula shown allows the exhaled air to flow from the endotracheal to the cranial side if the tracheal cannula inlet is closed either manually or by means of a valve mechanism. This makes laryngeal phonation possible (see schematic representation (c), right). To additionally improve phonation, a cannula smaller than the tracheal diameter (downsizing) is selected. During expiration, air can also flow cranially next to the cannula. If the fenestration of a tracheostomy tube is closed by an inner cannula without an opening or is not present (see a), right), ventilation occurs mainly through the tracheostoma opening (see schematic representation (c), left). Schematic representation (d) shows inhalation and exhalation through a blocked tube in the blocked and unblocked state.

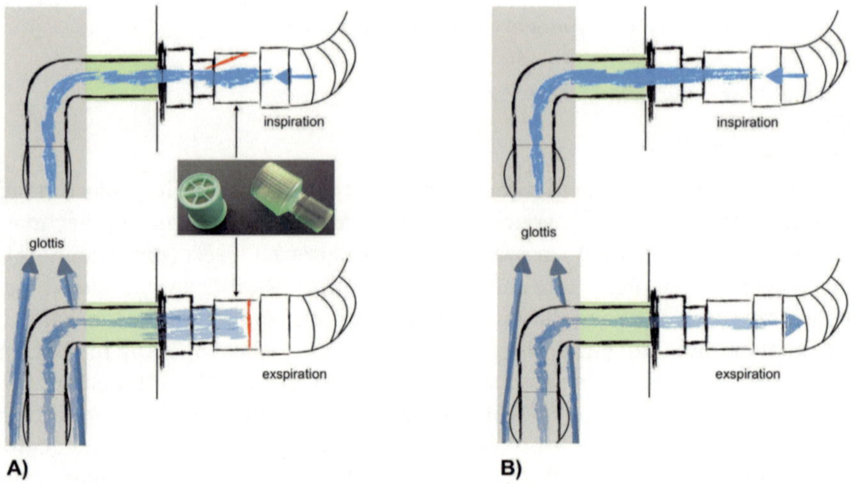

Figure 4.
Schematic representation of the creation of phonation conditions during ventilation. A: Using a Passy Muir® valve. The cuffed tracheostomy tube must be with the cuff deflated and not too large, at the top—start of inspiration—and at the bottom—expiration. B: Without valve, with an adapted unblocking that allows sufficient leakage in a cranial direction to enable phonation, at the top—start of inspiration—and at the bottom—expiration.

It is important to understand that a blockable cannula with a valve mechanism must always have a way of exhaling the inspired air again. Blocked speaking cannulas with an inserted valve mechanism are therefore life-threatening and absolutely contraindicated [22]. This should be borne in mind, as the wide range of tracheostomy tube sets on offer would make this possible in some cases (see **Figure 5**).

The tracheostomy tubes should be adapted to the depth of the tracheostoma shaft. This applies all the more if the perforation for phonation is to be located in the trachea and not in the tracheostoma shaft. The correct position of the fenestration can be controlled endoscopically. An appropriate cannula diameter is also necessary for voice production, which does not allow the expiratory airflow to escape from the tracheostoma next to the cannula but instead directs it cranially to the glottis.

Cannulas that are too large as well as blocking devices can damage the mucosa and thus lead to inflammation, endotracheal granulations, and pressure ulcerations. The latter can also lead to fistula formation (e.g., tracheoarterial). Pressure ulcerations can

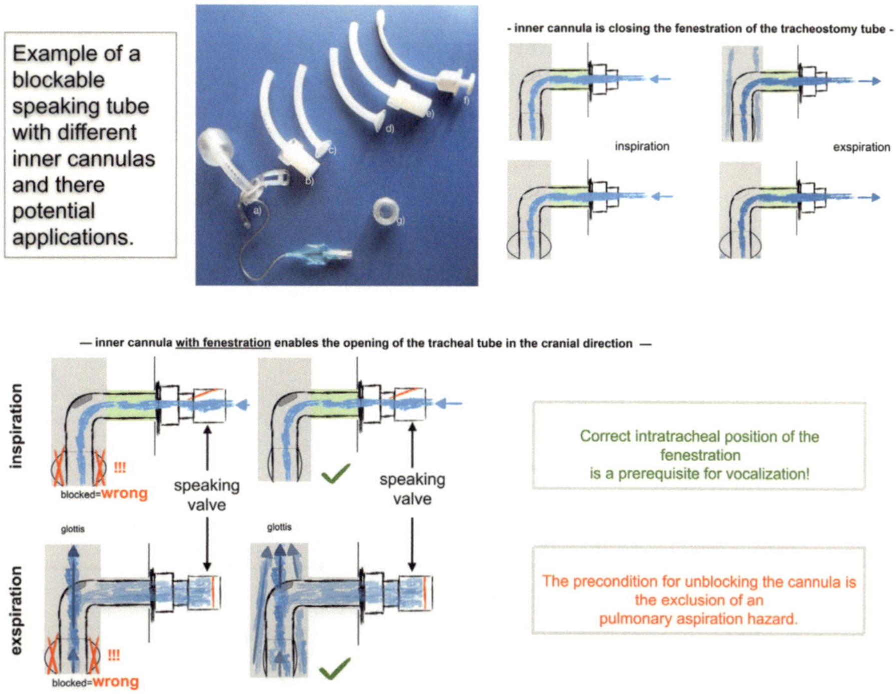

Figure 5.
Fenestrated blockable tracheostomy tube and its components. Due to the possible combinations, this cannula can lead to life-threatening events if used incorrectly. Photo: (a) fenestrated blockable tracheostomy tube, (b) fenestrated inner cannula with connector for connection to the speaking valve, (c) fenestrated inner cannula without connector, (d) inner cannula without opening for phonation connector, (e) inner cannula without opening for phonation with connector for connection to the respirator or a heat moisture exchanger, (f) inserter/obturator included in the set, (g) attachable speaking valve. Top right: Schematic representation of the respiratory flow during inhalation and exhalation with the fenestration closed in the blocked and unblocked state. Bottom: Schematic representation of the respiratory flow during inhalation and exhalation with open fenestration in the blocked and unblocked state. The illustration shows the need for adequate drainage of exhaled air in a cranial direction, as otherwise a systematic build-up of residual air would result, leading to barotrauma and life-threatening complications. Therefore, blocking with a speaking valve is absolutely contraindicated. For the time a speaking attachment is used, the cuff must be deflated, as shown in the adjacent figure. The risk of pulmonary aspiration should be excluded. The correct intratracheal position of the fenestration is a prerequisite for phonation. The position of the fenestration should ideally be checked endoscopically.

also be caused by an incorrect position, as shown in **Figure 2c**). In this case, the predetermined right-angled shape of a standard cannula and the deviating oblique angle of the tracheostoma shaft lead to permanent contact between the tracheal cannula and the tracheal wall. In certain cases, it is possible to adapt the cannula using flexible tracheostomy tubes or tracheostomy tubes specially made for the patient.

The size of the tracheostomy tube refers to the internal diameter (ID) in millimeters. A tracheotomy tube size 9 has a 9 mm ID. The information about the ID and external diameters is applied to the flange of the tube [23].

When changing a tracheostomy tube, it is to be expected that the removed tube is the property of the patient and should therefore not be discarded.

For all cannulas used, it is important to check whether a ventilator can be connected if necessary or whether a tracheostomy cannula would have to be changed. In circumstances where a tracheostomy tube change should be avoided, it may be possible to connect to a ventilator using attachments or adapters. Furthermore, the risk of changing the tracheostomy tube should be weighed against the option of intubation.

Double lumen tracheostomy tubes are also available for patients requiring one-lung ventilation or side-separated ventilation. This type of tracheostomy tube and further special cannulas have been summarized in **Figure 6**.

Patients with a subglottic obstruction are occasionally treated with a Montgomery tube or T-Tube (see **Figure 7**) to keep the lumen open. These cannulas are often in place for several weeks and can therefore adhere very firmly to the tracheal wall when

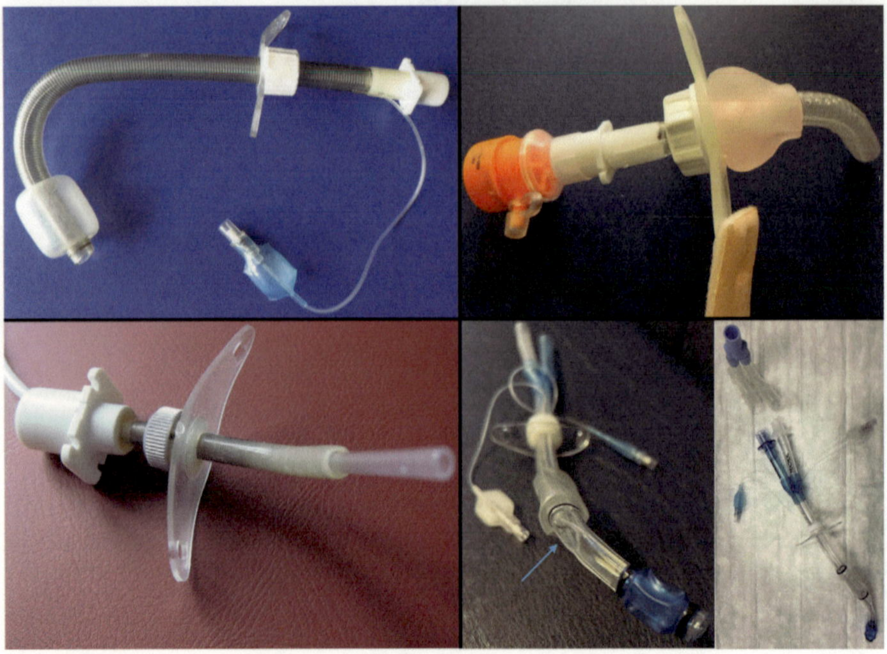

Figure 6.
Examples of special tubes. Top left: *Extra-long blockable tracheostomy tube that can be used with a long tracheostoma shaft.* Top right: *Non-blockable fenestrated tube with proximally adapted, custom-made seal (epithesis) for a pronounced funnel-shaped tracheostoma shaft entrance.* Bottom left: *non-occlusive pediatric tube. The suction catheter inserted here demonstrates that with smaller tube diameters, suctioning or endoscopy can lead to complete closure of the airway and must therefore be performed quickly.* Bottom right: *Double-lumen tracheostomy tube (DL-TK) for separate ventilation of the lungs on each side. The photo shows a left-sided DL-TK (see figure for close-up and overview). The blue arrow shows the tracheal opening below the tracheal blockage.*

they are changed. Changing the tracheostomy tube can therefore be associated with increased mucosal bleeding. It should therefore be checked whether any necessary ventilation can be established via the attachment. The resulting loss of inspiratory volume can be avoided. A laryngeal mask or a laryngeal tube can be inserted and clamped oropharyngeally for this purpose. If it is necessary to change the tracheostomy tube, the position of the Montgomery tube should be checked after reinsertion to prevent contact with the glottis [24–27].

Patients in whom access to the trachea is to be kept open sometimes no longer need a tracheal cannula. In these cases, a placeholder, plug, or so-called button is used. This is an inserted tube that can be closed at the front and has short T-shaped projections at the endotracheal end that serve as an abutment (see **Figure 7**). The closure enables intermittent suctioning in patients with limited muscle strength or in patients with weakened coughing impulses due to neuromuscular diseases or absent cough reflex of central origin, for example, and thus makes it possible to simulate the situation without a tracheostoma. In patients in or after weaning of the respirator with increased risk of respiratory exhaustion, for example, and thus makes it possible to simulate the situation without a

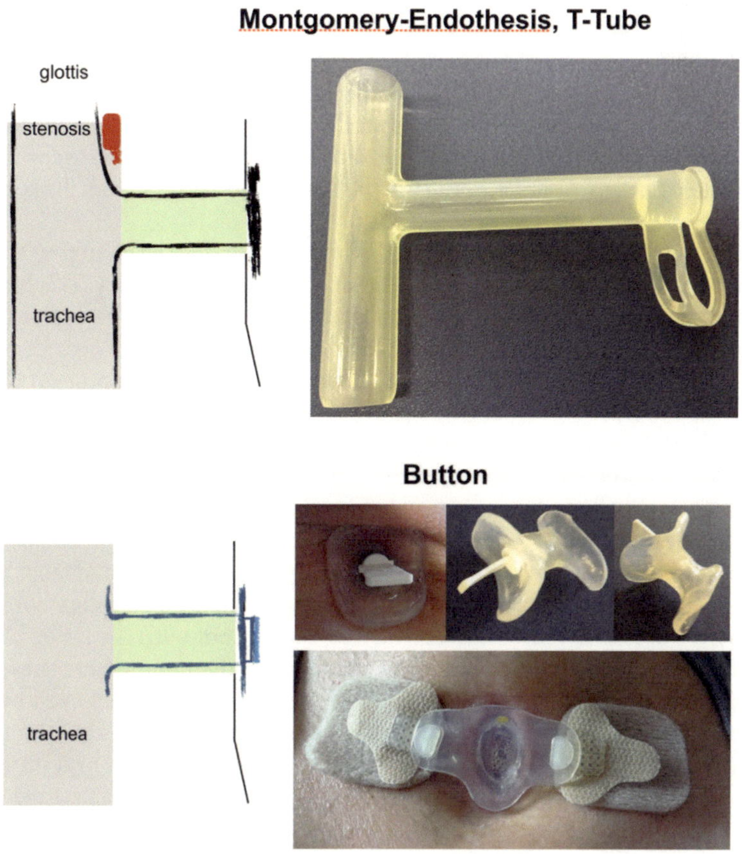

Figure 7.
Representation of a tracheal endothesis according to Montgomery (schematic, in sagittal section (top left)), photography (top right), which is used to splint tracheal stenoses. Bottom left: schematic representation of a placeholder in a sagittal section. Next to it is a photographic representation of individually adapted tracheostoma buttons that can be worn with or without attachment to the neck.

tracheostoma. By keeping the tracheostoma open, the button can be replaced with a tracheostomy tube at any time (e.g., if positive pressure ventilation is required).

In cases of repositioning during a procedure or operation, in the prone position, tracheal trauma, impaired ventilation, and an increased risk of dislocation may occur, necessitating a tracheostomy tube change. This may also be the case were a positive pressure ventilation is potentially required and there is only limited access to the airway during the procedure [28].

If a tracheostomy tube change is necessary, the following considerations should be made:

- Can I give the patient orotracheal ventilation/intubation if necessary?
- Is it necessary to optimize the positioning for the tracheostomy tube change?
- Are special additional instruments required?

Consecutively, appropriate preparations should be made.

The patient should be positioned accordingly. Insertion is simplified by moistening the tracheostomy tube with an appropriate lubricant, similar to intubation. If it is necessary to insert a cannula, the patient should lie flat on their back. Ideally, the patient should be able to change the tracheostomy tube themselves. Depending on the degree of difficulty, a Seldinger technique with a soft airway exchange catheter can be used. The more complicated the insertion of a tracheostomy tube is thought to be, the more likely it is that endoscopic confirmation of the correct tracheostomy tube position will be required. This option should therefore be available.

Adequate lighting and suction should always be available for changing tracheostomy tubes. The use of a speculum can be a useful aid if necessary. Tracheostomy tubes should also be available and provided in smaller sizes than the currently placed tube. In special cases, where the patient's position for a procedure does not allow the tracheostomy tube to remain in place, a flexible spiral tube (or others) can also be placed over the tracheostoma. Depending on the expected level of difficulty, it is recommended that two people carry out the tracheostomy tube change. The procedure should be secured by personnel in the same way as for an unexpectedly difficult intubation. That may include surgical support in appropriate cases (e.g., immature trachal shaft, T-tube exchange).

Preoxygenation can be achieved by connecting to the existing tracheostomy tube, by facemask (cupped tube), over the stoma (with pediatric facemask or soft laryngeal mask). Positive pressure ventilation can also be carried out with the latter [29–31]. This may be helpful in cases of tracheostomy tube dislodgement where the oxygenation of the patient has the top priority. Oxygenation can also be achieved by mask or supraglottic airway devices. Dislodged tracheostomy tube for patients with immature and highly instable tracheostoma shaft (within first week) attempt oral intubation first. Avoid passing rigid devices through the shaft, to prevent false passage [32], and do not perform high pressure ventilation in this case, to prevent emphysema or pneumothorax [33–35]. Obstruction of the tracheostomy tube can be due to secretions, blood, contact of the tip with the trachea, or other tissue structures (malposition). If the suction catheter cannot remove the obstacle and aspirate the obstructing material, an endoscopic control is recommended.

2.5 What does the tracheostoma look like?

To fully assess a tracheostoma, the tracheostoma entrance, the tracheostoma shaft, and the trachea must be examined.

The tracheostoma placement may already have been complicated by the following factors: fibrosis (prior radiation, prior tracheostomy, prior neck surgery), cancer, obstructing mass/edema, trauma, obese neck, low-lying trachea, and tracheal stenosis. Peri-procedural complications include hemorrhage, pneumothorax, and surgical site infection. Further complications include mucous plugging and accidental decannulation, which requires premature insertion of a tracheal cannula [36]. Even after successful decannulation, the following late complications should be considered: granulations, tracheal stenosis, tracheomalacia, and tracheoesophageal fistula [37, 38].

During the external assessment of the tracheostoma, particular attention should be paid to the cleanliness of the tracheostoma (wound secretions, saliva, pus), local signs of inflammation, granulation, bleeding, and the size of any cannula inserted.

A complete assessment of the tracheostoma is only possible without inserted material (e.g., tracheostomy tube, button). The same applies to the trachea, for example, for pressure damage caused by a blocked tracheal cannula. The assessment includes the external condition, deposits, mucosal irritation, inflammation, ulceration, granulation, and bleeding. In case of massive tracheostoma bleeding, hyperinflation of the tracheostomy cuff may prevent further airway contamination [8].

The length of the tracheostoma and its stability should also be assessed. Functional structural impairments are not always visible in patients with respiratory dependency. Instabilities of the trachea, such as tracheomalacia, usually only become apparent during spontaneous breathing. In the case of respirator dependency, the time window for assessment can also be extremely short. Abnormalities should always be evaluated with the treating colleagues and communicated to the subsequent specialist departments.

3. Conclusions

Patients with a tracheostoma are a heterogeneous group. This is reflected both in the type of underlying disease and in the way patients are equipped with aids. Before treating a patient with a tracheostoma, the indication, timing, and type of tracheostomy and the types of cannula care should be known. The treatment of these patients often requires a thorough anamnesis and interdisciplinary consultation. The positioning, length, and extent of the planned operation should be calculated to optimally organize tracheostomy care and avoid complications. If a tracheostomy tube exchange is necessary, the appropriate cannula must be selected based on the anatomical conditions, the planned procedure, and the nature and condition of the tracheostoma. The equipment and personnel requirements must be adjusted according to the risk to ensure adequate oxygenation.

Acknowledgements

I like to thank Dr. Susanne Sutarski (Department of otorhinolaryngeology, Bavaria Clinic Kreischa, Germany) for her insightful comments and for the support with the photographs. We are grateful for the support of the Open Access publication by the

Open Access Publication Fund of the Saxon State and University Library Dresden (SLUB Dresden).

Conflict of interest

The author declare no conflict of interest.

Author details

Torsten Richter
Department of Anesthesiology and Critical Care Medicine, University Hospital Carl Gustav Carus Dresden, Technische Universität Dresden, Dresden, Germany

*Address all correspondence to: torsten.richter@ukdd.de

References

[1] Epstein SK. Anatomy and physiology of tracheostomy. Respiratory Care. 2005;**50**(4):476-482

[2] Selekwa M, Maina I, Yeh T, Nkya A, Ncogoza I, Nuss RC, et al. Tracheostomy care quality improvement in low- and middle-income countries: A scoping review. PLOS Global Public Health. 2023;**3**(11):e0002294

[3] Bundesamt S. Statistischer Bericht-Fallpauschalbezogene Krankenhausstatistik (DRG-Statistik) - Operationen und Prozeduren der vollstationäüren Patientinnen und Patienten in Krankenhäusern (4-Steller) – 2023. Statistisches Bundesamt; 2024. Available from: https://www.destatis.de/DE/Themen/Gesellschaft-Umwelt/Gesundheit/Krankenhaeuser/Publikationen/Downloads-Krankenhaeuser/statistischer-bericht-operationen-prozeduren-5231401237015.html

[4] Strober W, Kallogjeri D, Piccirillo JF, Rohlfing ML. Tracheostomy incidence and complications: A national database analysis. Otolaryngology and Head and Neck Surgery. 2024;**171**(5):1379-1386

[5] Hulde N, Koppen M, Gratzke M, Kisch-Wedel H, Brenner P, Huge V. Hemorrhage of the innominate artery during percutaneous dilatation tracheotomy. Der Anaesthesist. 2018;**67**(6):448-451

[6] Cokis C, Towler S. Tracheo-innominate fistula after initial percutaneous tracheostomy. Anaesthesia and Intensive Care. 2000;**28**(5):566-569

[7] Grant CA, Dempsey G, Harrison J, Jones T. Tracheo-innominate artery fistula after percutaneous tracheostomy: Three case reports and a clinical review. British Journal of Anaesthesia. 2006;**96**(1):127-131

[8] Donaldson L, Raper R. Successful emergency management of a bleeding tracheoinnominate fistula. BML Case Reports. 2019;**12**(12):e232257

[9] Richter T, Sutarski S. Tracheostoma. Handling and complications. Der Anaesthesist. 2009;**58**(12):1261-1272; quiz 73-4

[10] Richter T, Gottschlich B, Sutarski S, Muller R, Ragaller M. Late life-threatening hemorrhage after percutaneous tracheostomy. International Journal of Otolaryngology. 2011;**2011**:890380

[11] Klemm E, Nowak A. Commentary: Percutaneous tracheostomy: Comparison of three different methods with respect to tracheal cartilage injury in cadavers-randomized controlled study. Pathology Oncology Research. 2023;**29**:1611451

[12] Tabaee A, Lando T, Rickert S, Stewart MG, Kuhel WI. Practice patterns, safety, and rationale for tracheostomy tube changes: A survey of otolaryngology training programs. The Laryngoscope. 2007;**117**(4):573-576

[13] Ardekian L, Barak M, Rachmiel A. Subcutaneous emphysema following emergent surgical conventional tracheostomy. Craniomaxillofacial Trauma & Reconstruction. 2014;**7**(4):290-293

[14] Luthra A, Chauhan R, Sabarwal P, Sahoo AK. To Be cautious or not: Tension pneumothorax after first tracheostomy tube exchange. Indian Journal of Otolaryngology and Head & Neck Surgery. 2019;**71**(Suppl 1):852-854

[15] Rajendram R, McGuire N. Repositioning a displaced tracheostomy tube with an aintree intubation catheter mounted on a fibre-optic bronchoscope. British Journal of Anaesthesia. 2006;**97**(4):576-579

[16] Kwon MA, Cho C, Park JH. Life-threatening tension pneumothorax after unsuccessful tracheostomy tube exchange in a trauma patient - a case report. Anesthesia and Pain Medicine. 2020;**15**(1):124-128

[17] Klemm E, Nowak AK. Tracheotomy-related deaths. Deutsches Ärzteblatt International. 2017;**114**(16):273-279

[18] Nowak A, Klemm E, Kunz T, Strametz R, Grundling M, Byhahn C. Letter to Kunz T et al. puncture tracheotomy in intensive care - update 2012. Anasthesiol Intensivmed Notfallmed Schmerzther 2012; 47(10): 598-604. Anästhesiologie, Intensivmedizin, Notfallmedizin, Schmerztherapie. 2013;**48**(1):4-5

[19] Shlugman D, Satya-Krishna R, Loh L. Acute fatal haemorrhage during percutaneous dilatational tracheostomy. British Journal of Anaesthesia. 2003;**90**(4):517-520

[20] Ayoub OM, Griffiths MV. Aortic arch laceration: A lethal complication after percutaneous tracheostomy. The Laryngoscope. 2007;**117**(1):176-178

[21] Furlow PW, Mathisen DJ. Surgical anatomy of the trachea. Annals of Cardiothoracic Surgery. 2018;**7**(2):255-260

[22] Selleng S, Antal M, Hansen T, Meissner K, Usichenko TI. Pneumothorax and cardiac arrest caused by speaking valve mistaken as moisture exchanger: An incident report. British Journal of Anaesthesia. 2013;**111**(2):297-298

[23] Hess DR, Altobelli NP. Tracheostomy tubes. Respiratory Care. 2014;**59**(6):956-971; discussion 71-3

[24] Montgomery WW. Manual for care of the Montgomery silicone tracheal T-tube. The Annals of Otology, Rhinology & Laryngology. Supplement. 1980;**89**(4 Pt 5):1-8

[25] Wahidi MM, Ernst A. The Montgomery T-tube tracheal stent. Clinics in Chest Medicine. 2003;**24**(3):437-443

[26] Guha A, Mostafa SM, Kendall JB. The Montgomery T-tube: Anaesthetic problems and solutions. British Journal of Anaesthesia. 2001;**87**(5):787-790

[27] Rewari V. Intraoperative airway management considerations for adult patients presenting with tracheostomy: Alternate techniques. Anesthesia and Analgesia. 2021;**133**(3):e41-ee2

[28] Rosero EB, Corbett J, Mau T, Joshi GP. Intraoperative airway management considerations for adult patients presenting with tracheostomy: A narrative review. Anesthesia and Analgesia. 2021;**132**(4):1003-1011

[29] Kannan S, Birch JP. Controlled ventilation through a tracheostomy stoma. Anaesthesia and Intensive Care. 2001;**29**(5):557

[30] Sharma R. Mask for stoma ventilation: Rescue using a Rendell-Baker-Soucek mask after a dislodged tracheostomy tube. Acta Anaesthesiologica Scandinavica. 2008;**52**(9):1305-1306

[31] Padley A. Yet another use for the laryngeal mask airway--ventilation of a patient with a tracheostomy stoma. Anaesthesia and Intensive Care. 2001;**29**(1):78

[32] Lewis RJ. Tracheostomies. Indications, timing, and complications. Clinics in Chest Medicine. 1992;**13**(1):137-149

[33] Cook TM, Woodall N, Harper J, Benger J, Audit FN, P. Major complications of airway management in the UK: Results of the fourth National Audit Project of the Royal College of Anaesthetists and the difficult airway society. Part 2: Intensive care and emergency departments. British Journal of Anaesthesia. 2011;**106**(5):632-642

[34] Seay SJ, Gay SL. Problem in tracheostomy patient care: Recognizing the patient with a displaced tracheostomy tube. ORL-Head and Neck Nursing. 1997;**15**(2):10-11

[35] Douglas WE, Flabouris A. Surgical emphysema following percutaneous tracheostomy. Anaesthesia and Intensive Care. 1999;**27**(1):69-72

[36] Murray M, Shen C, Massey B, Stadler M, Zenga J. Retrospective analysis of post-tracheostomy complications. American Journal of Otolaryngology. 2022;**43**(2):103350

[37] Shah RK, Lander L, Berry JG, Nussenbaum B, Merati A, Roberson DW. Tracheotomy outcomes and complications: A national perspective. The Laryngoscope. 2012;**122**(1):25-29

[38] Spataro E, Durakovic N, Kallogjeri D, Nussenbaum B. Complications and 30-day hospital readmission rates of patients undergoing tracheostomy: A prospective analysis. The Laryngoscope. 2017;**127**(12):2746-2753

Section 10

Drug (Ab)use and Anesthesiology

Chapter 12

Anesthesiologic Management of Patients with Opioids or Psychoactive Substance Use

Roberto Zoppellari, Milo Vason and Carlo Alessandro Locatelli

Abstract

This chapter focuses on the pharmacological interactions between opioids or psychoactive substances, such as cocaine, amphetamines, products containing tetrahydrocannabinol and cathinones with anesthetic drugs, and provides recommendations during the perioperative period for recognizing risks and reducing complications. Substance use can be suspected or confirmed in the preoperative phase via physical examination, anamnesis and toxicological tests. Assessment of appropriate timing of surgery is necessary, requiring, in case of opioid dependence, careful evaluation of treatment. Regional anesthesia is preferred in opioid users. General anesthesia could control cardiovascular alterations due to the central and peripheral neurotransmitter effects of psychostimulants. Indications and contraindications regarding anesthetic drugs and intraoperative strategies are discussed. Important postoperative implications include the use of intensive care unit; close respiratory and cardiovascular monitoring; multimodal analgesia and pain control; and withdrawal prevention. Finally, the review provides suggestions on how to approach the patient with other healthcare providers for offering opportunities to treat substance use disorder.

Keywords: opioids, psychoactive substances, anesthesiologic management, pharmacological interactions, sympathomimetic toxidrome

1. Introduction

A shocking augmentation in the use of opioids and psychoactive substances in the world increases the likelihood of surgical procedure for patients using these kinds of drugs. Therefore, anesthesiologists frequently encounter patients using drugs such as opioids, products with tetrahydrocannabinol, cocaine, amphetamines and similar-acting psychostimulants as well as new psychoactive substances. Nevertheless, despite this rising use, most anesthesiologists are not familiar regarding its implications with anesthetic agents and perioperative strategies. We think it is important to know the clinical presentations, the changes affecting the respiratory, cardiovascular and neurological systems of the user's body and the anesthetic implications of the above-mentioned drugs. These concerns represent an expanding area of perioperative medicine and necessitate a better understanding and management.

Anesthesiologic management of these patients during the perioperative period is a challenging task: individuals admitted to the operating room may be on chronic opioid therapy or may use a variety of diverse and illicit substances in continuous development. The use of these substances induces important changes in the human body, requiring appropriate knowledge to better manage the preoperative phase and the intraoperative and postoperative periods.

Recently, psychiatric literature has introduced the concept of substance use disorder, defined as substance abuse or substance dependence [1]. This is a widespread and increasing public health problem in the world.

Anesthesiologic considerations of patients using traditional or new opioids and psychoactive substances, such as cannabis, amphetamines and derivatives, cocaine and cathinones, may differ substantially from those of the typical patient. Therefore, we present suggestions regarding some strategies of management that may be used by anesthesiologists during the perioperative phase for this increasing subset of patients. The manuscript is divided into six sections: (1) pharmacological considerations of opioids and psychoactive substances; (2) preoperative phase; (3) intraoperative period; (4) postoperative implications; (5) a broader approach; and (6) conclusions.

A large body of literature has been published in this area. Nevertheless, this chapter is not an exhaustive review: the purpose of this chapter is to explore important pharmacological interactions of opioids and some of the most frequent psychoactive substances with anesthesiologic management and to provide a basic and brief overview to optimize care in the perioperative period.

2. Pharmacological considerations of opioids and psychoactive substances

The approach to potential implications of opioids and psychoactive substances during the perioperative period requires a brief summary of the pharmacology and toxicology of opioids, cannabis and psychostimulants, such as amphetamines, cocaine and cathinones.

Opioids include heroin, morphine, methadone, codeine, meperidine, buprenorphine, hydromorphone, tramadol and new synthetic opioids, such as fentanyl and its analogs. Heroin, or diacetylmorphine, is an opioid substance that is quickly hydrolyzed to morphine. Fentanyl analogs consist of benzimidazoles, benzimidazolones, piperidine and O-desmethyltramadol. Patients may be undergoing chronic therapy or may be using traditional or new opioids for recreational purposes. Common clinical manifestations of opioids include lethargy, neurocognitive effects, constipation, miosis and respiratory depression. Recently, a dizzying number of deaths in North America has been related to fentanyl [2]. This rapid emergency in public health has been complicated by adulteration of fentanyl and its analogs with xylazine, a nonopioid analgesic and sedative used in veterinary medicine and animal research [3]. To date, the contribution of xylazine to these deaths is unclear [4]. The European Union Early Warning and Response System (EWRS) operating on behalf of the European Union Drugs Agency (EUDA), a warning system that monitors fentanyls, nitazenes and adulterated opioids with xylazine, as well as new psychoactive substances such as synthetic cathinones and synthetic cannabinoids, has recently reported a significant increase in drug seizures [5].

Cannabis is the most common illicit drug in the world, but it is legal for recreational use in several states of America and Europe. It is derived from plants of the genus *Cannabis* and is also named marijuana or hashish. Cannabis contains more than 120 natural cannabinoids. The major psychoactive compound of cannabinoids is delta-9-tetrahydrocannabinol or THC [6]. Cannabinoids act by combining with specific receptors: CB1 (cannabinoid receptor 1) receptors, mainly located in the brain and CB2 (cannabinoid receptor 2) receptors, located in peripheral tissues [6]. It is important to note that the illegal market offers a growing number of new synthetic cannabinoids, such as synthetic cannabinoid receptor agonists, with increasing binding affinity and great potency at the CB1 (cannabinoid receptor 1) [7]. Products containing new synthetic cannabinoids, including cigarettes, cookies, liquids and jelly [6], present a highly varying range of different synthetic cannabinoid compounds. Thus, signs and symptoms, mainly psychoactive and cardiovascular, depend on the content and potency of cannabinoid compounds and route of delivery. Some acute physiological effects of cannabis include airway hyperreactivity, tachycardia, vasodilation, postural hypotension and abdominal pain [6]. Moreover, psychoactive effects may include euphoria, sedation, anxiety, altered sense of perception and psychosis [8]. Recent anecdotal reports, regarding a lethal case of myocardial infarction [9] and a fatal case of mesenteric ischemia [10], highlight the extreme severity of synthetic cannabinoids. Additionally, a review of 34 published case reports and case series has suggested a causal link between cannabis use and the occurrence of stroke [11]. These dramatic concerns are the tip of the iceberg, represented by the growing use of these recreational substances without knowledge of risks. Discontinuation of cannabis use may cause, in many heavy users, a withdrawal syndrome, characterized by tremors, chills, sweating, insomnia, anorexia, anxiety, irritability, fever, headache and abdominal pain [12]. In chronic users, cannabis withdrawal could persist up to some weeks [12].

Amphetamines are used to enhance cognitive or physical performance and to increase energy and euphoria. Toxic effects include tachypnea, tachycardia, hypertension, hyperthermia, sweating, rhabdomyolysis, hyperkalemia, agitation, confusion, seizures, delirium and psychosis [13]. The stimulant 3,4-methylenedioxymethamphetamine (also known as MDMA, or ecstasy) is a diffuse synthetic amphetamine derivative inducing distorted sensory perceptions and increasing sociability, communication, empathy and sexual arousal [14]. Many psychostimulants, such as amphetamines, cocaine and cathinones, increase the release or hinder the reuptake of dopamine, epinephrine, histamine and serotonin into synapses, or alter their neurotransmitter activity [14].

Cocaine derives from the leaves of *Erythroxylon coca*, a plant of South America. It is a local anesthetic that acts by blocking channels of sodium and is a psychostimulant drug that inhibits presynaptic reuptake of dopamine, epinephrine, norepinephrine and serotonin, leading to their enhanced availability. Toxic effects of cocaine include cardiac and peripheral vasoconstriction, arrhythmias, hyperthermia, euphoria, anxiety, irritability, mydriasis and seizures [14].

The United Nations Office on Drugs and Crime (UNODC) [15] has recently focused on the increasing use of new narcotic or psychotropic drugs, in pure form or in preparation, that are not controlled by the United Nations drug control conventions, but which may pose a public health threat comparable to that posed by substances listed in these conventions. These drugs, called new psychoactive substance (NPS) [16], include synthetic cannabinoids, synthetic cathinones, arylcyclohexylamine, phenethylamine, piperazine and tryptamine [17]. The use of new psychoactive substances, such as cathinones and amphetamine-type stimulants, e.g., arylcyclohexylamines, is expanding and is going to change the drug scene [18, 19]. In particular, illicit synthetic cathinones are emerging as substitutes of traditional and controlled drugs, such as cocaine, MDMA and amphetamines [20]. These substances are intentionally mislabeled, are hard to control by international laws and are sold online [20]. Once a new psychoactive substance is banned, a new compound with slight modification in the chemical formula is introduced into the market [19]. Governments are increasing their efforts to detect the ongoing synthesis and introduction into the illicit market of new psychoactive substances. In a recent Italian report, co-consumption of several new psychoactive substances was documented in 19.5% of intoxication cases, and 49.7% of biological samples were tested positive for abuse of traditional drugs too; the use of new psychoactive substances was common among males, particularly in the context of chemsex [18], the practice to increase and/or prolong sexual performance by intake of drugs, as users seek stimulant effects, an increase of empathy or hallucinations [21].

Synthetic cathinones are derivatives of the natural cathinone found in the leaves of the plant named *Catha edulis* or khat [19]. Synthetic cathinones act by interfering with the reuptake and release of dopamine, norepinephrine and serotonin and may cause severe psychostimulant effects and a sympathomimetic toxidrome [13]. Signs and symptoms of the intoxication of cathinones or new psychoactive substances can be variable and unpredictable [18]. Intensified alertness, communication, empathy, energy, libido increase and altered sensory experiences are among their psychostimulant effects [19]. The pattern of most clinical manifestations of sympathomimetic toxidrome includes psychomotor agitation, aggression, confusion, drowsiness, hallucinations, psychosis, seizures, rhabdomyolysis, tachycardia, hypertension, mydriasis, gastrointestinal symptoms, diaphoresis and hyperthermia. Benzodiazepines are the first-choice treatment for sympathomimetic toxidrome, resulting in the reduction of central nervous system (CNS) excitation, blood pressure, heart rate and muscle motor activity [13], due to their sympatholytic effect, despite pupil dilatation remaining unaffected [22]. In addition, symptomatic treatment to contrast sympathomimetic overdrive may include propofol, alpha-2 adrenergic receptor antagonists, such as phentolamine or doxazosin, nitroglycerine, nitroprusside, verapamil, morphine, cooling, dantrolene, careful infusion of fluids and mechanical ventilation [13, 19]. Due to the potential side effects of antipsychotics such as droperidol and haloperidol, including arrhythmias and hypotension, a prudent administration is recommended [13].

3. Preoperative phase

With the widespread and growing availability of opioids and psychoactive substances in the world population, it is expected that increasing numbers of drug-using patients will be admitted for both elective and emergent surgical procedures.

Clinical presentation may be characterized by different signs and symptoms and complicated situations may occur when patients are using multiple substances of abuse. The anesthesiologist should identify underdiagnosed patients who use opioids or psychoactive substances, but a detailed history may be unreliable. Substance use can be suspected or confirmed in the preoperative phase via physical examination, anamnesis and toxicological tests. Due to social stigma, an empathic and nonjudgmental approach is necessary to encourage openness about the type of substance they use, the recent intake, its frequency and route of administration. A comprehensive assessment of comorbid health conditions and an appropriate respiratory, cardiovascular, neurological and psychological evaluation are recommended.

Acute toxic effects of drugs, or withdrawal syndromes, could be observed. A withdrawal opioid syndrome consists of sympathoadrenergic reaction characterized by agitation, anxiety, nausea, vomiting, tremors, restlessness, runny nose, shivering, sweating, tremors and hypertension [23]. On the contrary, agitation, anxiety, restlessness, depressed mood and delirium are common symptoms of withdrawal syndrome by psychostimulants [14].

In chronic users of opioids, an assessment of appropriate timing of surgery should be defined. A screening risk index to predict respiratory depression due to opioids has been described: therefore, a prudent evaluation of several risk factors, such as dose and kind of used opioid, concomitant use of benzodiazepines or antidepressants, neuropsychiatric disorders, heart failure, pulmonary, cerebrovascular or renal diseases, should be carried out [24]. Patients with documented use of methadone, buprenorphine or naltrexone, drugs that are administered for opioid use disorder to decrease cravings driving drug-seeking behavior, should be cooperatively involved in an appropriate perioperative plan [25]. While methadone and buprenorphine are agonists at the μ-receptor opioid, naltrexone acts as a competitive antagonist at the μ-receptor. A multidisciplinary treatment strategy that involves the surgeon and mental health providers and/or experts of substance use disorder is recommended [25]. Elevated dose of methadone could increase QTc interval and facilitate a potential risk of arrhythmias, including torsades de pointes; this risk may increase in case of concomitant administration of other medications, such as amiodarone, clarithromycin, chlorpromazine, disopyramide, erythromycin and haloperidol [26]. While buprenorphine and methadone should be generally continued during the perioperative period, naltrexone administration should be discontinued about two or three days before elective surgery [25] considering its pharmacokinetics, accounting for five half-lives (the half-life is approximately 10 hours). On the contrary, the time interval from the last intramuscular injection of naltrexone depot and elective surgery is 28–30 days [27, 28]. Furthermore, when surgery is urgent or emergent, a higher intraoperative opioid requirement should be considered. Finally, planning strategies should include a tailored approach to involve the patient in an individualized treatment [27, 28]. Further studies are needed to define best practices regarding perioperative management of buprenorphine [29] and naltrexone [30].

Fever, tachycardia, hypertension, severe agitation and troponin increase, due to the acute effects of cannabis containing high concentration of psychoactive compound, have been described [31]. Both during withdrawal and after intake of cannabinoid products with elevated content of THC, symptoms of altered sensorium, such as anxiety, aggression and irritability, could preclude physical examination and complete anamnesis. Moreover, cannabis withdrawal may be similar to withdrawal of other psychoactive substances. In these situations, urine drug screening may be an important aid. In chronic cannabis users, dehydration, electrolyte derangement and hypovolemia have been reported; these pathological manifestations may be caused by intractable emesis, due to cannabinoid hyperemesis syndrome, a complex clinical disorder requiring treatment with benzodiazepines or butyrophenones, such as haloperidol or droperidol [32]. It is important to recognize that significant hypovolemia may also be observed due to hyperthermia caused by amphetamines. Cannabis smoking may cause respiratory disorders such as oropharyngitis, bronchitis and emphysema [33], as well as cardiovascular activation. A delay of at least one hour before surgery has been proposed, especially if anamnesis reports angina, to reduce the risk of myocardial infarction; this suggestion has been proposed by a retrospective study of 3882 cases showing the determinant effect of cannabis smoking immediately before myocardial infarction [34]. Consensus recommendations have been proposed on tapering or discontinuing cannabis use more than a week before surgical procedure in heavy users; if the surgical procedure is planned within that time frame, abrupt stopping of drug without adequate therapy may enhance the risk of cannabis withdrawal syndrome [35]. In synthetic cannabinoid users, a bleeding condition that was difficult to treat and explain has been reported [36]. In addition, two poison centers (Illinois, USA; Israel) have published on large outbreaks of severe coagulopathy in users of synthetic cannabinoids adulterated with anticoagulant [37, 38].

Due to a recent systematic review evidencing the occurrence of acute coronary syndrome in patients using amphetamines and cathinones, preoperative assessment should be carried out with the utmost care [39]. The choice of optimal timing of surgery may be challenging for the surgical team. Cardiovascular activation and acute agitation due to toxic effects of psychostimulants require postponing surgery, if possible. In chronic users, the decision to stop or taper psychostimulants in elective surgery should be evaluated by the surgical team, with the aid of expert providers of substance use, to balance risks and benefits [40]. In patients using cocaine, a delay of one week before elective surgery has been suggested [41]. Likewise, in acutely opioid-intoxicated patients, optimal timing to perform a tailored perioperative management is essential.

Finally, preoperative cooperation and informed consent may be problematic with intoxicated patients [6, 42]; sometimes, when patients under the psychoactive effect of substances are admitted for emergent surgical procedures, an informed consent from them may be impossible. Nevertheless, when feasible, a delay in surgery is essential to let patients regain the capacity to consent.

If new psychoactive substance use is suspected and surgery is not urgent, a preoperative drug screening may provide useful information to guide and optimize effective anesthesiologic management [43].

4. Intraoperative period

Indications and contraindications to regional anesthesia should be considered, depending on the kind of drug. Neuraxial and regional anesthesia, when possible, is preferred in opioid users. On the contrary, in psychostimulant users, general anesthesia could reduce metabolic demands, decrease body temperature and control cardiovascular alterations better. Nevertheless, regional anesthesia is not contraindicated, but requires adequate cooperation of the patient using psychostimulants.

Moreover, two issues related to respiratory function in opioid users need to be considered: the first is the risk of aspiration owing to reduced gastric emptying; the second is the occurrence of pulmonary edema from overdose [27]. In contrast, severe opioid withdrawal can induce sympathetic stimulation resulting in risks of hypertensive crisis and/or myocardial infarction. In chronic users of opioids, the occurrence of intraoperative awareness during general anesthesia has been reported [44]. The choice of opioid-free anesthesia is controversial, since it is not associated with postoperative opioid underprescription, or reduced consumption postdischarge [45, 46]. In opioid users, intraoperative infusion of remifentanil has been disputed: its effects to induce acute opioid tolerance, defined as an augmentation in the required dose to provide adequate analgesia, and hyperalgesia, defined as the reduction of pain threshold after chronic opioid therapy, have been questioned [47]. Based on short duration of action and μ-receptors' affinity, fentanyl and sufentanil are indicated. Long exposure induces tolerance, which requires large doses of opioids during the intraoperative period and consequent possible hemodynamic alterations [48]. Infusions of ketamine [49] and alpha-2-agonist dexmedetomidine have been proposed during maintenance of anesthesia [27].

Hyperemesis may occur due to chronic use of cannabis [32] or cannabis withdrawal [8], but an aspiration risk during induction of anesthesia has not been proven [8]. Due to the large prevalence of cannabis use, the literature reports several complications for patients with the use of anesthetic drugs. Cases regarding occurrence of laryngospasm [50] and uvular edema during anesthesia have been reported [51]. Smoking cannabis may increase airway hyperreactivity [41]. Activation of the sympathetic nervous system may induce important tachycardia; especially in patients with cardiac failure, tachycardia contraindicates administration of drugs that increase heart rate, such as ketamine and atropine [41]. Cannabis use increases the need for sedation during esophagogastroduodenoscopies and colonoscopies: in a review of 250 medical records from one center and one endoscopist, patients regularly using cannabis required a higher amount of fentanyl, midazolam and propofol than nonusers; these data were reported as statistically significant [52]. A prospective study, regarding the induction with propofol to insert a laryngeal mask airway with a bispectral index value lower than 60, reported a dose of anesthetic significantly higher in 30 patients using cannabis than in 30 nonusers [53]. Case reports have suggested that cannabis use prior to surgery may induce inhaled anesthetic tolerance intraoperatively and consequent need to increase anesthetics administration [54, 55]. In addition, a retrospective study on intraoperative consumption of sevoflurane in 97 patients operated for tibia fracture suggests that preoperative cannabis use requires higher dose of volatile anesthetic agent to maintain adequate anesthesiologic plan, supporting the hypothesis of increased tolerance [56]. Recommendations derived from an expert panel consensus have drawn attention to considering an increased administration of anesthetics during anesthesia induction and maintenance [35].

Hyperkalemia due to rhabdomyolysis, caused by muscle activity and resulting from psychostimulants such as amphetamines, contraindicates succinylcholine administration for intubation [43]. In these patients, actions such as insertion of tracheal and gastric tube should be carried out with judicious care, due to possible destruction of nasal septum and soft palate [41]. In patients using psychostimulants, anesthetic drugs such as benzodiazepines and propofol are recommended [14]. Dexmedetomidine use has been reported [14, 57]. In addition, a recent review of the medical literature supported the beneficial role of dexmedetomidine as treatment for patients intoxicated by psychostimulants, due to its counteracting effect toward norepinephrine release [58]. Psychostimulants induce sympathetic excitation resulting in tachycardia and peripheral depletion of catecholamines: therefore, prudence in administering ketamine for induction, due to its depressive effects on cardiac performance, is suggested [59]. Sympathetic excitation also includes agitation, seizures, hyperthermia, vasospasm, arrhythmia and hypertension, increasing the risk of myocardial infarction and non-cardiogenic pulmonary edema [13, 43]. Hypertension treatment is a matter of discussion: propranolol, a beta-blocker, and particularly labetalol, an alpha-and-beta-blocker, are generally contraindicated due to their effect on unopposed alpha-receptor activation [60, 61]; calcium channel blockers, such as nitroglycerin, nitroprusside and alpha-adrenergic blocker, phentolamine, may be beneficial [14, 41]. Therefore, careful monitoring of invasive pressure and continuous measurement of temperature are recommended. The treatment of intraoperative hypotension requires the administration of direct-acting vasopressors, such as epinephrine, norepinephrine and phenylephrine [40, 41, 57], whereas ephedrine administration is contraindicated, due to its powerful sympathetic stimulation [62]. Finally, acute exposure to psychostimulants may enhance minimum alveolar concentration of inhaled anesthetic [14].

5. Postoperative implications

Important postoperative implications include possible prolonged mechanical ventilation; use of intensive care unit; close cardiovascular, metabolic and agitation or delirium monitoring; avoidance of pain and precipitation of withdrawal; monitoring and management of possible postoperative agitation and cardiovascular alterations.

Intensive care unit admission may be considered when large doses of opioids and/or infusion of dexmedetomidine or ketamine should be administered as adjuvants to achieve adequate analgesia [63]. When a high dose of postoperative methadone is required, to reduce risks of respiratory depression [64] or fatal arrhythmias [65, 66], especially for patients treated with antiretroviral drugs [67], postoperative monitoring in adequate setting is mandatory. Additionally, to monitor and manage severe postoperative agitation and cardiovascular alterations in cannabis, amphetamine and cathinone users, prolonged mechanical ventilation and use of intensive care unit, as an alternative to monitored setting, could be a possible choice [13].

The impact on the cardiovascular system in patients using cannabis has been reported in a study of 4,186,622 patients presented for major elective surgeries [68]. In this large retrospective cohort analysis, cannabis use disorder was statistically associated with an increase in postoperative risk of myocardial infarction. Considering these data, which describe the adjusted odds of myocardial infarction 1.88 times higher in patients with an active cannabis use disorder compared with individuals without an active cannabis use disorder, the authors recommend postoperative cardiac monitoring.

A multimodal analgesic plan is crucial for patients using opioids and psychoactive substances to avoid pain, assure patient satisfaction, facilitate recovery and enhance discharge. Furthermore, postoperative pain is a major concern and multimodal analgesic care should be included in a thorough perioperative strategy.

In opioid users, neuraxial or regional analgesia and continuous blocks of peripheral nerve are preferred to avoid pain [69]. Even when general anesthesia is indicated, regional anesthesia may be preferred to reduce opioid consumption [23]. In addition, an armamentarium of analgesic drugs may be used: administration of acetaminophen and nonsteroidal anti-inflammatory drugs, such as ketorolac, is a viable option [70]; infusion protocols of low doses of ketamine [27], dexmedetomidine or lidocaine have also been proposed [28]. Nevertheless, caution must be observed in administering postoperative ketamine: despite its known benefits, the potential to induce a new drug addiction in predisposed patients should be considered [48]. As chronic users of opioids present tolerance and potential hyperalgesia, a pain protocol should be defined to avoid both overdosing and underdosing risks. Patients require careful monitoring to evaluate the risk of pain due to tolerance or, on the contrary, the appearance of respiratory depression, depending on the dose. Moreover, many patients using opioids still experience significant pain following surgery [48]. A prudent evaluation of opioid weaning is suggested, but caution on opioid sparing strategy should be taken. It is important to note that opioid therapy represents a cornerstone of acute postoperative pain planning [69]. While a daily dose of methadone is used to maintain therapy in chronic users to avoid withdrawal, fractionated doses may be administered as the duration of analgesia is typically 6–8 hours [28]. This approach is associated with methadone kinetics, which presents a distribution phase of about 8–12 hours, corresponding with analgesia, and a long elimination phase (30–60 hours), which generally prevents withdrawal syndrome [26]. To avoid withdrawal, if methadone is continued, no administration of buprenorphine should be considered: methadone is a full agonist at the μ-receptor opioid, whereas buprenorphine is both an agonist at the μ-receptor and an antagonist at the kappa-receptor. Thus, since buprenorphine has a tight binding affinity at the μ-receptor opioid, but a partial activation compared with other opioids, it induces displacement of other μ-receptor agonists. Moreover, in case of buprenorphine reduction, a full dose of μ-agonist agent must be used to assure adequate analgesia [63, 69]. Preventing occurrence of withdrawal (consisting of craving use of opioids, chills, cramps, diaphoresis and diarrhea) is paramount. Recent protocols and guidelines of treatment have been published [25, 27, 71].

In cannabis users, both withdrawal and increased pain perception are reported during the postoperative period [6, 8]: thus, higher administration of analgesics may be required [35]. Postoperative strategies include regional or local analgesia; in addition, acetaminophen and nonsteroidal anti-inflammatory drugs administration, such as ibuprofen, may provide adequate analgesic effect [72, 73].

The appearance of signs of withdrawal from psychostimulants, such as agitation, depression and delirium, requires quick treatment with benzodiazepines and antidepressants [14].

6. A broader approach

The use of opioids and psychoactive substances is a rapidly evolving cause of social concern, which poses a wide problem to world health.

The anesthesiologist plays an important role in the multidisciplinary team caring for patients in the perioperative setting [69], whose responsibilities should include identification of patients using recreational drugs through an appropriate approach; family counseling; engaging the patient in shared options; and referral to expert healthcare providers. Therefore, the perioperative period may be an opportunity to encourage the patient to engage in recovery [74, 75]. These concerns are particularly important for people with substance use disorder, defined by reiterated patterns of drug use associated with functional impairment. The definition of substance use disorders has been referred to opioids, psychostimulants and cannabis [1, 8].

We put forward some suggestions on how to approach the patient together with other healthcare providers, aiming to offer opportunities to treat substance use disorder. Indeed, the shame associated with opioid or psychoactive substance use and the fear of punishment [15] or adverse judgment still induce patients to refuse opportunities for treatment [74]. Due to a real risk of criminalization, this special population may suffer from self-stigma [74]. Additionally, patients using opioids or psychoactive substances may have prior negative experiences with healthcare providers and may regard the multidisciplinary team with suspicion [23]. Finally, preoperative assessment must avoid the stigmatization of ethnic, social and racial factors characterizing patients [69]. The anesthesiologist may play a key role in the perioperative period; this approach consists of clinical discretion and farsighted referral to a multidisciplinary team. Some experiences of motivational and behavioral interventions by anesthesiologists to encourage patient cooperation for tapering postoperative opioid consumption have been reported [69]. Multidisciplinary team, including toxicologists, practice providers to prescribe medications, psychiatrists, cognitive-behavioral counselors, peer support specialists and social workers, is essential to provide individualized treatments and tailored recovery [76]. For example, detoxification from opioids may be carried out with medications (such as methadone, buprenorphine or naltrexone) and nonpharmacologic approaches. Nonpharmacologic strategies consist of cognitive-behavioral therapy, contingency management, motivational interviewing, support groups, relaxation techniques and physical therapy [27].

This is a new opportunity for anesthesiologists, as they may demonstrate their value in the healthcare system, making a positive impact on the patients' lives [69]. Thus, an increased awareness toward possibilities of recovery with people using opioids and psychoactive substances must be fostered and encouraged, with specific knowledge and training [76], overcoming stereotypes and barriers [14, 74].

7. Conclusions

This chapter on the pharmacological interactions between opioids or psychoactive substances and anesthetic practice requires further studies in the field of analgesia and anesthesia, due the continuous introduction in the illegal market of new substances. There is a noteworthy concern that is on the rise, because adequate data regarding chemistry, pharmacology and toxicology of new psychoactive substances are limited compared to traditional drugs of abuse [21]. In addition, the stigma due to use of illicit substances may alter the reliability of described observations [8].

To date, thorough consensus guidelines about optimal anesthesiologic strategies for substances users are insufficient, also in the case of individuals using opioids [23, 69]. Nevertheless, we think that our suggestions for optimizing anesthetic plan, recognizing risks and reducing complications in opioid or psychoactive-using patients, are significant. Anesthesiologists should be familiar with concerns regarding these patients and be able to manage the appropriate anesthetics and avoid contraindicated drugs. A good knowledge of the pharmacology and toxicology of opioids and psychoactive substances may improve perioperative management of patients. In the operating room, anesthesiologists already routinely manage potential poisons, such as hypnotic, sedative, analgesic and neuromuscular blocking drugs, titrate their effects and avoid their possible toxicity; additionally, then, they ought to increase their knowledge on the pharmacological interactions of anesthetics with recreational drugs or medications used for nonmedical purposes [57].

For patients who undergo elective or emergent surgery, there are some perioperative challenges, including: suspicion and recognition of the drug, knowledge of risks, appropriate anesthesiologic technique, management of tolerance during anesthesia, careful postoperative monitoring, prevention of withdrawal and, finally, use of multimodal analgesia. A tailored anesthesiologic approach is essential. Furthermore, anesthesiologists, as leaders of perioperative medicine, play a paramount role in facilitating access and treatment of patients with substance use disorder to healthcare providers. It is crucial to stress that this approach may change the patient's life.

In conclusion, a safe perioperative management that takes into account the pharmacological implications of anesthetics with recreational drugs, or medications used for nonmedical purposes, as well as a motivational action for improving the health of people who use opioids and psychoactive substances, should be considered. Caring for this expanding segment of the patient population is a new challenging frontier for anesthesiologists in the coming years.

Acknowledgements

We are grateful to Barbara Palazzi, Department of Anesthesia and Intensive Care, Ferrara Sant'Anna Hospital, Azienda Ospedaliero Universitaria di Ferrara, Italy, for her precious help.

Conflict of interest

The authors declare no conflict of interest.

Author details

Roberto Zoppellari[1*], Milo Vason[2] and Carlo Alessandro Locatelli[3]

1 Medical and Surgical Society of Ferrara, Ferrara, Italy

2 Department of Anesthesia and Intensive Care, Ferrara Sant'Anna Hospital, Azienda Ospedaliero Universitaria di Ferrara, Italy

3 Toxicology Unit, Pavia Poison Centre and National Toxicology Information Centre, Laboratory of Clinical and Experimental Toxicology, Pavia Hospital, Istituti Clinici Scientifici Maugeri IRCCS, Pavia, Italy

*Address all correspondence to: roberto.zoppellari1955@gmail.com

References

[1] Hasin DS, O'Brien CP, Auriacombe M, Borges G, Bucholz K, Budney A, et al. DSM-V criteria for substance use disorders: Recommendations and rationale. The American Journal of Psychiatry. 2013;**170**:834-851. DOI: 10.1176/appi.ajp.2013.12060782

[2] Mowry JB. Forty years of National Poison Data System Annual Reports. Clinical Toxicology (Philadelphia, Pa.). 2023;**61**(10):713-716. DOI: 10.1080/15563650.2023.2286200

[3] Solanki PK, Yellapragada S, Lynch B, Eibel M, Viscusi ER, Emerick T. Emergence of xylazine as a public health threat: What does the anesthesiologist need to know for perioperative care? Regional Anesthesia and Pain Medicine. 2024. DOI: 10.1136/rapm-2023-105190

[4] Hoffman RS. Closing the xylazine knowledge gap. Clinical Toxicology (Philadelphia, Pa.). 2023;**61**(12):1013-1016. DOI: 10.1080/15563650.2023.2294619

[5] De Morais J, Evans-Brown M, Gallegos A, Christie R, Jorge R, Planchuelo G, et al. Update from the EU early warning system on new psychoactive substances. Clinical Toxicology (Philadelphia, Pa.). 2024;**62**(51,S1):3. DOI: 10.1080/15563650.2024.2333651

[6] Alexander JC, Joshi JP. A review of the anesthetic implications of marijuana use. Baylor University Medical Center Proceedings. 2019;**32**(3):364-371. DOI: 10.1080/08998280.2019. 1603034

[7] Waters ML, Dargan PI, Yates C, Dines AM, Eyer F, Giraudon I, et al. Clinical effects of cannabis compared to synthetic cannabinoid receptor agonists (SCRAs): A retrospective cohort study of presentations with acute toxicity to European hospitals between 2013 and 2020. Clinical Toxicology (Philadelphia, Pa.). 2024;**62**(6):378-384. DOI: 10.1080/15563650. 2024.2346125

[8] Ladha KS, Manoo V, Virji A-F, Hanlon JG, Mclaren-Blades A, Goel A, et al. The impact of perioperative cannabis use: A narrative scoping review. Cannabis and Cannabinoid Research. 2019;**4**(4):219-230. DOI: 10.1089/ can.2019.0054

[9] Simon G, Tóth D, Heckmann V, Kuzma M, Mayer M. Lethal case of myocardial ischemia following overdose of the synthetic cannabinoid ADB-FUBINACA. Legal Medicine (Tokyo, Japan). 2022;**54**:102004. DOI: 10.1016/j. legalmed.2021.102004

[10] Hakimian D, Tomer O, Hiller N, Heyman SN, Israel S. Fatal mesenteric ischemia induced by synthetic cannabinoids: A case report and literature review. Case rep. Emergency Medicine. 2017;**2017**:6964078. DOI: 10.1155/2017/6964078

[11] Hackam DG. Cannabis and stroke. Systematic appraisal of case reports. Stroke. 2015;**46**:852-856. DOI: 10.1161/ STROKEAHA.115.008680

[12] Budney AJ, Hughes JR, Moore BA, Vandrey R. Review of the validity and significance of cannabis withdrawal syndrome. The American Journal of Psychiatry. 2004;**161**:1967-1977. DOI: 10.1176/ appi.ajp.161.11.1967

[13] Greene SL, Kerr F, Braitberg G. Amphetamines and related drugs of abuse. Emergency Medicine Australasia. 2008;**20**:391-402. DOI: 10.1111/j.1742-6723.2008.01114.x

[14] Emerick TD, Martin TJ, Ririe DG. Perioperative considerations for patients exposed to psychostimulants. Anesthesia and Analgesia. 2023;**137**:474-487. DOI: 10.1213/ANE.0000000000006303

[15] UNODC. Synthetic Drug Strategy. 2021. Available from: https://www.drugsandalcohol.ie/35191/1/UNODC_Synthetic_Drugs_Strategy_2021. p. 1-8. pdf [Accessed: 11 2021]

[16] Crulli B, Dines AM, Blanco G, Giraudon I, Eyer F, Liechti ME, et al. Dargan PI and on behalf of the euro-DEN plus research group. Novel psychoactive substances-related presentations to the emergency departments of the European drug emergencies network plus (euro-DEN plus) over the six-year period 2014-2019. Clinical Toxicology (Philadelphia, Pa.). 2022;**60**(12):1318-1327. DOI: 10.1080/15563650.2022.2137524

[17] Locatelli CA, Lonati D, Petrolini VM. New drugs of abuse and cardiovascular function. In: Govoni S, Politi P, Vanoli E, editors. Brain and Heart Dynamics. Cham: Springer; 2020. pp. 1-27. DOI. DOI: 10.1007/978-3-319-90305-7_55-1

[18] Buscaglia E, Lonati D, Papa P, Giardini I, Simeoni E, Schicchi A, et al. Prevalence of new psychoactive substance (NPS) intoxications from the beginning of COVID-19 pandemic in Italy. Clinical Toxicology (Philadelphia, Pa.). 2024;**62**(51,S1):26. DOI: 10.1080/15563650.2024.2333651

[19] Mas-Morey P, Visser MH, Winkelmelen L, Touw DJ. Clinical toxicology and management of intoxications with synthetic cathinones ("bath salts"). Journal of Pharmacy Practice. 2013;**26**:353-357. DOI: 10.1177/0897190012465949

[20] Karila L, Megarbane B, Cottencin O, Lejoyeux M. Synthetic cathinones: A new public health problem. Current Neuropharmacology. 2015;**13**:12-20. DOI: 10.2174/1570159X13666141210224137

[21] Assi S, Gulyamova N, Ibrahim K, Kneller P, Osselton D. Profile, effects, and toxicity of novel psychoactive substances: A systematic review of quantitative studies. Human Psychopharmacology: Clinical and Experimental. 2017;**32**:e2607. DOI: 10.1002/hup.2607

[22] Hou RH, Scaife J, Freeman C, et al. Relationship between sedation and pupillary function: Comparison of diazepam and diphenhydramine. British Journal of Clinical Pharmacology. 2006;**61**:752-760. DOI: 10.1111/j.1365-2125.2006.02632.x

[23] Shah S, Kapoor S, Durkin B. Analgesic management of acute pain in opioid tolerant patients: A growing challenge. Current Opinion in Anaesthesiology. 2015;**28**:398-402. DOI: 10.1097/ACO.0000000000000218

[24] Zedler BK, Saunders WB, Joyce AR, et al. Validation of a screening risk index for serious prescription opioid-induced respiratory depression or overdose in a US commercial health plan claims database. Pain Medicine. 2017;**19**:68-78. DOI: 10.1093/pm/pnx009

[25] Anitescu M. The patient with substance use disorder. Current Opinion in Anaesthesiology. 2019;**32**(3):427-437. DOI: 10.1097/ACO.0000000000000738

[26] Peng PWH, Tumber PS, Gourlay D. Review article: Perioperative pain management of patients on methadone therapy. Canadian Journal of Anaesthesia. 2005;**52**:513-523. DOI: 10.1007/BF03016532

[27] Barreveld AM, Mendelson A, Deiling B, Armstrong CA, Viscusi ER,

Kohan LR. Caring for our patient with opioid use disorder in the perioperative period: A guide for the anesthesiologist. Anesthesia and Analgesia. 2023;**137**:474-487. DOI: 101213/ANE.0000000000006280

[28] Harrison TK, Kornfeld H, Aggarwal AK, Lembke A. Perioperative considerations for the patient with opioid use disorder on buprenorphine, methadone or naltrexone maintenance therapy. Anesthesiology Clinics. 2018;**36**:345-359. DOI: 10.1016/j.anclin.2018.04.002

[29] Goel A, Azargive S, Weissman JS, Shanthanna H, Hanlon JG, Samman B, et al. Perioperative pain and addiction interdisciplinary network (PAIN) clinical practice advisory for perioperative management of buprenorphine: Results of a modified Delphi process. The British Journal of Anaesthesia. 2019;**123**(2):e333-e342. DOI: 10.1016/j.bja.2019.03.044

[30] Goel A, Kapoor B, Wu M, Iyayi M, Englesakis M, Kohan L, et al. Perioperative naltrexone management: A scoping review by the perioperative pain and addiction interdisciplinary network. Anesthesiology. 2024;**141**:388-399. DOI: 10.1097/ALN.0000000000005040

[31] Rickner SS, Cao D, Kleinschmidt K, Fleming S. A little "dab will do ya" in: A case report of neuro-and cardiotoxicity following use of cannabis concentrates. Clinical Toxicology (Philadelphia, Pa.). 2017;**55**(9):1011-1013. DOI: 10.1080/15563650.2017.1334914

[32] Richards JR. Cannabinoid hyperemesis syndrome: Pathophysiology and treatment in the emergency department. The Journal of Emergency Medicine. 2018;**54**:354-363. DOI: 10.1016/j.jemermed. 2017. 12.010

[33] Ashton CH. Adverse effects of cannabis and cannabinoids. British Journal of Anaesthesia. 1999;**83**:637-649. DOI: 10.1093/bja/83.4.637

[34] Mittleman MA, Lewis RA, Maclure M, Sherwood JB, Muller JE. Triggering myocardial infarction by marijuana. Circulation. 2001;**103**:2805-2809. DOI: 10.116/ 01.cir.103.23.2805

[35] Ladha KS, McLaren-Blades A, Goel A, Buys MJ, Farquhar-Smith P, Haroutounian S, et al. Perioperative pain and addiction interdisciplinary network (PAIN): Consensus recommendations for perioperative management of cannabis and cannabinoid-based medicine users by a modified Delphi process. British Journal of Anaesthesia. 2021;**126**(1):304-318. DOI: 10.1016/j.bja.2020.09.026

[36] US Department of Veterans' Affairs. National PBM Bulletin. Synthetic Marijuana and Potential Risk for Bleeding 2019. Available from: https://www.pbm.va.gov/PBM/vacenterformedicationsafety/nationalpbmbulletin/

[37] Devgun JM, Rasin A, Kim T, Mycyk MB, Bryant SM, Wahl MS, et al. An outbreak of severe coagulopathy from synthetic cannabinoids tainted with long-acting anticoagulant rodenticides. Clinical Toxicology (Philadelphia, Pa.). 2020;**58**(8):821-828. DOI: 10.1080/15563650.2019.1690149

[38] Lurie Y, Nadir Y, Hoffman R, Miller A, Efrati E, Ring G, et al. An outbreak of severe coagulopathy in northern Israel among users of illicit synthetic cannabinoids adulterated with brodifacoum. Clinical Toxicology (Philadelphia, Pa.). 2023;**61**(6):429-435. DOI: 10.1080/15563650.2023.2215402

[39] Gresnigt FMJ, Smits ES, den Haan C, Riezebos RK, Franssen EJF,

de Lange DW. The association of amphetamines and cathinones with acute coronary syndrome – A systematic review. Clinical Toxicology (Philadelphia, Pa.). 2023;**61**(5):336-345. DOI: 10.1080/15563650.2023.2191819

[40] Fischer SP, Healzer JM, Brook MW, Brock-Utne JG. General anesthesia in a patient on long-term amphetamine therapy: Is there cause for concern? Anesthesia and Analgesia. 2000;**91**:758-759. DOI: 10.1097/00000539-200009000-00050

[41] Hernandez M, Birnbach DJ, Van Zundert AA. Anesthetic management of the illicit-substance-using patient. Current Opinion in Anaesthesiology. 2005;**18**:315-324. DOI: 10.1097/01.aco.0000169241.21680.0b

[42] Martel ML, Klein LR, Miner JR, et al. A brief assessment of capacity to consent instrument in acutely intoxicated emergency department patients. The American Journal of Emergency Medicine. 2018;**36**:18-23. DOI: 10.1016/j.ajem.2017.06.043

[43] Beaulieu P. Anesthetic implications of recreational drug use. Canadian Journal of Anaesthesia. 2017;**64**:1236-1264. DOI: 10.1007/s12630-017-0975-0

[44] Huxtable CA, Roberts LJ, Somogyi AA, Macintyre PE. Acute pain management in opioid-tolerant patients. Anaesthesia and Intensive Care. 2011;**39**(5):804-823. DOI: 10.1177/0310057X1103900505

[45] Kharash ED, Clark JD. Opioid-free anesthesia: Time to regain our balance. Anesthesiology. 2021;**134**:509-514. DOI: 10.1097/ALN.0000000000003705

[46] Shanthanna H, Ladha KS, Kehlet H, Joshi GP. Perioperative opioid administration: A critical review of opioid-free versus opioid-sparing approaches. Anesthesiology. 2021;**134**:645-659. DOI: 10.1097/ALN.0000000000003572

[47] Kim NS, Stoicea N, Soghomonyan S, Bergese SD. Intraoperative use of remifentanil and opioid induced hyperalgesia/acute opioid tolerance: A systemic review. Frontiers in Pharmacology. 2014;**5**:1-9. DOI: 10.3389/fphar.2014.00108

[48] Thomas DA, Boominathan P, Goswami J, Mukherjee S, Vadivelu N. Perioperative management of patients with addiction to opioid and nonopioid medications. Current Pain and Headache Reports. 2018;**22**:52. DOI: 10.1007/s11916-018-0704-6

[49] Schwenk ES, Viscusi ER, Buvanendran A, Hurley RW, Wasan AD, Narouze S, et al. Consensus guidelines on the use of intravenous ketamine infusions for acute pain management from the American Society of Regional Anesthesia and Pain Medicine, the American Academy of pain medicine, and the American Society of Anesthesiologists. Regional Anesthesia and Pain Medicine. 2018;**43**(5):456-466. DOI: 10.1097/AAP.0000000000000806

[50] White SM. Cannabis abuse and laryngospam. Anaesthesia. 2002;**57**:606-625. DOI: 10.1046/j.1365-2044.2002.265824.x

[51] Mallat A, Roberson J, Brock-Utne JG. Preoperative marijuana inhalation—An airway concern. Canadian Journal of Anaesthesia. 1996;**43**:691-693. DOI: 10.1007/BF03017953

[52] Twardowski MA, Link MM, Twardowski NM. Effects of cannabis use on sedation requirements for endoscopic procedures. The Journal of

the American Osteopathic Association. 2019. DOI: 10.7556/jaoa.2019.052

[53] Flisberg P, Paech MJ, Shah T, Ledowski T, Kurowski I, Parsons R. Induction dose of propofol in patients using cannabis. European Journal of Anaesthesiology. 2009;**26**(3):192-195. DOI: 10.1097/EJA.0b013e328319be59

[54] Symons IE. Cannabis smoking and anaesthesia. Anaesthesia. 2002;**57**(11):1142-1143. DOI: 10.1046/j.1365-2044.2002.288312.x

[55] Richtig G, Bosse G, Arlt F, von Heymann C. Cannabis consumption before surgery may be associated with increased tolerance of anesthetic drugs: A case report. International Journal of Case Reports and Images. 2015;**6**(7):436-439. DOI: 10.5348/ijcri-201573-CR-10534

[56] Holmen IC, Beach JP, Kaizer AM, Gumidyala R. The association between preoperative cannabis use and intraoperative inhaled anesthetic consumption: A retrospective study. Journal of Clinical Anesthesia. 2020;**67**:1-2. DOI: 10.1016/j.jclane.2020.109980

[57] Wong GT, Irwin MG. Poisoning with illicit substances: Toxicology for the anaesthetist. Anaesthesia. 2013;**68**(suppl 1):117-124. DOI: 10.1111/anae.12053

[58] Baumgartner K. Doering M, Mullins ME and on behalf of the Toxicology Investigators Consortium. Dexmedetomidine in the treatment of toxicologic conditions: A systematic review and review of the toxicology investigators consortium database. Clinical Toxicology (Philadelphia, Pa.). 2022;**60**(12):1356-1375. DOI: 10.1080/15563650.2022.2138761

[59] Waxman K, Shoemaker WC, Lippmann M. Cardiovascular effects of anesthetic induction with ketamine. Anesthesia and Analgesia. 1980;**59**:355-358

[60] Moran S, Isa J, Steinemann S. Perioperative management in the patient with substance abuse. The Surgical Clinics of North America. 2015;**95**:417-428. DOI: 10.1016/j.suc.2014.11.001

[61] Hall AP, Henry JA. Acute toxic effects of "ecstasy" (MDMA) and related compounds: Overview of pathophysiology and clinical management. British Journal of Anaesthesia. 2006;**96**(6):678-685. DOI: 10.1093/bja/ael078

[62] Kuczkowski KM. Anesthetic implications of drug abuse in pregnancy. Journal of Clinical Anesthesia. 2003;**15**:382-394. DOI: 10.1016/S0952-8180(03)00056-4

[63] Anderson TA, Quaye AN, Ward EN, Wilens TE, Hilliard PE, Brummett CM. To stop or not, that is the question. Acute pain management for the patient on chronic buprenorphine. Anesthesiology. 2017;**126**:1180-1186. DOI: 10.1097/ALN.0000000000001633

[64] Bryson EO. The perioperative management of patients maintained on medications used to manage opioid addiction. Current Opinion in Anaesthesiology. 2014;**27**:359-364. DOI: 10.1097/ACO.0000000000000052

[65] Behzadi M, Joukar S, Beik A. Opioids and cardiac arrhythmia: A literature review. Medical Principles and Practice. 2018;**27**(5):401-414. DOI: 10.1159/000492616

[66] Chou R, Weimer MB, Dana T. Methadone overdose and cardiac arrhythmia potential: Findings from a review of the evidence for an American pain society and college on

problems of drug dependence clinical practice guideline. The Journal of Pain. 2014;**15**(4):338-365. DOI: 10.1016/j.jpain.2014.01.495

[67] Kao D, Bucher Bartelson B, Khatri V, Dart R, Mehler PS, Katz D, et al. Trends in reporting methadone-associated cardiac arrhythmia, 1997-2011: An analysis of registry data. Annals of Internal Medicine. 2013;**158**(10):735-740. DOI: 10.7326/0003-4819-158-10-201305210-00008

[68] Goel A, McGuinness B, Jivraj NK, Wijeysundera DN, Mittleman MA, Bateman BT, et al. Cannabis use disorder and perioperative outcomes in major elective surgeries. Anesthesiology. 2019;**132**(4):625-635. DOI: 10.1097/ALN.0000000000003067

[69] Larach DB, Hah JM, Brummet CM. Perioperative opioids, the opioid crisis, and the anesthesiologist. Anesthesiology. 2022;**136**:594-608. DOI: 10.1097/ALN.0000000000004109

[70] White PF. The changing role of nonopioid analgesic techniques in the management of postoperative pain. Anesthesia and Analgesia. 2005;**101**(5 Suppl):5-22. DOI: 10.1213/01.ANE.0000177099.28914.A7

[71] Kohan L, Potru S, Barreveld AM, Sprintz M, Lane O, Aryal A, et al. Guidelines for the use of buprenorphine for opioid use disorder in the perioperative setting. Regional Anesthesia and Pain Medicine. 2021;**46**:860-861. DOI: 10.1136/rapm-2021-103092

[72] Joshi GP, Kehlet H. PROSPECT working group. Guidelines for perioperative pain management: Need for re-evaluation. British Journal of Anaesthesia. 2017;**119**:703-706. DOI: 10.1093/bja/ aex304

[73] Thybo KH, Hägi-Pedersen D, Dahl JB, Wetterslev J, Nersesjan M, Jakobsen JC, et al. Effect of combination of paracetamol (acetaminophen) and ibuprofen vs either alone on patient-controlled morphine consumption in the first 24 hours after total hip arthroplasty: The PANSAID randomized clinical trial. JAMA. 2019;**321**:562-571. DOI: 10.1001/jama.2018.22039

[74] Ward EN, Quaye AN, Wilens TE. Opioid use disorders:Perioperative management of a special population. Anesthesia and Analgesia. 2018;**127**:539-547. DOI: 10.1213/ANE.0000000000003477

[75] Goel A, Lamba W. Nothing about us without us: A solution to iatrogenic perioperative morbidity and mortality in people who use drugs. Anesthesia and Analgesia. 2023;**137**:470. DOI: 10.1213/ANE.0000000000006571

[76] Ruiz FJ, Warner NS, Acampora G, Coleman JR, Kohan L. Substance use disorders: Basic overview for the anesthesiologist. Anesthesia and Analgesia. 2023;**137**:508-520. DOI: 10.1213/ANE.0000000000006281